Textbook of

MICROBIOLOGY

FOR GNM STUDENTS

Textbook of

MICROBIOLOGY

FOR GNM STUDENTS

As per the INC Syllabus

Second Edition

Darshan Panda MSc PhD
Senior Researcher
Indian Council of Agricultural Research (ICAR)
National Rice Research Institute (NRRI)
Cuttack, Odisha, India

Sandeep Dhuper MSc PhD
Lecturer in Microbiology
LearnEx Academy
8504 Clearbrook Drive, Fort Worth
Texas, US

Ashutosh Debata MSc PhD
Former Director
DRIEMS School and College of Nursing
Cuttack, Odisha, India

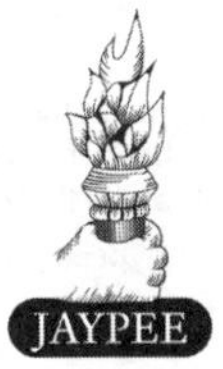

JAYPEE BROTHERS MEDICAL PUBLISHERS
The Health Sciences Publisher
New Delhi | London

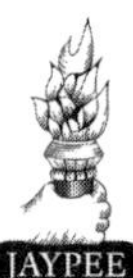

JAYPEE **Jaypee Brothers Medical Publishers (P) Ltd**

Headquarters
EMCA House
23/23-B, Ansari Road, Daryaganj
New Delhi - 110 002, India
Landline: +91-11-23272143, +91-11-23272703
+91-11-23282021, +91-11-23245672
E-mail: jaypee@jaypeebrothers.com

Corporate Office
4838/24, Ansari Road, Daryaganj
New Delhi - 110 002, India
Phone: +91-11-43574357
Fax: +91-11-43574314
E-mail: jaypee@jaypeebrothers.com

Overseas Office
J.P. Medical Ltd
83 Victoria Street, London
SW1H 0HW (UK)
Phone: +44 20 3170 8910
E-mail: info@jpmedpub.com

EU GPSR Authorised Representative
Logos Europe, 9 rue Nicolas Poussin
17000, La Rochelle, France
Phone: +33 (0) 6 67 93 73 78
E-mail: contact@logoseurope.eu

Website: www.jaypeebrothers.com
Website: www.jaypeedigital.com

Inquiries for bulk sales may be solicited at: jaypee@jaypeebrothers.com

Textbook of Microbiology for GNM Students

First Edition: 2015

Second Edition: 2023

Reprint: **2026**

ISBN: 978-93-5465-953-9

Printed at: Samrat Offset Pvt. Ltd.

Dedicated to...

My father *Mr Narendra Panda*, who inculcated the spirit of hardship and discipline in me, and my mother *Mrs Mita Panda*, who honed up my spirit while drafting the second edition of this book.

My Late paternal grandmother *Mrs Shreemati Devi* and Late grandfather *Mr Bharat Panda*, who are still showering their blessings.

My maternal grandmother *Mrs Chabbirani Dash*, and grandfather Late *Mr Pramothesh Dash*, who infused a sense of dedication in my temperament.

Preface to the Second Edition

Microbiology is like sand blowing away a lifeline. Microorganisms proved to be more vitally important to mankind than could be thought of earlier. During the past few years, the application of microorganisms to the environment and health industry has enhanced vigorously. Due to such development, wc felt the need to revise the text of the first edition of *Textbook of Microbiology for GNM Students*.

A new chapter and laboratory exercises are added to this and the first edition has been reshuffled a bit. Hope the scholars would find the necessary information appropriate to the requirements. This will serve as the most informative handbook for nursing/medical students according to the current syllabus.

Darshan Panda
Sandeep Dhuper
Ashutosh Debata

Preface to the First Edition

Many of the health problems in developing countries like India aré different from those of developed countries. Bacterial diseases still play a considerable role in our country. Nurses form the backbone of any medical services or patient care in the health sector. Nursing encompasses autonomous and collaborative care of individuals of all ages, families, groups and communities, sick or well and in all settings. It aims at promotion of health, prevention of illness and the care of ill, disabled and dying people. Knowledge of microbiology is indispensably linked with nursing practice. It is one of the fundamental basis of knowledge that governs how every nurse interacts with patients in many settings. Nurses apply knowledge of microbiology in methods of infection control, keeping instruments clean and free of contamination, how to dress wounds safely in a way that minimizes the possibility of infection, and also in identifying types of infections.

Textbook of Microbiology for GNM Students delves into ever demanding, thoughtful necessity of an absolutely well documented compilation of factual details related to theoretical principles and point wise explanation catering to the needs of GNM students. The entire course content presented in the GNM Microbiology syllabus has been developed meticulously and painstakingly. It has been designed and expanded as per the **Indian Nursing Council (INC) Syllabus.** Each chapter has duly been enumerated in a simple, lucid and crisp language easily comprehensible by its readers. An innovative and widely acceptable style of presentation has been adopted encompassing introduction, labeled diagrams, graphics, descriptions, explanations, possible questions, model answers and suggested reading. It is assumed that this edition will be useful for nursing students and faculties.

Darshan Panda
Sandeep Dhuper
Ashutosh Debata

Acknowledgments

On the Eve of the publication of the second edition of the *Textbook of Microbiology for GNM Students*, we would like to first offer our obeisances to the supreme universal energy that has blessed the spirit of our entire team during the manifestation of this book. We acknowledge Professor Baishnab C Tripathy, School of Life Sciences, Jawaharlal Nehru University, New Delhi, Dr Padmini Swain, Ex-Director, Indian Council of Agricultural Research–National Rice Research Institute (ICAR–NRRI), Cuttack, Odisha, Dr MJ Baig, Head, Crop Physiology and Biochemistry Division, ICAR–NRRI, and Dr Lambodar Behera, Principal Scientist, Crop Improvement Division, ICAR-NRRI, for their incessant guidance, encouragement, inspiration, and support. We have derived subtle guidance from Dr Kutubuddin Molla, Scientist, Crop Improvement Division, ICAR-NRRI, who has advised us to frame the flow of the chapters by infusing creativity and the essence of "elementary fractions".

Our sincere gratitude to Dr Ponnu Kangeswari, Principal DRIEMS School and College of Nursing, Tangi, Cuttack, Odisha, and Mrs N Premlata Devi, Vice-Principal, DRIEMS School and College of Nursing for their constant support in providing opportunities to research and understand the fundamental needs of the GNM students while studying microbiology. Further, we extend our special thanks to Dr Soumya Mohanty, Dr Goutam Kumar Dash, Dr Samarendra Narayan Mallick, and Dr Sagar Banerji for their incessant support and help during the development of this edition.

We take this opportunity to express our profound gratitude and sincere regards to Dr Dhirendra Kumar Singh, Professor, Kalinga Institute of Dental Sciences, KIIT (deemed to be University), Bhubaneswar, and Dr Mamta Jena, Research Scientist I, Multi-disciplinary Research Unit, Srirama Chandra Bhanja Medical College and Hospital (SCBMCH), Cuttack, Odisha to provide us with a scientific aegis to accomplish our writing goals.

We feel deeply obliged and indebted to Mr Pitamber Acharya, Dr Bandita Dash, Mrs Sudipta Kar, Mr Omprakash Dash, and Ms Srishti Acharya for consistent motivation, well wishes, and blessings. Further, we owe special gratitude to our science teacher Mrs Smita Das for sowing the seed of analytical thinking in our temperament.

We should also thank Ms Akankhya Mohanty, Mr Jasprit Swain, Mr Pratik Panda, Mr Rohit Santra, Ms Pujarini Biswal,

Ms Suma Karmakar, Ms V Ramya, Mr Sonit Patanaik, Ms Manisha Mahapatra and Ms Subhasmita Sahoo for their assistance in the development of questions.

Additionally, we extend our thanks to Mrs Chandamuni Tudu, Dr Deeptirekha Behera, Dr Alaka Swain, Dr Kamal Ruhil, Dr Prajjal Dey, Dr Deepali Dash, Mrs Monalisha Biswal, Ms Swagatika Das, Mrs Baneeta Mishra, Mrs Manaswini Dash, Mr Santanu Nayak, Mr Jitendra Kumar Das, and Mr Pradeep Nayak for their consistent support and assistance. We must also mention our, mentor and unconditional supporter our best friend, Mr Avijeet Rathsharma, who has always been there with us during the entire development of this edition. We also want to express our sincere thanks to Mr Viraj Basu, Mr Anirban Choudhury, Mr Anish Mishra, Mr Umesh Chandra Lenka, and Md Khalid who have provided us with ideas for figures and tables for this edition. Special thanks to our confidants Mr Navpreet Arora, Mrs Souvagini Arora, and Mr Rohit Das for their spectacular ideas for the beautification of the book. We duly accede to the enthusiasm of Dr Sarthak Patra in extending a helping hand for the completion of this edition. Above all, we would also like to thank our family, Late Mr Shyamasundar Panda, Mr Madhusudan Panda, Dr Prasanna Panda, Mr Dhirendra Panda, Dr Samarendra Panda, Mr Raghunath Panda, Mr Abhinash Panda, Mrs Ruchi Tiwari, Dr Aishwarya Panda, Dr Archayan Panda, Mr Amaresh Panda, Mr Nursingha Panda, Mr Srinivas Panda, Mrs Chinmayee Panda, Mrs Satarupa Panda, and Mr Shaktishankar Panda, for their support and motivation.

We are immensely appreciative to Shri Jitendar P Vij (Group Chairman) and Mr Ankit Vij (Managing Director) of M/s Jaypee Brothers Medical Publishers (P) Ltd, New Delhi, India, for believing in us and providing us with an opportunity to edit a book written by a renowned author. We are highly obliged to Mr MS Mani (Group President), Dr Madhu Choudhary (Director-Educational Publishing), Ms Pooja Bhandari (Production Head), Ms Sunita Katla (Executive Assistant to Group Chairman and Publishing Manager), Ms Samina Khan (Executive Assistant to Director–Educational Publishing), Mr Rajesh Sharma (Production Coordinator), Ms Seema Dogra (Cover Visualizer) Mr Binay Kumar and Mr Rahul Jadli (Proofreaders), Mr Deep Kumar Dogra (Typesetter), Mr Sumit Kumar (Graphic Designer) and their team members, for all their support to work in this project and make it a success.

Contents

Contents

INC Syllabus

Course Description

This course is designed to help students gain knowledge and understanding of the characteristics and activities of micro-organisms, how they react under different conditions and how they cause different disorders and diseases. Knowledge of these principles will enable student to understand and adopt practices associated with preventive and promotive health care.

General Objectives

Upon completion of the course, the students shall be able to:

1. Describe the classifications and characteristics of micro-organisms.
2. List the common disease producing microorganisms.
3. Explain the activities of microorganism in relation to the environment and the human body.
4. Enumerate the basic principles of control and destruction of microorganisms.
5. Apply the principles of microbiology in nursing practice.

Total Hours - 30

Unit No.	Learning Objectives	Content	Hr.	Teaching learning activities	Assessment methods
1.	Describe evolution of microbiology and its relevance in nursing	**Introduction** • History of bacteriology and microbiology • Scope of microbiology in nursing	3	Lecture-cum-discussions	Objective type Short answer
2.	Classify the different types of micro-organism	**Microorganisms** • Classification, characteristics, (Structure, size, method and rate of reproduction)	8	Lecture-cum-discussions	Short answer

Contd...

Contd...

Unit No.	Learning Objectives	Content	Hr.	Teaching learning activities	Assessment methods
	Describe the normal flora and the common diseases caused by pathogens Explain the methods to study microbes	• Normal flora of the body. • Pathogenesis and common diseases. • Methods for study of microbes culture and isolation of microbes		Explain using slides, films, videos, exhibits, models Staining and fixation of slides	Objective type Essay type
3.	Describe the sources of infection and growth of microbes. Explain the transmission of infection and the principles in collecting specimens	**Infection and its transmission** • Sources and types of infection, nosocomial infection • Factors affecting growth of microbes • Cycle of transmission of infection portals of entry, exit, modes of transfer • Reaction of body to infection, mechanism of resistance • Collection of specimens	4	Lecture Demon-strations Specimens Explain using charts	Short answer Objective type Essay type
4.	Describe various types of immunity, hyper-sensitivity auto-immunity and immunizing agents	**Immunity** • Types of immunity — innate and acquired • Immunization schedule Immuno-prophylaxis (vaccines, sera, etc.) • Hypersensitivity and auto-immunity • Principles and uses of serological tests	5	Lecture-cum-discussions Demon-stration Exhibits	Short answer Objective type Essay type

Contd...

Contd...

Unit No.	Learning Objectives	Content	Hr.	Teaching learning activities	Assessment methods
5.	Describe the various methods of control and destruction of microbes	**Control and destruction of microbes** • Principles and methods of microbial control ▪ Sterilization ▪ Disinfection ▪ Chemotherapy and antibiotics ▪ Pasteurization • Medical and surgical asepsis • Bio-safety and waste management	5	Lecture, Demon-stration Videos visit to the CSSD	Short answer Objective type Essay type
6.	Demonstrate skill in handling and care of microscopes Identify common microbes under the microscope	**Practical Microbiology** • Microscope—Parts, uses, handling and care of microscope • Observation of staining procedure, preparation and examination of slides and smears • Identification of common microbes under the microscope for morphology of different microbes	5	Lecture, Demon-strations Specimens Slides	

Color Plate 1

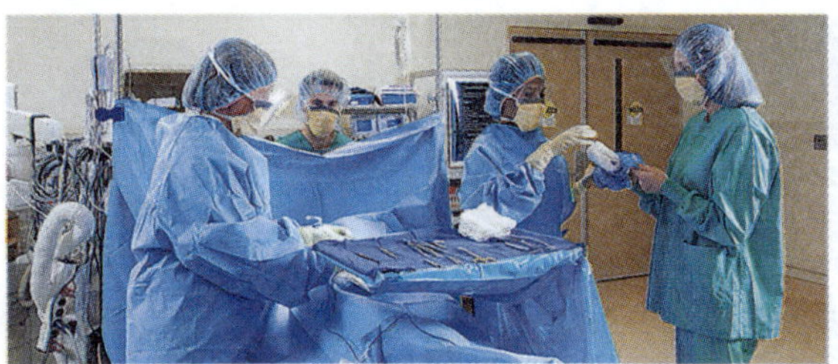

Figure 1.1.13: Maintain a sterile field.

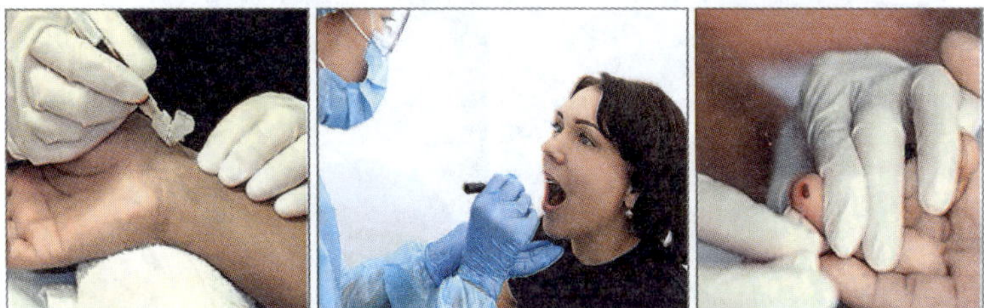

Figure 1.1.14: Collection of patient's samples.

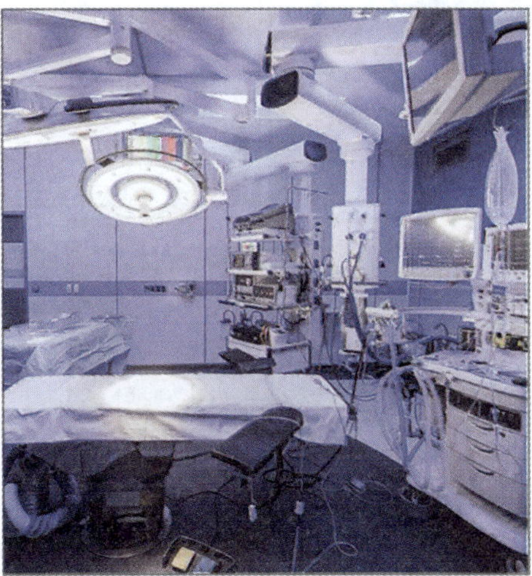

Figure 1.1.15: Controlling microbial growth.

Color Plate 2

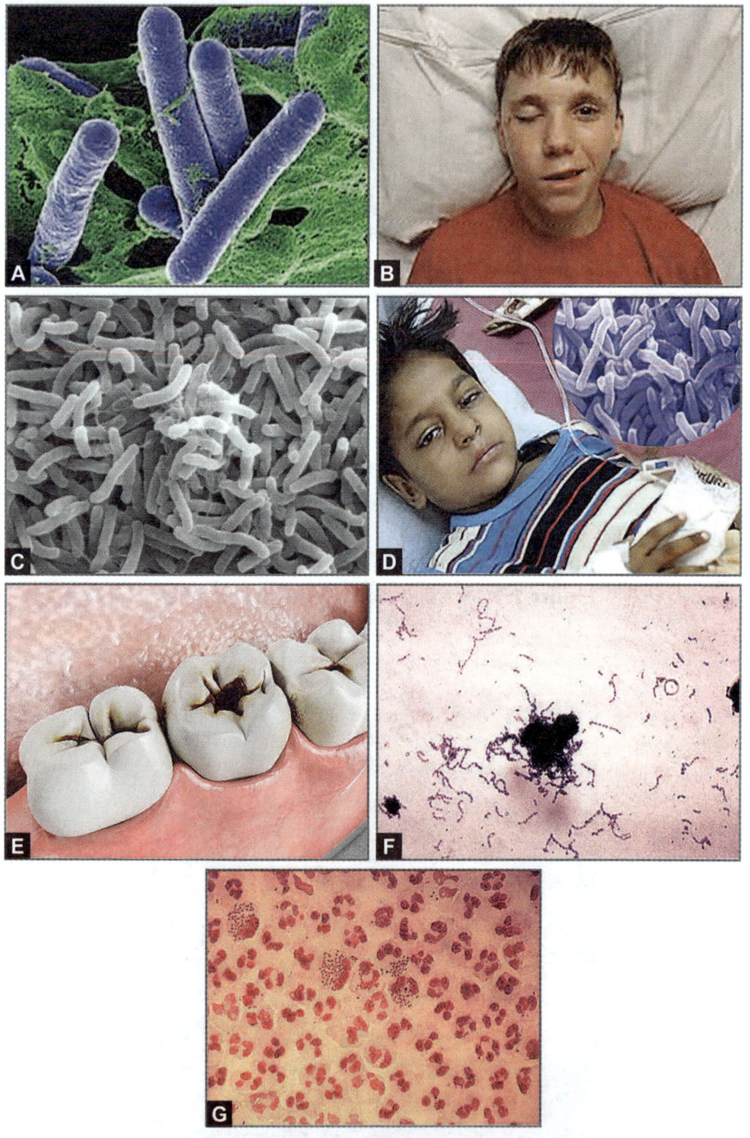

Figures 2.9.1A to G

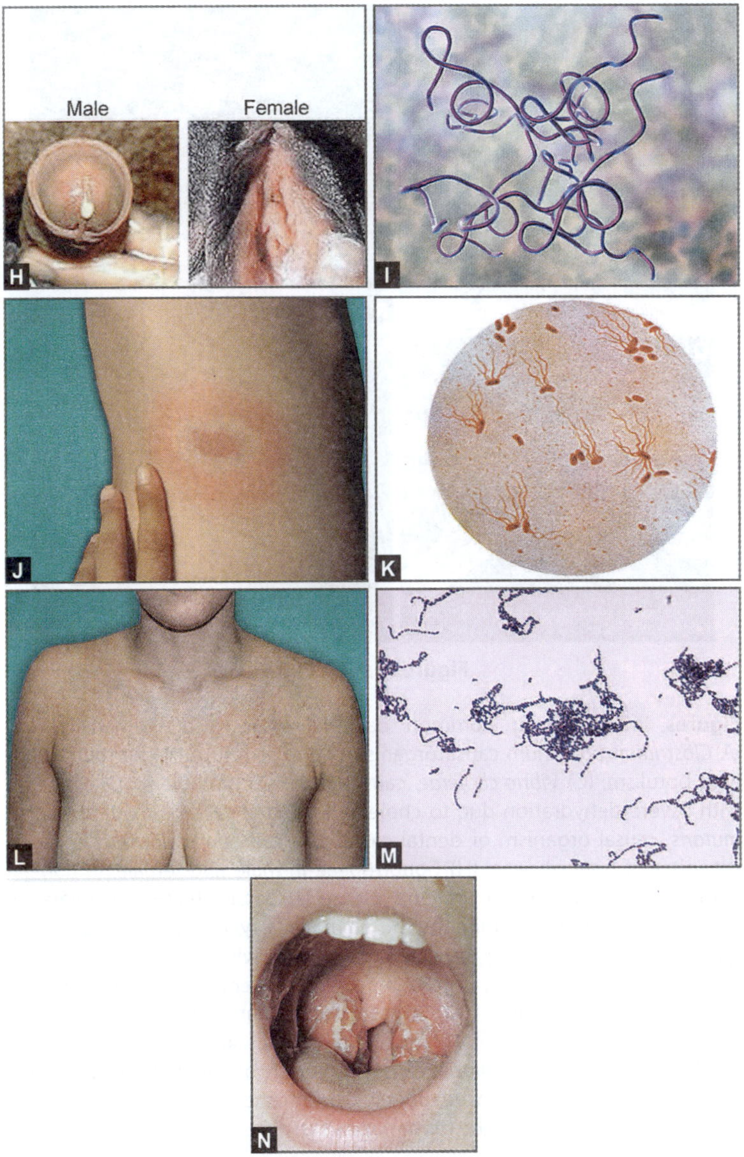

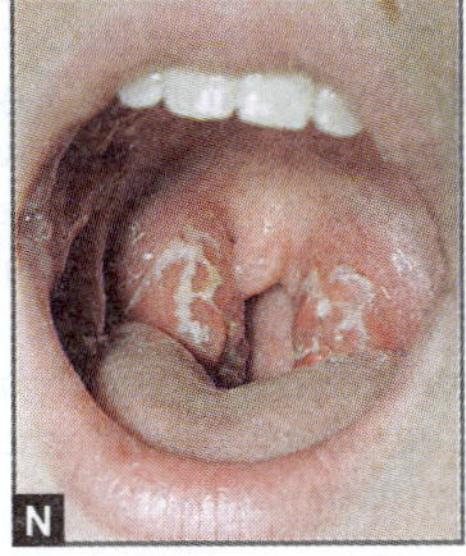

Figures 2.9.1H to N

Color Plate 4

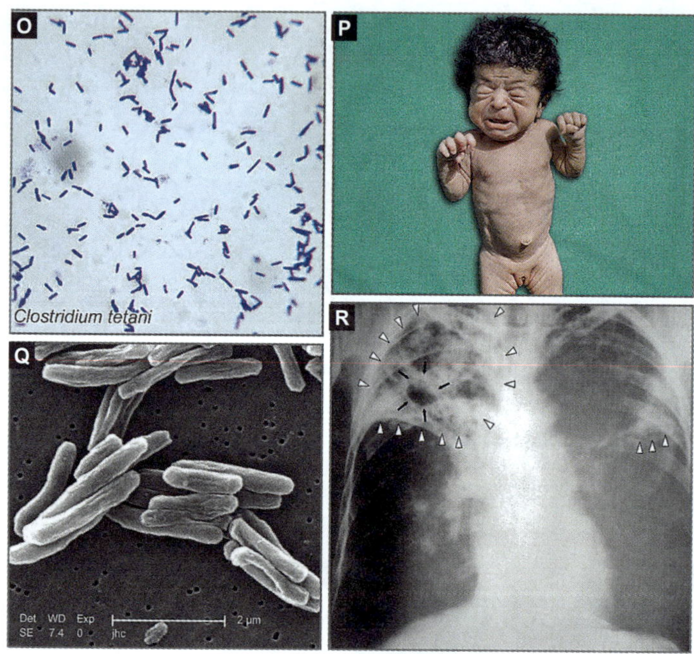

Figures 2.9.1O to R

Figures 2.9.1A to R: Common bacterial diseases of human beings. (A) *Clostridium botulinum*, causal organism of botulism; (B) A 14-year-old patient with botulism; (C) *Vibrio cholerae,* causal organism of cholera; (D) A person with severe dehydration due to cholera; (E) Dental caries; (F) *Streptococcus mutans*, causal organism of dental caries; (G) *Neisseria gonorrhoeae*, causal organism of gonorrhoeae; (H) Gonorrhoeae in male and female; (I) *Borrelia burgdorferi*, causal organism of lyme disease; (J) Classic bull's-eye appearance is also called erythema migrans; (K) *Salmonella typhi*, causal organism of typhoid; (L) Rose spots on the chest of a patient with typhoid fever due to the bacterium *Salmonella*; (M) *Streptococcus pyogenes,* causal organism of streptococcal pharyngitis; (N) Streptococcal pharyngitis; (O) *Clostridium tetani*, causal organism of tetanus; (P) A child suffering from tetanus; (Q) *Mycobacterium tuberculosis*, causal organism of tuberculosis; (R) Chest X-ray of a person with advanced tuberculosis: Infection in both lungs is marked by white arrow-heads and the formation of a cavity is marked by black arrows.

Color Plate 5

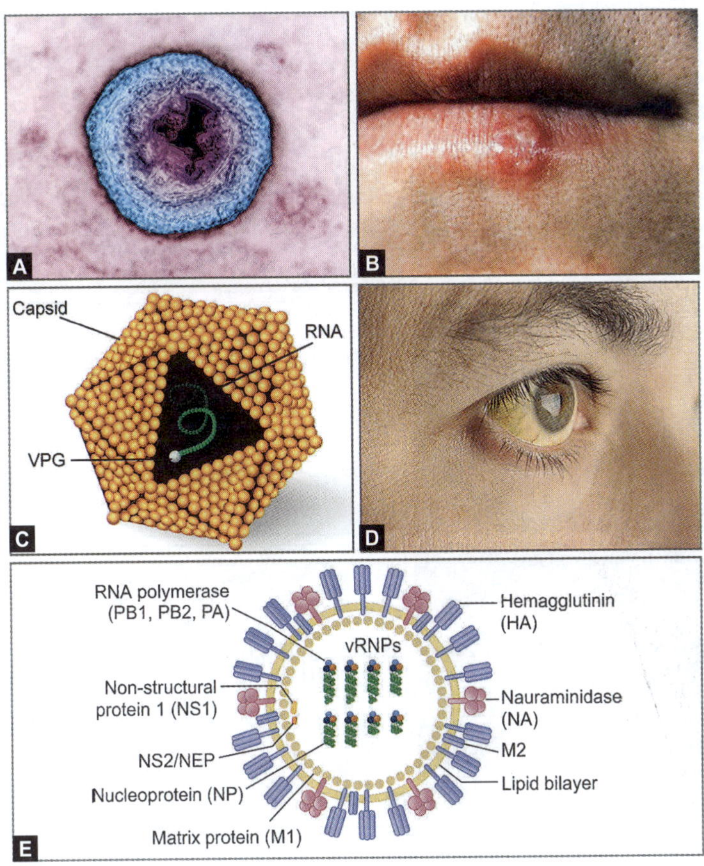

Figures 2.9.2A to E

Color Plate 6

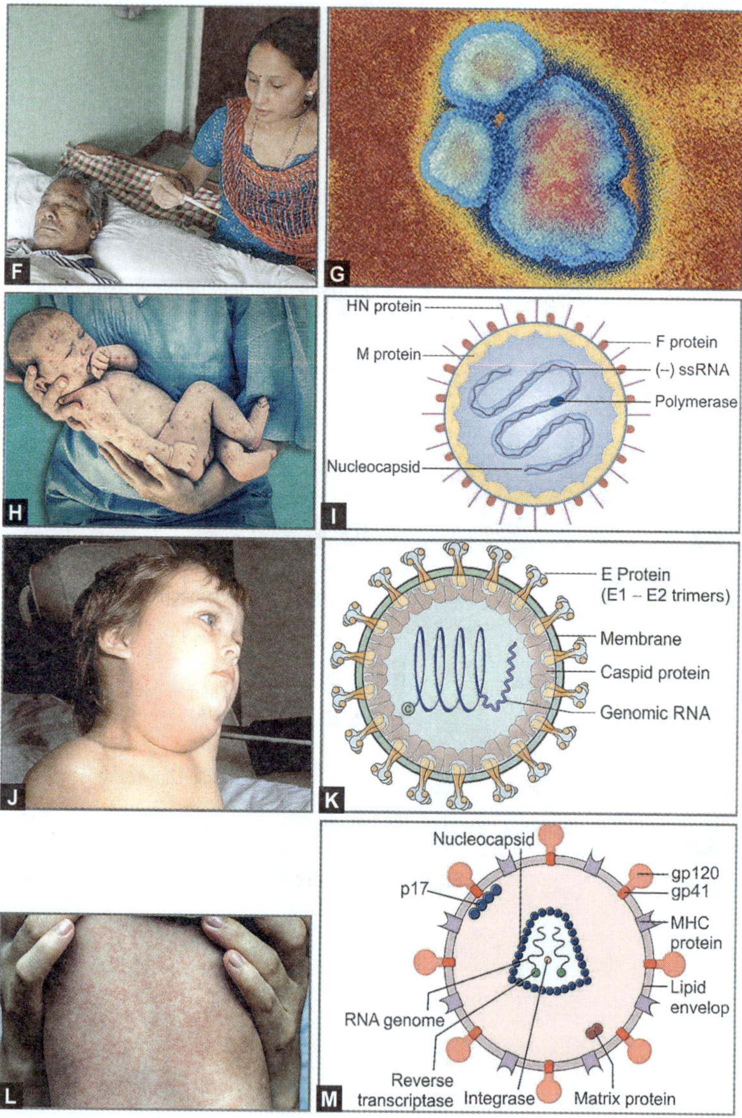

Figures 2.9.2F to M

Color Plate 7

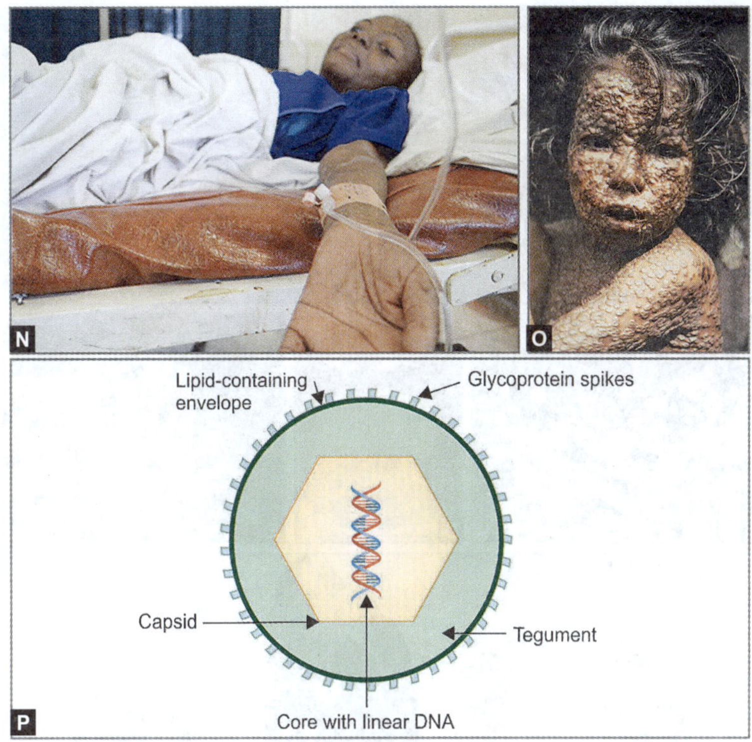

Figures 2.9.2N to P

Figures 2.9.2A to P: Common viral diseases in human beings. (A) Herpes virus; (B) Herpes labialis (blister) of the lower lip in a herpes patient; (C) Hepatitis A virus; (D) A case of jaundice caused by hepatitis A; (E) Influenza virus; (F) A patient suffering from influenza; (G) Measles virus; (H) A patient suffering from measles; (I) Mumps virus; (J) A patient suffering from mumps; (K) Rubella virus; (L) A patient suffering from Rubella (German fever); (M) Human immunodef iciency virus (HIV); (N) A patient suffering from acquired immunodeficiency syndrome (AIDS); (O) *Varicella zoster* virus; (P) A child suffering from smallpox.

Color Plate 8

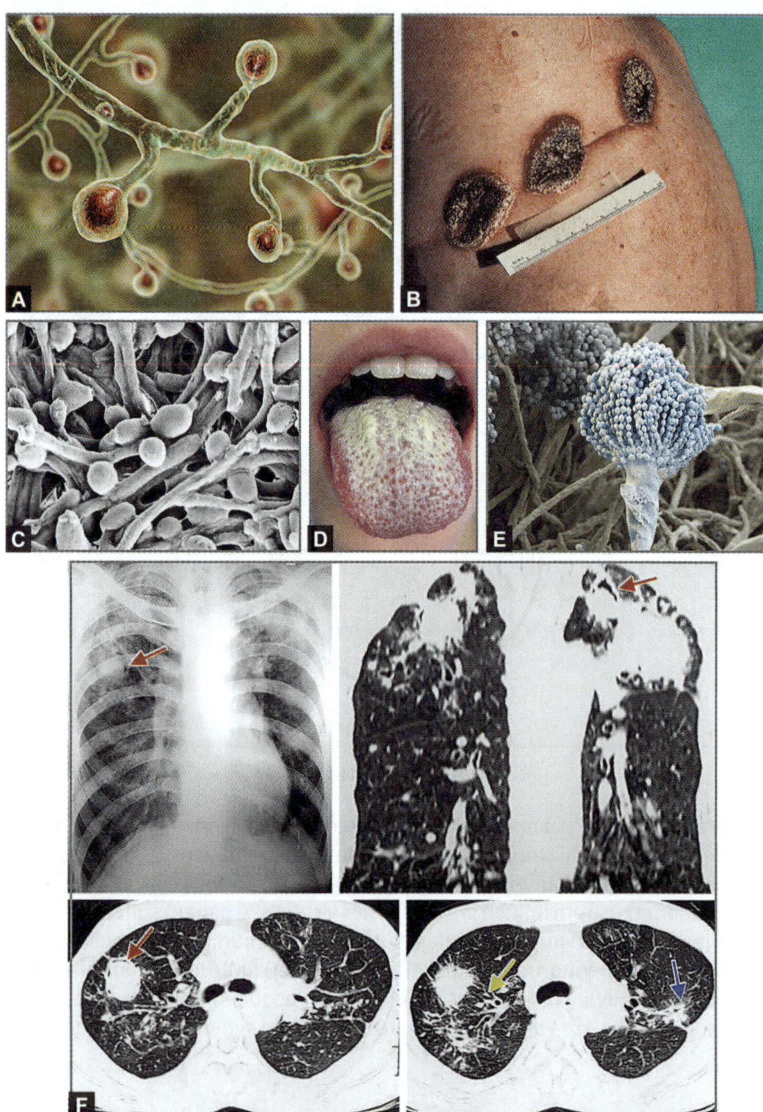

Figures 2.9.3A to F

Color Plate 9

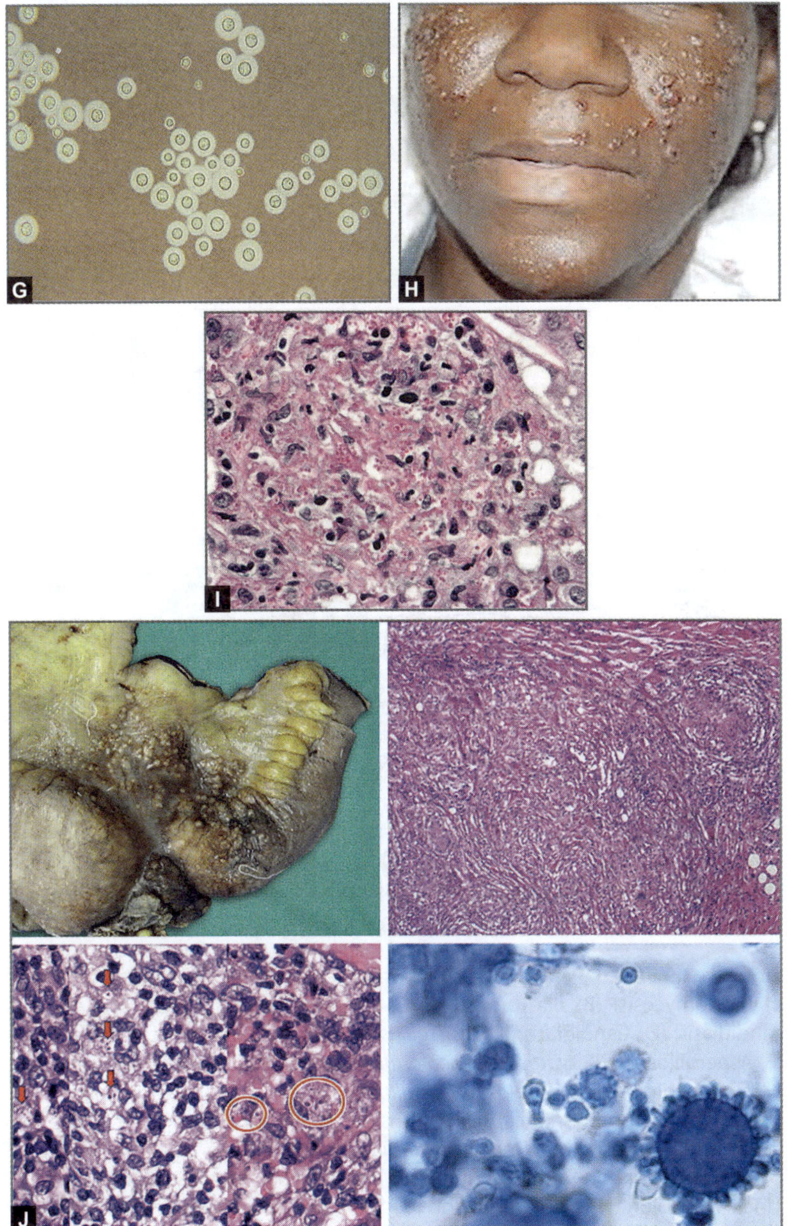

Figures 2.9.3G to J

Color Plate 10

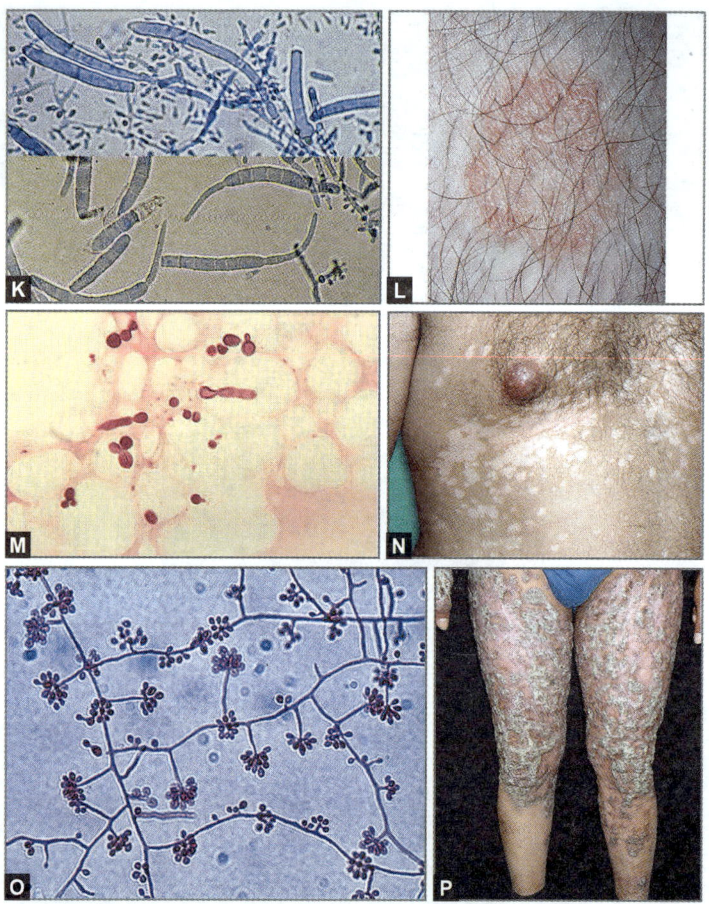

Figures 2.9.3 K to P

Figures 2.9.3A to P: Mycosis: (A) *Blastomyces dermatitidis*, causal organism of Blastomycosis; (B) Blastomycosis; (C) *Candida albicans*, causal organism of candidiasis; (D) Candidiasis; (E) *Aspergillus* spp., causal organism of Aspergillosis; (F) Aspergillosis; (G) *Cryptococcus neoformans*, causal organism of Cryptococcosis; (H) Cryptococcosis; (I) *Histoplasma capsulatum*, causal organism of Histoplasmosis; (J) Colony of *Histoplasma capsulatum* inside the lungs of the patient suffering from Histoplasmosis; (K) *Tricophyton rubrum* (Dermatophyte), causal organisms of Dermatophytosis; (L) Dermatophytosis; (M) *Malassezia furfur*, causal organisms of Tinea versicolor; (N) Tinea versicolor; (O) *Sporothrix schenckii*, causal organism of Sporotrichosis; (P) Sporotrichosis.

Color Plate 11

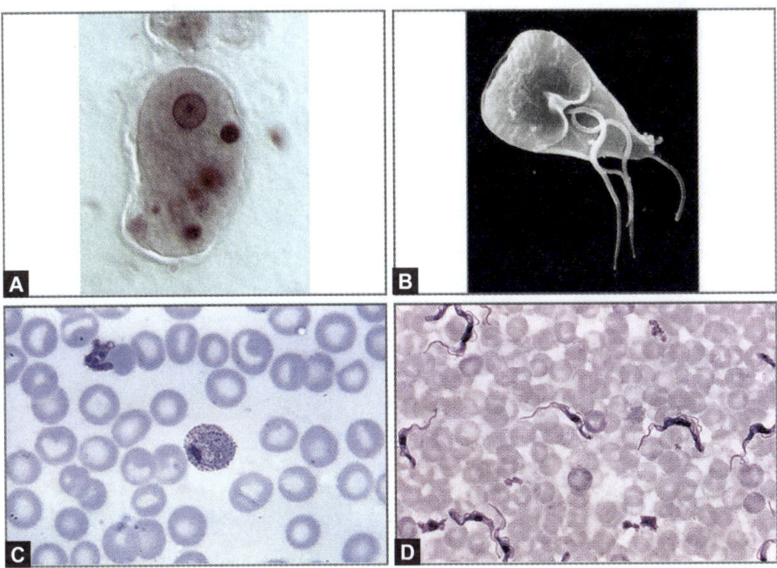

Figures 2.9.4A to D: Common protozoan parasites of human beings. (A) *Entamoeba histolytica*, causal organism of amoebiasis; (B) *Giardia lamblia*, causal organism of giardiasis; (C) *Plasmodium vivax*, causal organism of malaria; (D) *Trypanosoma brucei*, causal organism of African sleeping sickness.

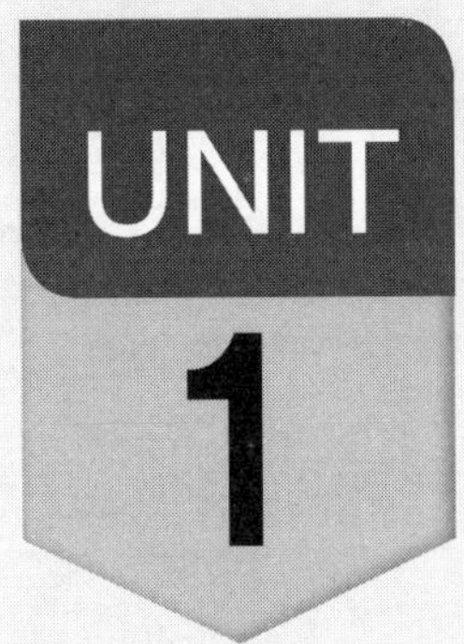

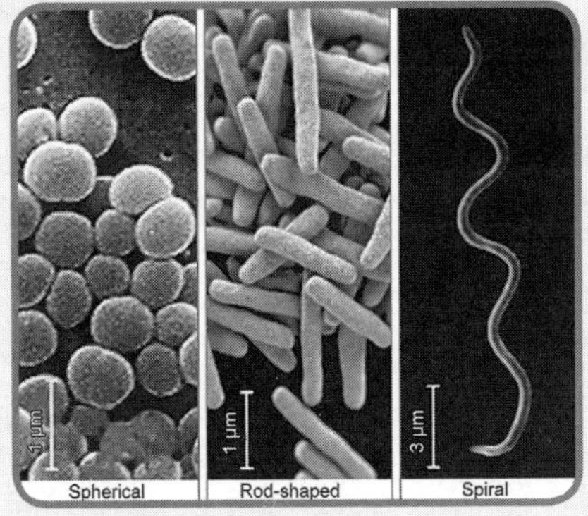

Introduction to Microbiology

Learning Objectives

- Understanding microorganisms
- History of microbiology
- Evolution of microorganisms
- Scope of microbiology in nursing

Understanding Microorganisms

WHAT ARE MICROORGANISMS?

Microorganisms are microscopic organisms (very small and can only be seen by microscope). These may be unicellular (having a single cell) or multicellular (having more than one cell). **The general characteristics of microorganisms are discussed in below Table.**

Table 1.1.1: General characteristics of microorganisms.

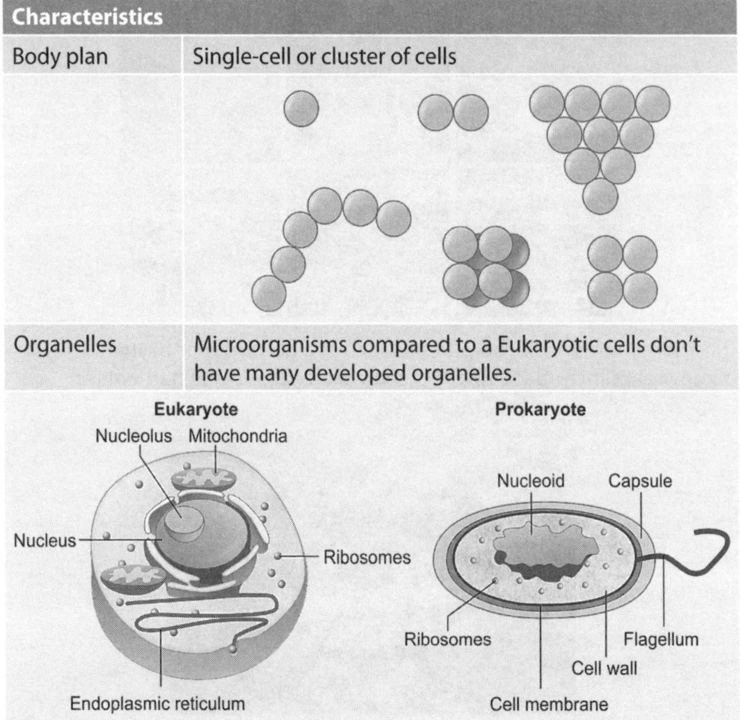

Characteristics	
Body plan	Single-cell or cluster of cells
Organelles	Microorganisms compared to a Eukaryotic cells don't have many developed organelles.

Contd...

Contd...

Characteristics	
Size	Dimensions of microscopic organisms fall within the range of micrometers, sometimes nanometers Most microbes extend from the smallest viruses to much bigger protozoans

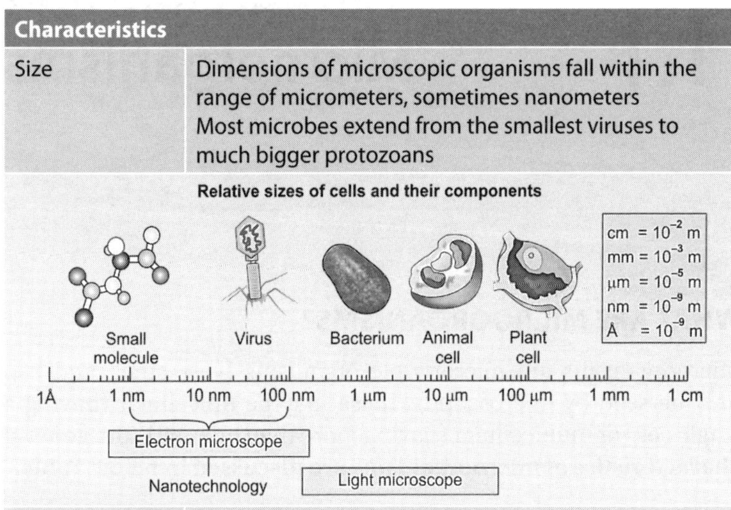

Habitat	They are ubiquitous (found everywhere)

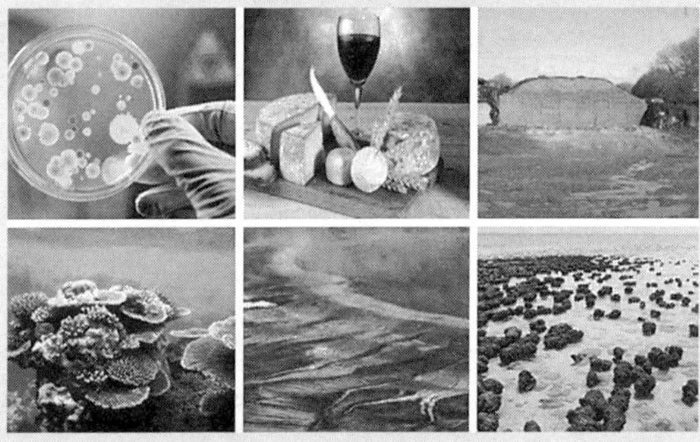

Microorganisms to environment	Microorganisms such as algae produce oxygen. They decompose organic material, provide nutrients for plants, etc.

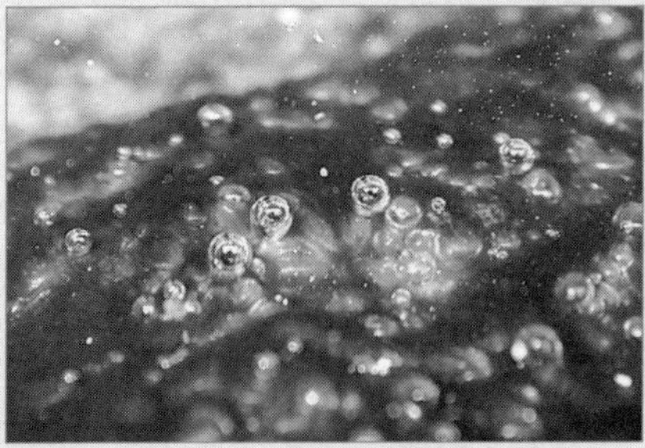

Contd...

Contd...

Characteristics	
Micro-organisms to humans	Some microorganisms are good for human health, and some are pathogenic (causing severe diseases in humans and animals)

Harmful microorganisms	Beneficial microorganisms
Salmonella found on raw chicken	Penicillin
E coli found on row meat	Blue cheese
Ringworm	Bacteria that turns milk to yogurt (YOGURT)
Athletes foot	Yeast for making bread
Red algae	Bacteria is a cow's stomach that allows the cow to digest gross
Streptococcus bacteria	Bacteria in your intestines used in digestion

Factors affecting growth of microorganisms	Nutrients, oxygen, water, temperature, acidity, light, and chemicals affect the growth of microorganisms. Specific organisms require an optimum growth factor to survive and grow

Moisture	Oxygen	Carbon dioxide
Temperature	pH	Light
Osmotic effect	Mechanical and sonic stress	

MICROBIOLOGY: STUDY OF MICROORGANISMS

Microbiology is the scientific study of microorganisms. Various branches of Microbiology include:

- Bacteriology: The study of bacteria.
- Mycology: The study of fungi.
- Protozoology: The study of protozoa.
- Phycology (or algology): The study of algae.
- Parasitology: The study of parasites.
- Virology: The study of viruses.
- Nematology: The study of the nematodes.

Categories of Microorganisms

Depending on their cell type, microorganisms are divided in below **Flowchart**.

Flowchart 1.1.1: Categories of microorganisms depending on their cell type.

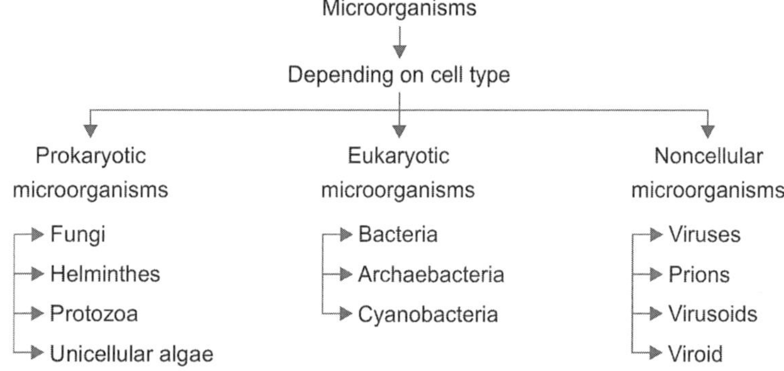

Prokaryotic Microorganisms (Fig.1.1.2)

They are simple, self-sufficient, unicellular organisms having primitive nuclei and mitochondria being capable of leading independent lives.

Examples

- Bacteria: *E.coli, Vibrio cholerae*
- Archaebacteria: *Thermobacillus* SPS
- Cyanobacteria: *Spirulina* SPS

Eukaryotic Microorganisms

They have a complex cellular structure. The cells have defined nuclei and membrane-bound organelles. They are self-sufficient and capable of leading independent lives.

Examples

- Fungi: Molds and yeasts
- Helminths: Tapeworm, Hookworms
- Protozoa: *Plasmodium*
- Unicellular algae: *Chlamydomonas*

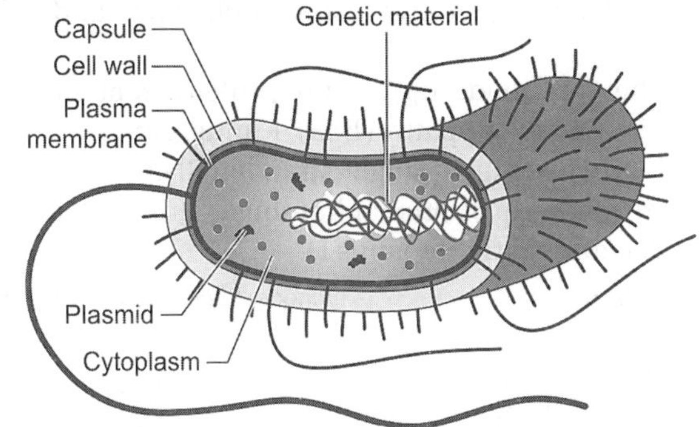

Figure 1.1.1: Prokaryotic microorganisms.

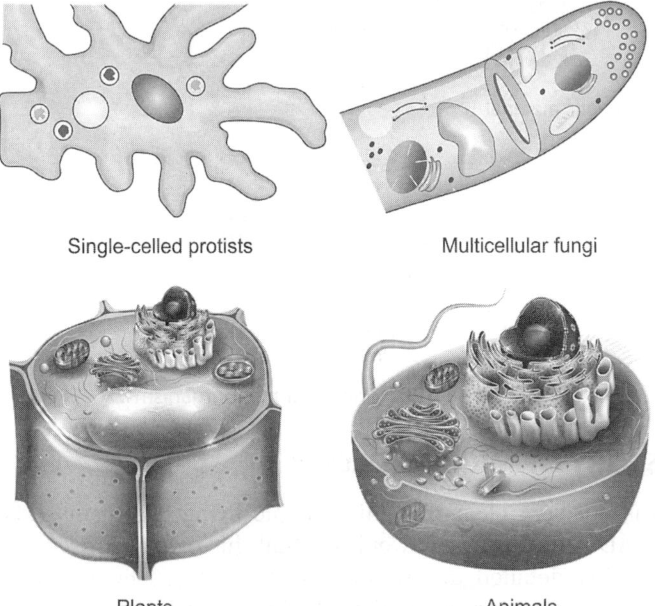

Figure 1.1.2: Eukaryotic microorganisms.

Noncellular Microorganisms

They are without any cell forms and are called acellular. They are of the following types:

- Viruses: They consist of DNA or RNA and proteins. They are not capable of leading independent lives. They grow and multiply by infecting cells of higher organisms (prokaryotic and eukaryotic cells).
- Prions: They are made up of only proteins that cause Bovine Spongiform Encephalopathy (BSE), Kunue, etc.
- Virusoids are made up of single-stranded RNA.
- Viroids are made-up of circular but single-stranded RNA without protein. It causes Viral Hepatitis D

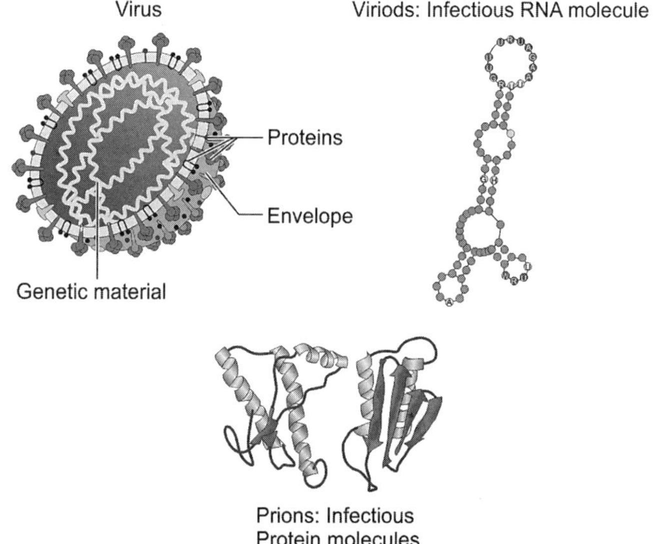

Figure 1.1.3: Noncellular microorganisms.

HISTORY OF MICROBIOLOGY

It was not very clear that microscopic living organisms exist. In 1600 AD Anton van Leeuwenhoek built his own microscopes and made first detailed descriptions of microscopic living creatures. Leeuwenhoek observed a variety of things like rain water, pond water and scrapings from his own teeth under the lens of his so-called microscope. He saw minute moving objects and called them as "Little animalcules", such as protozoa, yeasts and bacteria. He made accurate sketches and communicated his findings to "Royal Society of London". He had most likely observed single celled eukarytoic microbes. With this observation the Science of Microbiology was started. For this reason Anton van Leeuwenhoek is called as the father of Microbiology.

CONTRIBUTION OF EMINENT SCIENTISTS TO MICROBIOLOGY

Edward Jenner (1749–1823)

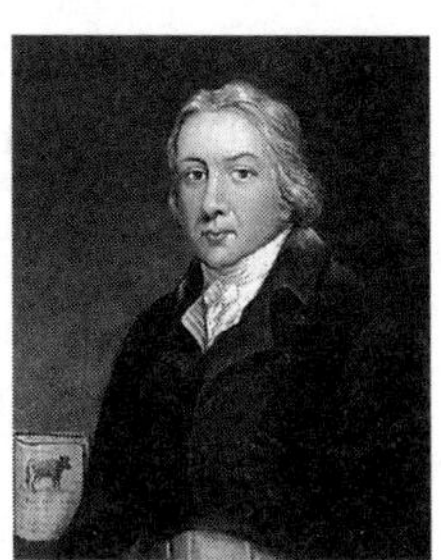

Figure 1.1.4: Edward Jenner (1749–1823).

- Jenner was an English doctor who discovered vaccination against smallpox. This ultimately led to eradication of smallpox.
- He observed that dairy workers exposed to occupational (from their dairy job) cowpox infection were naturally immune to smallpox.
- In 1796, he experimentally proved that resistance to smallpox can be induced by injecting cow pox material from disease pustules into man.
- Jenner published his findings in 1798 in a pamphlet "An inquiry into the cause and effect of variole vaccine".

LOUIS PASTEUR (1822–1895)

Era	Discoverer	Important Events
Eighteenth Century	Edward Jenner (1729–1799)	Discovery of smallpox vaccine
Nineteenth Century	Justus von Liebig (1803–1873)	Conceptualized the physicochemical theory of fermentation
	Philipp Semmelweis (1818–1865)	First and foremost introduced the application of antiseptics
	Joseph Lister (1827–1912)	Developed aseptic techniques: Isolated bacteria in pure culture
	Fanny Hesse (1850–1934)	Suggested use of agar as a solidifying material for the preparation of microbiological media
	Paul Ehrlich (1854–1915)	Developed modern concept of chemotherapy and chemotherapeutic agents

Contd...

Contd...

Era	Discoverer	Important Events
	Hans Christian Gram (1853–1933)	Invented vital and important procedure for differential staining of microorganisms, i.e., the well-known Gram stain
Twentieth Century	August von Wassermann (1866–1925)	Developed complement-fixation test for syphilis
	Martinus Willem Beijerinck (1851–1931)	Employed the principles of enrichment cultures: Confirmed finding of the very first virus
	Félix d'Hérelle (1873–1949)	Discovered independently the bacteriophages, i.e., viruses that destroy bacteria

- He was a Professor of Chemistry at the University of Lille, France.
- He is also called as "father of Modern Microbiology".
- Generation"(Abiogenesis), experimentally by using swan-necked flasks experiment.
- He experimentally showed that souring of wine and beer is due to the growth of undesirable organisms.
- He also showed that the desirable microorganisms produce alcohol by a chemical process called "Fermentation".
- He introduced the technique of "Pasteurization" and proposed the "Germ theory of disease".

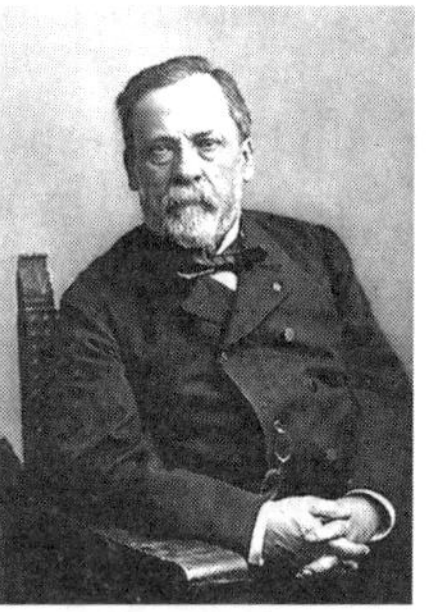

Figure 1.1.5: Louis Pasteur (1822–1895).

Germ Theory of Disease

- This theory was developed in 1860's, by Louis Pasteur.
- It states that tiny living beings are the cause of infectious diseases.
- While doing his research in puerperal fever or child bed fever Louis Pasteur proposed this theory.
- This disease for the first time supports that pathogenic microorganisms such as bacteria and viruses could cause disease.
- The term "germ" here stands for microscopic organisms that causes infectious diseases.
- Apart from the pathogen itself, certain environmental and hereditary factors may cause severity of the disease.

Pasteurization

- This is a special technique of heat sterilization developed by Louis Pasteur.
- Originally, it was used to kill undesirable microorganisms that cause souring of wine.
- This technique is now extensively used to kill disease causing germs in milk.
- The process of pasteurization of milk includes heating it to 60–65°C (140–150°F) for 30 mins followed by a rapid cooling.
- This decreases the rapid curdling of milk due to the action of microorganisms.

- He developed **steam sterilization technique**, today popularly called as **autoclaving**.
- He experimentally differentiated between aerobic and anaerobic bacteria and coined the term "**anaerobic**" to refer the organisms that do not require oxygen for growth.
- He developed **anthrax vaccine**.
- He also developed a **vaccine against rabies** (Hydrophobia).

Robert Koch (1843–1912)

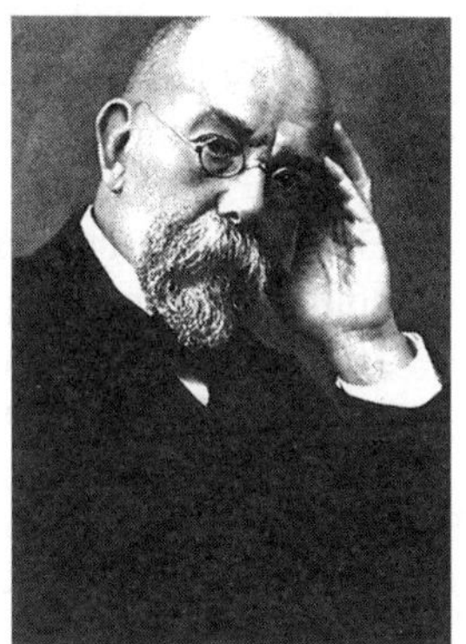

Figure 1.1.6: Robert Koch (1843–1912).

- He was a German doctor who later became the Professor of Hygiene and Director of Institute of Infective Diseases at Berlin.
- He is known as father of Practical Bacteriology.
- He is also regarded as "father of Medical Microbiology and Bacteriology".
- He discovered *Bacillus anthracis,* the causal organism of the disease Anthrax.
- He introduced staining techniques for the study of disease causing microorganisms.
- He discovered *Mycobacterium tuberculosis* which causes tuberculosis in human beings.
- He also discovered *Vibrio cholerae,* the causative agent of Cholera disease.

- He developed pure culture techniques by introducing solid media.
- He had a great contribution in the development of pure culture techniques.
- He gave Koch's Postulates.

Koch's Postulates

- A specific organism should be found constantly in association with disease.
- The organisms should be isolated and grown in a pure culture in the laboratory.
- The pure culture when inoculated into a healthy susceptible animal should produce symptoms/lesions of the same disease.
- From the inoculated animals, the microorganism should be isolated in pure culture.
- An additional criterion introduced is that specific antibodies to the causative organisms should be demonstrable in patient's serum.

Joseph Lister (1827–1912)

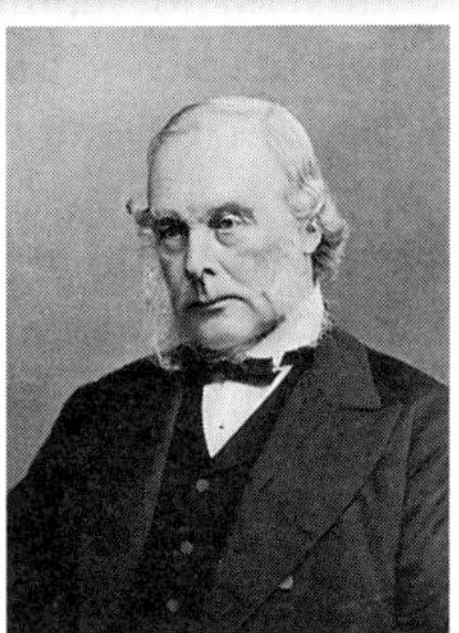

Figure 1.1.7: Joseph Lister (1827–1912)

- He was a Professor of Surgery at University of Glasglow and Edinburgh and later at King's College, London.
- He is also known as "Father of Antiseptic Surgery".
- He was the first person to use an antiseptic solution during the process of surgery.
- He used carbolic acid (phenol) on the wound during surgery which successfully prevented sepsis (infection) after operation.
- He also introduced application of carbolic acid during wound dressing.
- Lister's antiseptic surgery later led to the development of aseptic surgery.

Elie Metchnikoff (1845–1916)

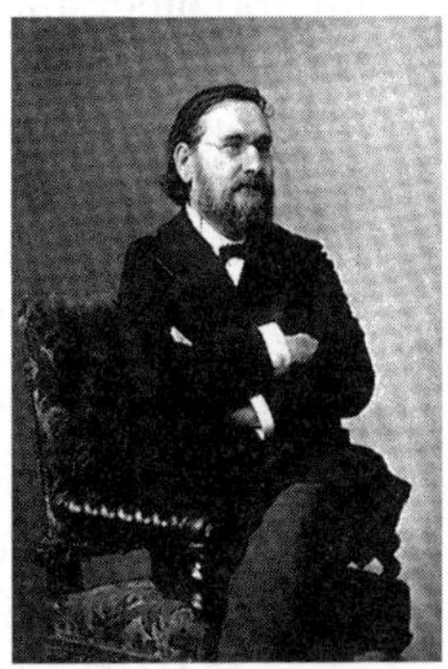

Figure 1.1.8: Elie Metchnikoff (1845–1916).

- Elie Metchnikoff, a Russian-French Biologist, discovered the phenomenon of phagocytosis.
- He discovered the process of phagocytosis in the transparent larvae of starfish.

- The cells which carry out phagocytosis are called as phagocytes.
- While working at Pasteur Institute in Paris, he found that in human blood leukocytes carry out phagocytosis against invading bacteria.
- Large number of leukocytes gather in the infected area which results in swelling, reddening and pain due to dead phagocytes forming pus.

Alexander Fleming (1881–1955)

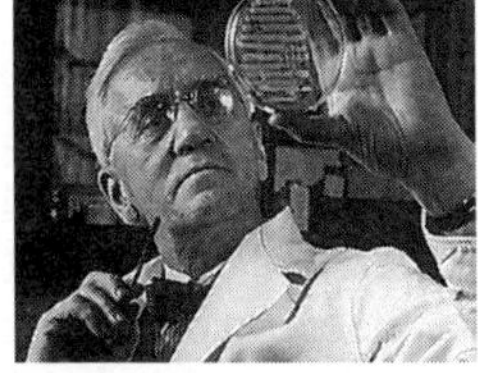

Figure 1.1.9: Alexander Fleming (1881–1955).

- He was an English Scientist who worked at St Marry's Hospital in London.
- He discovered lysozyme in 1922 by demonstrating that nasal secretion (fluid from nose) has the power of killing certain bacteria.
- Lysozymes are enzymes present in body fluids such as tears, sweat, and nasal fluid that have the power to kill certain bacteria.
- In 1929, he made an accidental discovery of the antibiotic Penicillin from the fungus Penicillium notatum.
- In 1945 Fleming, Florey and Chain shared the Nobel Prize in physiology and medicine for the discovery of Penicillin.

Paul Ehrlich (1854–1915)

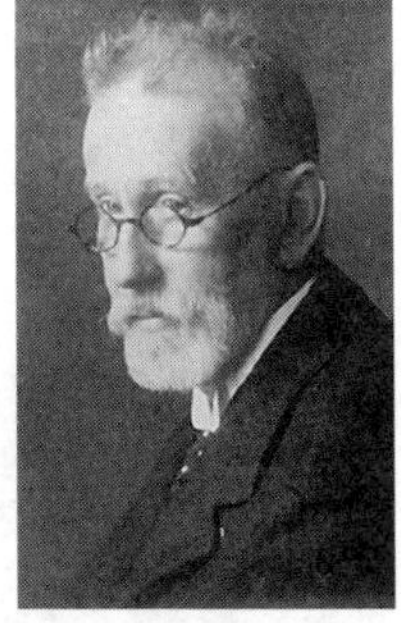

Figure 1.1.10: Paul Ehrlich (1854–1915).

- He was a German Bacteriologist who invented the technique of Chemotherapy in medicine.
- He is also called as "father of Chemotherapy".
- The very concept of Chemotherapy is based on the fact that organisms causing diseases could selectively be killed with chemical drugs without harming the host.
- He produced the first synthetic drug - arsphenamine to control the Syphilis disease.
- He also observed that drug would undergo certain changes in the body after it would produce desired action.

EVOLUTION OF MICROORGANISMS

What is Evolution?

Evolution is the process by which different kinds of living organisms are believed to have developed from earlier forms during the history of the earth.

The evolution of microorganisms is deeply connected with the evolution of life on planet earth.

- Scientific evidence suggests that life began on Earth some 3.5 billion years ago.
- Since then, life has evolved into a wide variety of forms, which biologists have classified into a hierarchy of taxa.
- Some of the oldest cells on earth are single-cell organisms called archaea and bacteria. Fossil records indicate that mounds of bacteria once covered young earth.
- Some began making their food using carbon dioxide in the atmosphere and energy they harvested from the sun.
- This process (called photosynthesis) produced enough oxygen to change earth's atmosphere.
- Soon afterward, new oxygen-breathing life forms came onto the scene. With a population of increasingly diverse bacterial life, the stage was set for more life to form.
- There is compelling evidence that mitochondria and chloroplasts were once primitive bacterial cells.

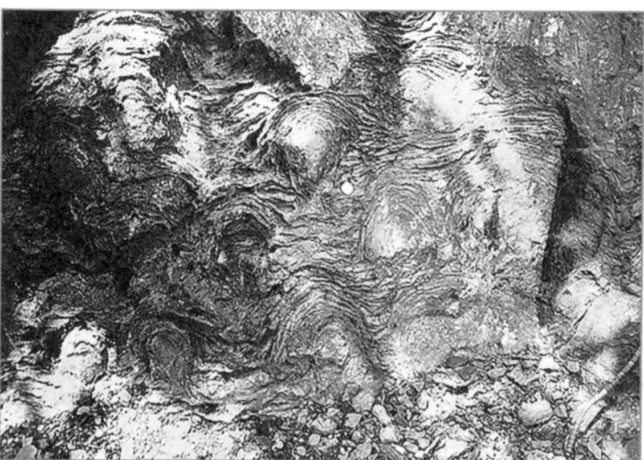

Figure 1.1.11: Extremophiles: Photosynthetic fossilized cyanobacteria in a billion-year-old rock formation of Glacier National Park, Montana, USA.

- This evidence is described in the endosymbiotic theory. Symbiosis occurs when two different species benefit from living and working together.
- When one organism lives inside the other it's called endosymbiosis.
- The endosymbiotic theory describes how a large host cell and ingested bacteria could easily become dependent on one another for survival, resulting in a permanent relationship.
- Over millions of years of evolution, mitochondria and chloroplasts have become more specialized and today they cannot live outside the cell. Mitochondria and chloroplasts have striking similarities to bacteria cells.
- They have their DNA, which is separate from the DNA found in the nucleus of the cell. And both organelles use their DNA to produce many proteins and enzymes required for their function.
- A double membrane surrounding both mitochondria and chloroplasts is further evidence that each was ingested by a primitive host.
- The two organelles also reproduce like bacteria, replicating their DNA and directing their division.

SCOPE OF MICROBIOLOGY IN NURSING

The Profession of Nursing

Nursing care focuses on distributing superior quality health care to the patients. This goal requires the nurse to perform the following tasks:

- Assessment
- Diagnosis
- Outcome identification
- Planning
- Implementation
- Evaluation

Nurses assess patients' conditions by observation and examination of individuals. After collecting the data, nurses analyze the situation and generate a diagnosis. This is the reason why they should have good knowledge of microbiology.

The knowledge of microbiology for nursing students also plays an important role to make them understand the principles of the personal, hospital, and community hygiene, basic procedures in hospitals and health care centers, and the prevention of diseases.

Nursing students need to study the microbes that infect humans, the disease they cause, and their diagnosis, prevention, control, and treatment. The job of a nurse is to deal with all these aspects and be aware so that she can perform their duties safely and healthy.

Following are the important scope of microbiology in nursing

- **To prevent the spread of Nosocomial infections:** These are the types of infections that can be acquired in hospitals or health care centers. Knowledge about specific infections within a hospital can help Nurses prevent their spread among patients of different age groups. Patients affected with microbial diseases are mostly admitted to communicable diseases wards. Nurses take care of these patients by following strict protocols, aseptic techniques, and using PPE kits to prevent the transmission of infections to other individuals.
- **To follow the Immunization schedule:** The process of giving a vaccine to a person to protect them from diseases is called immunization. Nurses must have proper knowledge of the vaccines and the immunization schedule used in the prevention of dreadful diseases. Handling and storage of vaccines is also an important task that is taken care of by Nurses. Vaccines if carelessly handled may affect an individual with severe illness. The knowledge of specific immune responses and lab techniques is also a crucial part of the system. Hence Nurses need to understand the basics of types of immunity, microbial antigens, different classes of antibodies, and related reactions such as agglutination and precipitation in serological tests.

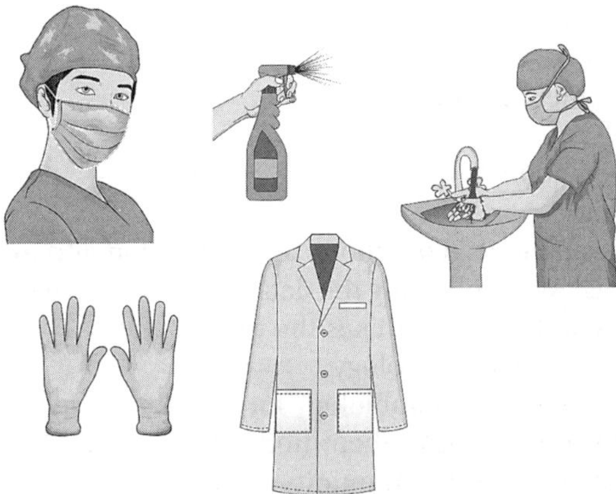

Figure 1.1.12: Hospital infection control.

Beneficiary	Age	Vaccine
Infants	Birth	BCG* and OPV**
	6 weeks	DPT and OPV
	10 weeks	DPT and OPV
	14 weeks	DPT and OPV
	9 months	Measles vaccine
	18 months	DPT and OPV (Booster dose)
Children	5 years	DT vaccine
	10 years	Tetanus Toxoid
	16 years	Tetanus Toxoid

* At birth or at the time of DPT/OPV.
** Dose called as zero dose and can be given till 14 days of age, if missed early.
(BCG: bacillus Calmitte-Guerin; DPT: diphtheria, pertussis and tetanus OPV: oral polio vaccine; DT: diphtheria and tetanus vaccine)

- **To maintain a sterile field**: Nurses usually work with respirators, catheters, transfusions, and gastronomy feeds in the intensive care units and with surgical equipment such as knives, needles, scissors, etc., in the operation theaters. Hygienic use of these medical instruments by Nurses following proper sterilization measures will maintain a safe and healthy environment for patients, attendants as well as health workers.

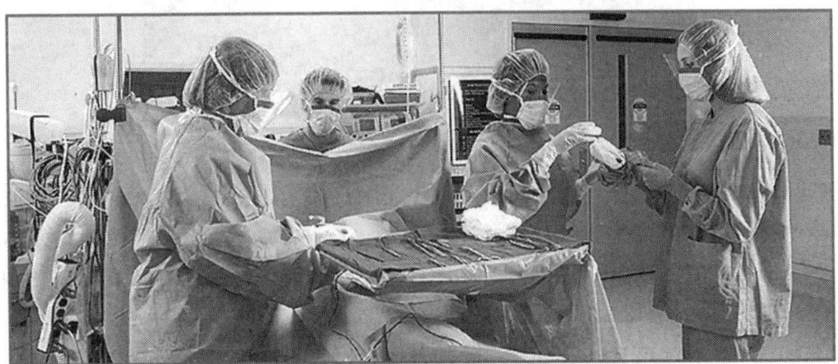

Figure 1.1.13: Maintain a sterile field *(For color version see Plate 1).*

- **Collection of patient's samples**: Nurses often need to collect patient's blood, sputum, fecal, or urine samples for examination and diagnosis. They should be well trained in the aseptic collection of samples in sterile vials and storing them for lab examinations. They should also have a sound knowledge of serological tests conducted with patients' blood samples.

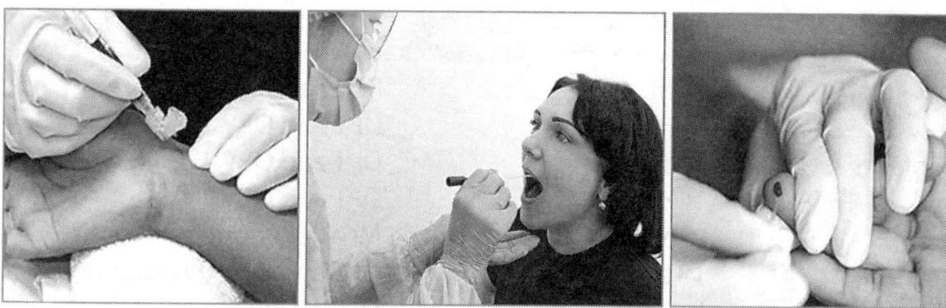

Figure 1.1.14: Collection of patient's samples *(For color version see Plate 1)*.

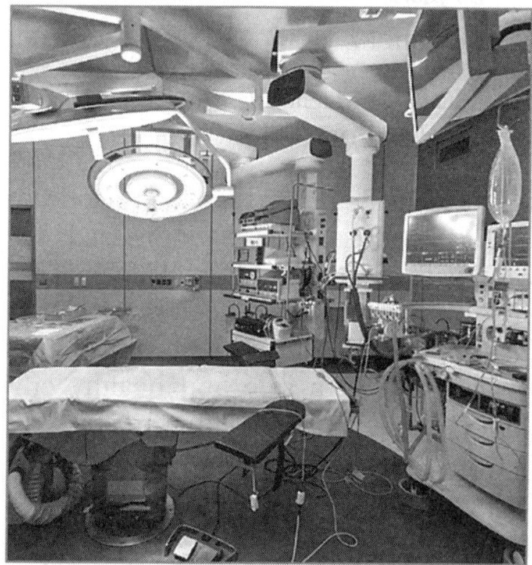

Figure 1.1.15: Controlling microbial growth *(For color version see Plate 1)*.

- **Controlling microbial growth**: Nurses should be well versed in controlling microbial growth either by physical methods such as heat, filtration, or ultra-radiation or by chemical methods – using alcohol, antibiotics, etc.
- **Microbes versus diseases information**: Nurses need to know about common diseases caused and the organs affected by the microbial infections.

POSSIBLE QUESTIONS

Objective Type or Fill in the Blanks

1. The study of algae is known as _______.
   a. Mycology b. Protozoology
   c. Phycology d. Virology

2. Which of the following microorganism has complex cellular structure?
   a. *Spirulina SPS* b. *Plasmodium*
   c. *E. coli* d. *Vibrio cholerae*
3. Prion is made up of _________.
   a. DNA b. RNA and DNA
   c. Protein d. Both a and b
4. Virusoids are made up of _______.
   a. dsDNA b. dsRNA
   c. ssDNA d. ssRNA
5. Hepatitis-D is caused by ____.
   a. Virus b. Bacteria
   c. Viroidis d. Protozoa
6. Kunue occurs due to _____.
   a. Yeast b. Bacteria
   c. Thermobacillus SPS d. Prions
7. Father of microbiology is known as_______.
   a. Gregor Johann Mendel b. Anton Van Leeuwenhoek
   c. T. H. Morgan d. Edward Jenner
8. Who discovered vaccination against smallpox ?
   a. Anton Van Leeuwenhoek b. Louis Pasture
   c. Edward Jenner d. Felix H.d' Herelle
9. Jenner published his experiment in which year?
   a. 1798 b. 1797
   c. 1796 d. 1799
10. Father of modern microbiology ________.
    a. Louis Pasture b. Edward Jenner
    c. TH Morgan d. Bateson
11. "Germ theory of disease" was proposed by _________.
    a. Louis Pasture b. August Von Wassermann
    c. Paul Ehrlich d. Fenny Hesse
12. A special technique of heat sterilization is called as ________.
    a. Pasteurization b. Heat Sterilization
    c. Denaturation d. Rolling Boil
13. Pasteurization of milk includes heating it with the temperature _______.
    a. 60°–65°C b. 140°–150°F
    c. 70°–90°C d. Both a and b
14. Autoclaving refers to ________.
    a. Steam and heat sterilization technique
    b. Heat sterilization
    c. Steam sterilization
    d. Dry heat sterilization
15. Louis Pasture developed vaccine against ____________.
    a. Rabies b. Anthrax
    c. Both a and b d. Alzheimer

16. Anaerobic refers to the organism that __________.
    a. Requires oxygen
    b. Don't require oxygen
    c. Requires oxygen in small amount
    d. None of the above
17. Who is the father of medical microbiology and bacteriology____________.
    a. Robert Koch b. Joseph Lister
    c. Elie Metchnikoff d. MacCarthy
18. Tuberculosis in human being is caused by _________.
    a. Tobacco Mosaic Virus b. *Mycobacterium tuberculosis*
    c. *Entamoeba histolytica* d. *Vibrio cholerae*
19. Which statement is correct about Koch's Postulate?
    a. Organism should be isolated and grown in pure culture medium
    b. Specific organism should constantly associated with disease
    c. It decreases the rapid curdling of milk
    d. Both a and b
20. Common name of phenol is ____________.
    a. Carbolic acid b. Carboxylic acid
    c. Acetic acid d. Formic acid
21. Who discovered phenomenon of phagocytosis?
    a. Alexander Fleming b. Elie Metchnikoff
    c. Paul Ehrlich d. Robert Koch
22. Phagocytosis was discovered in ___________.
    a. Pus cell b. Larvae of Star fish
    c. Both a and b d. None of the above
23. The cell that carryout phagocytosis are called as__________ .
    a. Phagosome b. Phagocytes
    c. Phagocyst d. None of the above
24. Swelling, reddening, and pain in the affected areas is due to __________.
    a. WBC b. RBC
    c. Leukocyte d. Phagocyte
25. Tears, sweat and nasal fluid have enzyme __________.
    a. Lysozyme b. Amylase
    c. Lipase d. Trypsin
26. Penicillin was discovered by _________.
    a. Joseph Lister b. Alexander Fleming
    c. Justus von Liebig d. None of the above
27. Penicillin was discovered in the year ________.
    a. 1929 b. 1999
    c. 1927 d. 1928
28. Who is regarded as the Father of Chemotherapy?
    a. Paul Ehrlich b. Aristotle
    c. Horace Mann d. None of the above
29. Identify the first synthetic drug.
    a. Arsphenamine b. Paracetamol
    c. Morphine d. Codeine

30. Syphilis disease can be controlled by the use of drug _______.
    a. Arsphenamine
    b. Aspirin
    c. Amlodipine
    d. Dopamine

Answers

1. c	2. b	3. c	4. d	5. b
6. d	7. b	8. c	9. a	10. a
11. a	12. a	13. d	14. c	15. c
16. b	17. a	18. b	19. d	20. a
21. b	22. b	23. b	24. c	25. a
26. b	27. a	28. a	29. a	30. a

Short Type Questions

1. What was the contribution of Louis Pasteur in microbiology?
2. What do you understand by Germ theory of Disease?
3. Explain in brief the process of Pasteurization?
4. Who is called as the "Father of Medical Microbiology and Bacteriology"? What was his contribution to the field of microbiology?
5. List out the postulates given by Robert Koch.
6. What was Edward Jenner's discovery and why is it considered to be the most important discovery in the history of microbiology?
7. What was Joseph Lister's contribution to microbiology?
8. Who invented the technique of Chemotherapy? What was his contribution in the field of medical microbiology?
9. Name some of the vaccines developed by Louis Pasteur.
10. Who is called as the "Father of Antiseptic Surgery" and what was his role in the field of medical microbiology?
11. Which was the first antibiotic discovered by Alexander Fleming? From which organisms was it discovered?
12. What is the role of Lysozyme against bacteria?
13. How do nurses play an important role in prevention of nosocomial infections?
14. What do you mean by immunization schedule? Why is it important for nurses to have a detail knowledge about immunization schedule?
15. How do nurses work on maintaining a sterile environment within the hospital premises?
16. Why is it important for nurses to know the correct procedure for patient's sample collection?
17. How can nurses control microbial growth in hospitals?
18. Mention five characteristic features of microorganisms.
19. What is the scope of microbiology in the field of nursing?

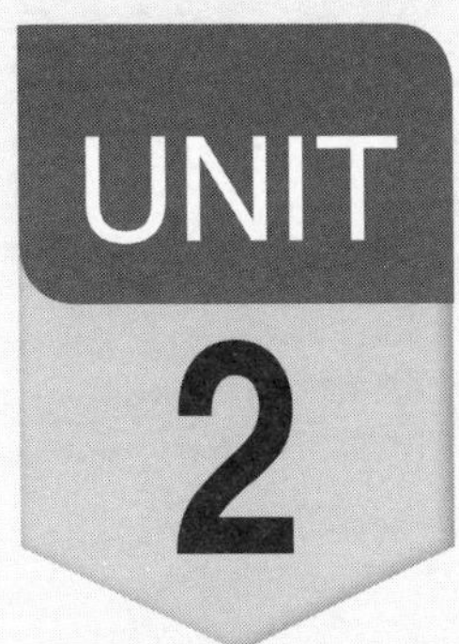

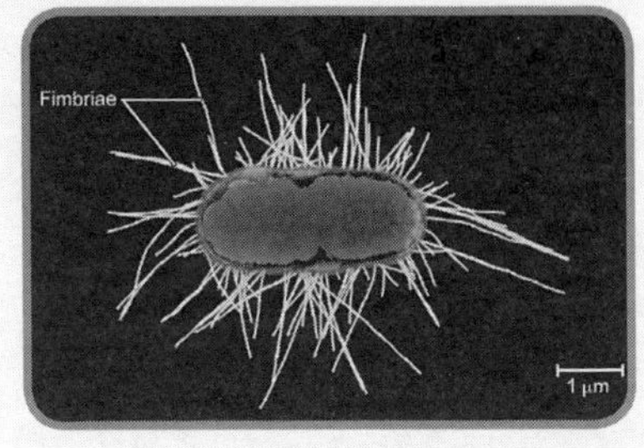

Classification, Structure, Growth and Pathogenesis

Learning Objectives

- Classification of microorganisms
- Structure of bacteria
- Structure of viruses
- Growth of microorganisms
- Normal flora of the human body
- Bacterial reproduction
- Bacterial culture and its types
- Isolation of microbes
- Pathogenesis and common diseases

Classification of Microorganisms

WHAT IS THE CLASSIFICATION OF MICROORGANISMS?

Biological Classification, or Taxonomy is a method of classifying and categorizing living organisms into groups which share similar characteristic features. There are different types of microorganisms, each differing in its characteristic features. In order to have a systematic study they can be classified under various groups.

WHY WE NEED TO CLASSIFY MICROORGANISMS?

More than five million species of microorganisms have already been reported. Thousands more are added to the list every year. It would be difficult to describe and name each one individually. If any microorganism is picked up randomly it would not be possible to describe its basic properties and features so easily. But if their groups are made based on similarities of characteristics then it would be easy to identify them and understand their basic characteristic features.

BASIS OF CLASSIFICATION

We classify microorganisms on the following basis:

- Cell type: Eukaryotic or prokaryotic
- Cellular or acellular
- Biochemical properties

MAJOR GROUPS OF MICROORGANISMS

Eukaryotic Microorganisms

Basic Features of Eukaryotic Cells

- Contain nucleus bounded by nuclear membrane
- Contain complex phospholipids, sphingolipids, histones and sterols

- Have multiple diploid linear (straight) chromosomes and nucleosomes
- Have 80s ribosomes
- Have membrane bound cell organelles, such as vacuoles, mitochondria, etc.

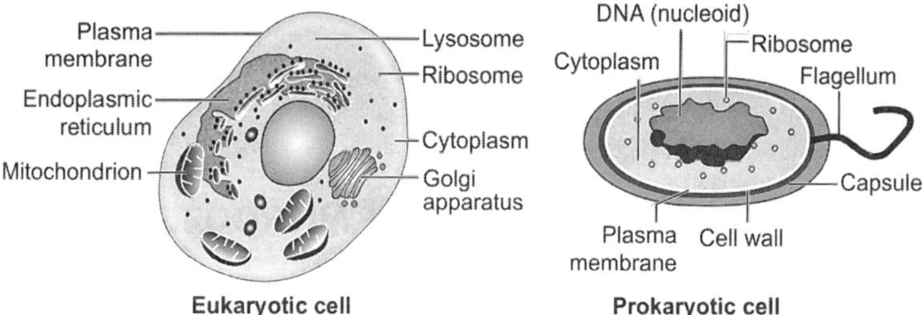

Figure 2.1.1: Eukaryotic and prokaryotic cells.

The following are the types of eukaryotic microorganisms:

Protozoa

- Protozoa are eukaryotic microorganisms.
- Protozoa lack the capability for photosynthesis, although the genus Euglena is renowned for motility as well as carrying out photosynthesis and is, therefore, considered both as alga and protozoan.
- Although most protozoa reproduce by asexual methods, sexual reproduction has been observed in several species.
- Most protozoa species are aerobic but some anaerobic species have been found in the human intestine and animal lumen.
- Protozoa are located in most moist habitats. Free-living species inhabit freshwater and marine environments and terrestrial species inhabit decaying organic matter. Some species are parasites of plants and animals.
- Protozoa play an important role as **zooplankton,** the free-floating aquatic organisms of the oceans.
- Their cells have no cell walls and therefore can assume an infinite variety of shapes.
- Most protozoa have a single nucleus but some have both macronucleus and one or more micronuclei. Contractile vacuoles may be present in protozoa to remove excess water and food vacuoles are often observed.
- Protozoa are **heterotrophic** microorganisms and most species obtain large food particles by **phagocytosis.**

- Many protozoa species move independently by one of three types of locomotor organelles: flagella, cilia and pseudopodia.
- *Example: Entamoeba histolytica* causes amoebiasis in human beings.

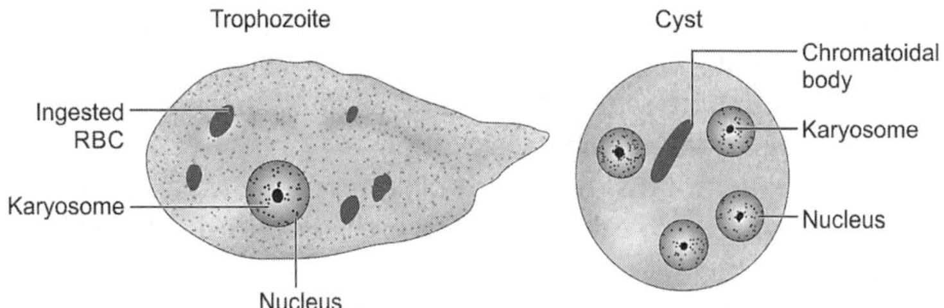

Figure 2.1.2: *Entamoeba histolytica*, the causal agent of amoebiasis in human beings.

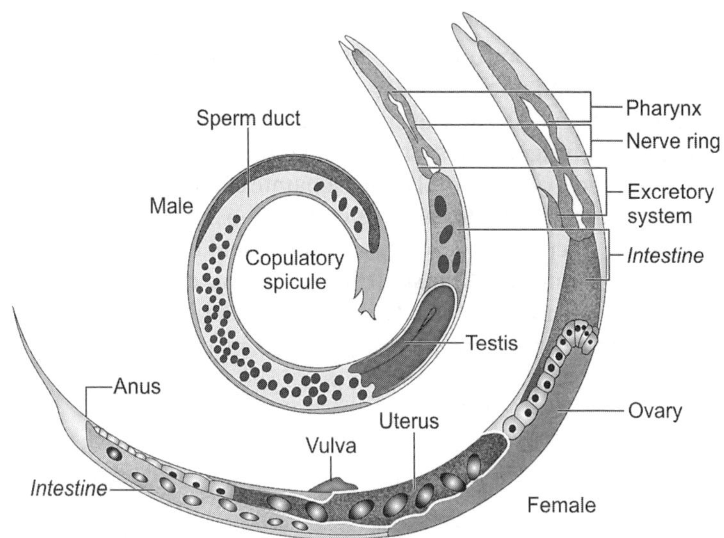

Figure 2.1.3: *Ascaris lumbricoides* (roundworm), the causal agent of ascariasis in humans.

Helminths

- Helminths are parasitic, multicellular eukaryotic animals.
- The majority of these animals belong to phyla Platyhelminthes and Nematoda.

- Many parasitic helminths do not have a digestive system and instead absorb nutrients from the food that is consumed by their host organisms, the host's body fluids and tissues.
- Parasitic helminths have very simple nervous system because they have to respond to very few changes in their host's environment.
- They lack or have reduced means of locomotion because they are transferred from one host to another.
- Parasitic helminths have complex reproductive system that produces fertilized eggs (zygotes) which infect the host organism.
- Examples:
  - *Taenia solium* (Pork tapeworm) causes Taeniasis
  - *Ascaris lumbricoides* (roundworm) causes Ascariasis

Fungi

- Fungi are **eukaryotic** and have membrane-bound cellular organelles and nuclei.
- They have no plastids of any kind (and no chlorophyll). The hyphae of fungi are of two general kinds: Some are **septate** and are divided by **septa** (walls) that separate cylindrical hyphae into cells; in **nonseptate** fungi, the hypha is one long tube.
- Mitosis occurs in nonseptate hyphae, but there is no accompanying **cytokinesis** (division of the cytoplasm) so the hyphae are **multinucleate** (with many nuclei).

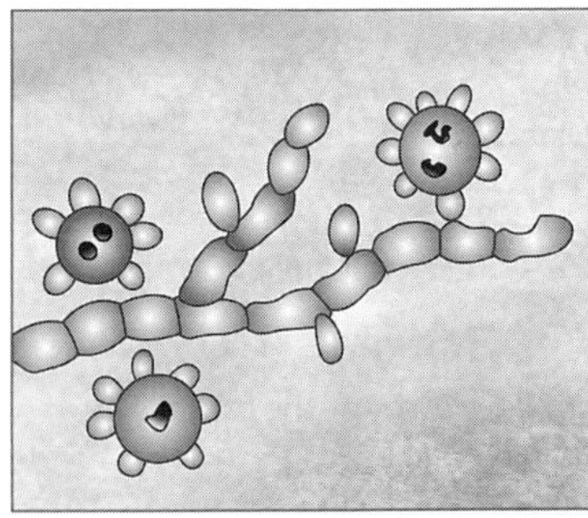
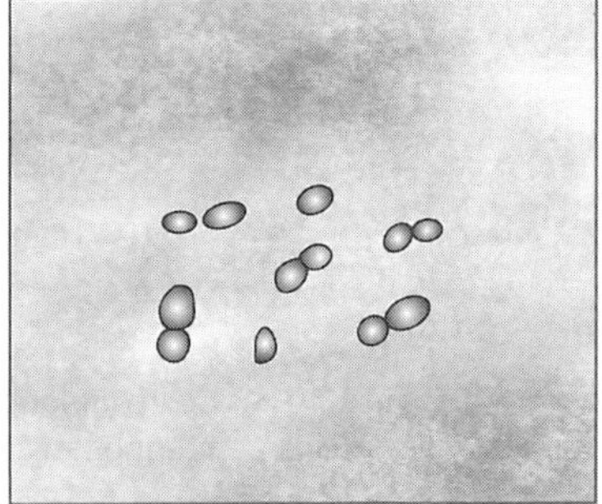

Figure 2.1.4: *Histoplasma capsulatum*, the causal agent of histoplasmosis in human beings.

- An organism or part of an organism with many nuclei not separated by walls or membranes—is termed as **coenocytic** and the organism is a coenocyte.

- Fungi are **heterotrophic** but unlike animals and many other heterotrophs can ingest their nutrients as bits or bites of food, the fungi secrete digestive enzymes into their surroundings and in effect digesting their food outside of their bodies.
- They can absorb smaller particles and incorporate nutrients into their own cells. Some are **parasites** obtaining nutrients from living organisms but more are **saprobes (saprotrophs)** that digest and recycle materials from dead organisms.
- *Example: Histoplasma capsulatum* causes histoplasmosis in human beings.

Algae

- **Algae** are eukaryotic organisms that have no roots, stems, or leaves but do have chlorophyll and other pigments for carrying out photosynthesis.
- Algae may be unicellular or multicellular.
- **Unicellular algae** occur most frequently in water especially in plankton.
- **Phytoplankton** is the population of free floating microorganisms composed primarily of unicellular algae.
- Algae establish symbiosis with fungi to form lichen.
- Reproduction in algae occurs in both asexual and sexual forms. Asexual reproduction occurs through fragmentation of colonial and filamentous algae or by spore formation (as in fungi). Spore formation takes place by mitosis. Binary fission also occurs (as in bacteria).
- *Example: Prototheca cutis* causes skin infection in human beings.

Prokaryotic Microorganisms

Basic Features of Prokaryotic Cells

- Lack nuclei.
- Have single circular chromosome. Some also contain plasmids.
- Have 70s ribosomes.
- Lack membrane bound cell organelles, such as vacuoles, mitochondrias, etc.
- Bacteria
  - Bacteria are prokaryotic organisms.
  - They are microscopic, unicellular, may occur singly or in aggregations to form colonies.

- They possess rigid cell walls. **Cell wall** is made up of **peptidoglycan (Mureins) and Lipopolysaccharides**.
- **Ribosomes** are scattered in cytoplasmic matrix and are of **70s type.**
- Most of the bacteria are heterotrophic. Some bacteria are autotrophic, possess **bacteriochlorophyll** which is not in plastids and instead it is found to be scattered.
- Motile bacteria possess one or more **flagella.**
- The common method of multiplication is **binary fission.**
- True sexual reproduction is lacking but **genetic recombination** occurs by conjugation, transformation and transduction.
- *Examples:*
  - *Vibrio cholerae* causes Cholera
  - *Salmonella typhi* causes Typhoid
  - *Mycobacterium tuberculosis* causes Tuberculosis

Some special categories of bacteria are as follows:

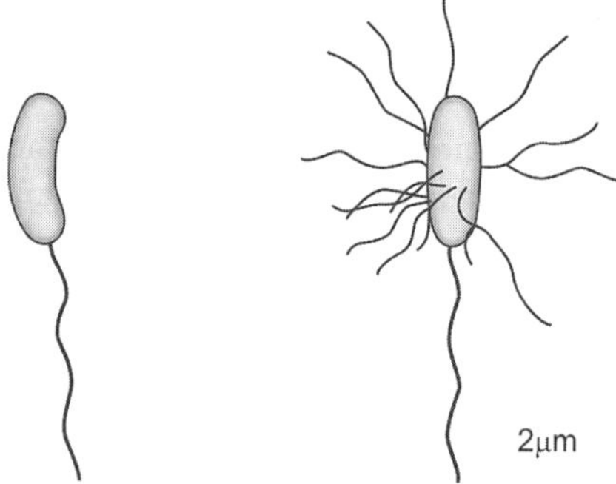

Figure 2.1.5: *Vibrio cholerae*, the causal agent of cholera in human beings.

Chlamydia

- *Chlamydia* are Gram-negative bacteria.
- They are obligate intracellular parasites. They can survive only by establishing "residence" inside the infected cells.
- They need their host's ATP as energy source for their own cellular activity.
- They are coccoid in shape and non-motile.
- They can be transmitted from person-to-person contact or by airborne respiration.

- *Examples:*
  - *Chlamydia trachomatis* causes trachoma
  - *C. pneumoniae* causes mild form of pneumonia in adolescence
  - *C. psittaci* causes psittacosis

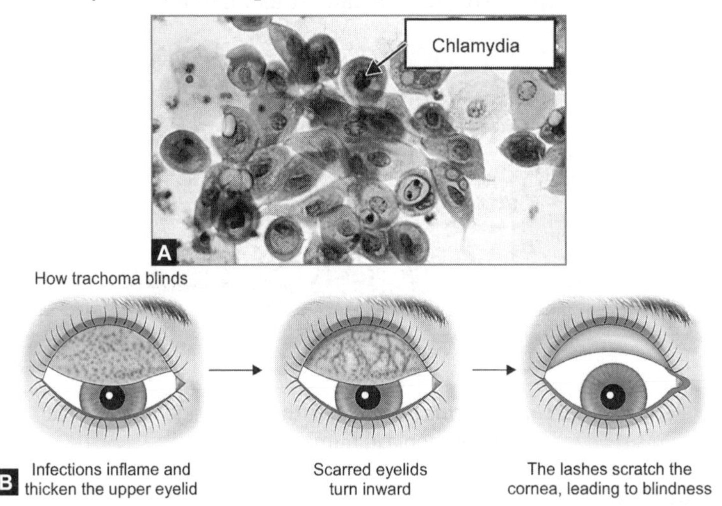

Figures 2.1.6 A and B: *Chlamydia trachomatis*, the causal agent of trachoma in human beings.

Mycoplasma

- The *Mycoplasma* are tiny free-living organisms capable of self-replication.
- They are smaller than some of larger viruses.
- They lack cell walls.
- Are only prokaryotes that contain sterols.
- They are facultatively anaerobic bacteria.
- Take on many shapes (pleomorphic).
- Mycoplasmas can also resemble fungi because some Mycoplasmas produce filaments that are commonly seen in fungi. It is these filaments that led scientists to name it Mycoplasma. Myco means "fungus."
- Mycoplasma are unable to move by themselves because they do not have flagella but some are able to glide on a wet surface.

- *Examples*:
  - *Mycoplasma pneumonia* is the cause of atypical pneumonia commonly referred to as walking pneumonia.
  - *Ureaplasma urealyticum* is a bacterium that is found in urine and one that can cause urinary tract infection.

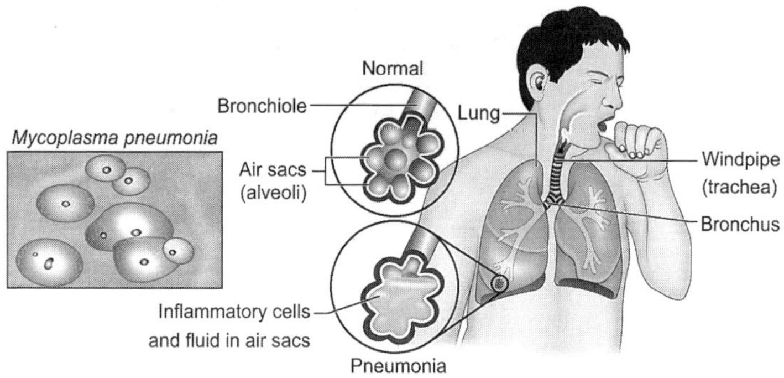

Figure 2.1.7: *Mycoplasma pneumonia*, the causal agent of atypical pneumonia in human beings.

Rickettsia

- Rickettsias are small rod-shaped or spherical bacteria that live in the cells of ticks, lice, fleas, mites (arthropods) and can be transmitted to humans when bitten by arthropods.
- They are small, Gram-negative, non-motile, rod to coccoid-shaped bacteria.
- Rickettsias reproduce by binary fission.
- It is similar to Chlamydia in that they both are of the size of large viruses.

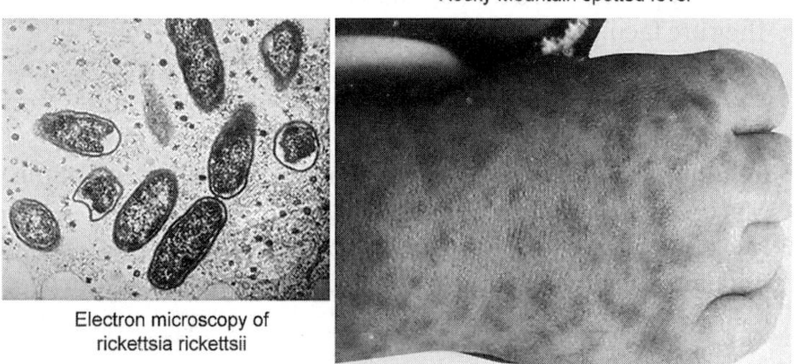

Figure 2.1.8: *R. rickettsii*, the causal agent of Rocky Mountain spotted fever in human beings.

- Like Chlamydia they are obligate intracellular parasites who can't produce ATP and depend for the same on attacked host cell.
- *Examples:*
  - *Rickettsia prowazekii* is transmitted by lice and causes endemic typhus.
  - *R. rickettsii* is transmitted by ticks and causes Rocky Mountain spotted fever.

Siprochaetes

- Spirochaetes are tiny Gram-negative organisms that look like corkscrews.
- They move in a unique spinning motion via 6 thin endoflagella called axial filaments.
- These organisms replicate by transverse fission.
- They cannot be cultured in ordinary media.
- They are too small to be seen using light microscope. Special procedures are required to view these organisms, including darkfield microscopy, immunofluorescence and silver stains.
- *Examples:*
  - *Treponema pallidum* causes syphilis
  - *Borrelia burgdorferi* causes Lyme disease

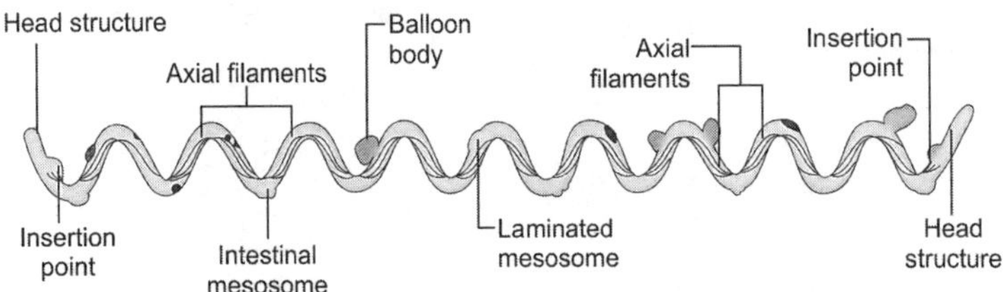

Figure 2.1.9: *Treponema pallidum,* the causal agent of syphilis.

Archaebacteria

- Cell wall is not made up of peptidoglycan.
- Cell membrane contains long-chain branched alcohols (phytanols) bound to glycerol by ethereal linkages.
- They are extremophiles as they can grow in extreme habitats such as at high temperature, under high pressure.
- The major categories of archaebacteria comprise essentially of:
  - *Methanogenic bacteria:* example, *Methanococcus*
  - *Extreme halophiles:* example, *Halobacterium*
  - *Thermophiles:* example, *Thermoplasma*
  - *Acidophiles:* example, *Sulfolobus*

Acellular Microorganisms

Basic Features of Acellular Microbes

- These are neither prokaryotic nor eukaryotic.
- Do not contain cell wall, cell membrane of any cell organelles.
- Do not behave as living organisms outside the host cells.
- They are made-up of nucleic acid and protein (e.g. virus), only nucleic acid (e.g. viroids) or only protein (e.g. prions).

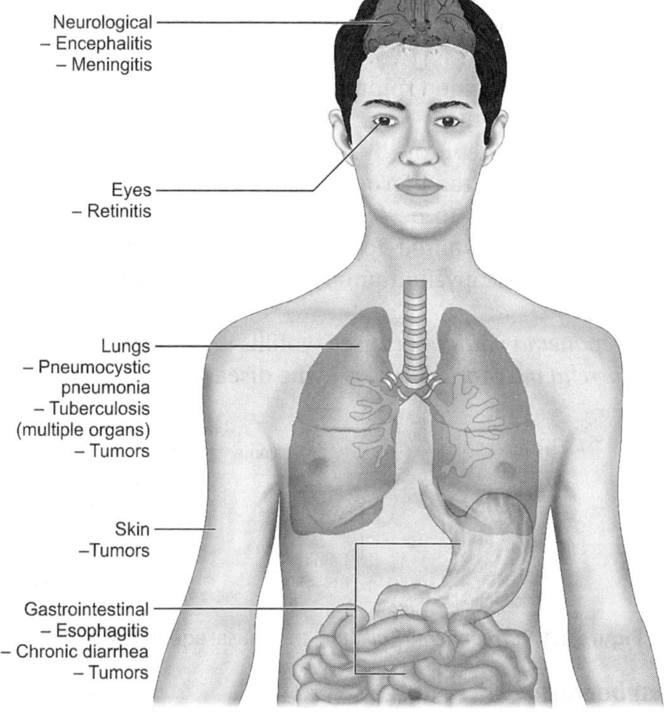

Figure 2.1.10: Symptoms of AIDS.

Viruses

- Are acellular and are not visible with light microscope.
- Are obligate intracellular parasites.
- Contain no organelles or biosynthetic machinery except for few enzymes.
- Contain either RNA or DNA as genetic material.

- Are called as bacteriophages (or phages) if they have bacterial host.
- *Examples:*
  - Poxviridae causes pox (pus-filled lesions) diseases such as smallpox
  - Poliovirus causes poliomyelitis
  - Human immunodeficiency virus (HIV) causes acquired immunodeficiency syndrome (AIDS)

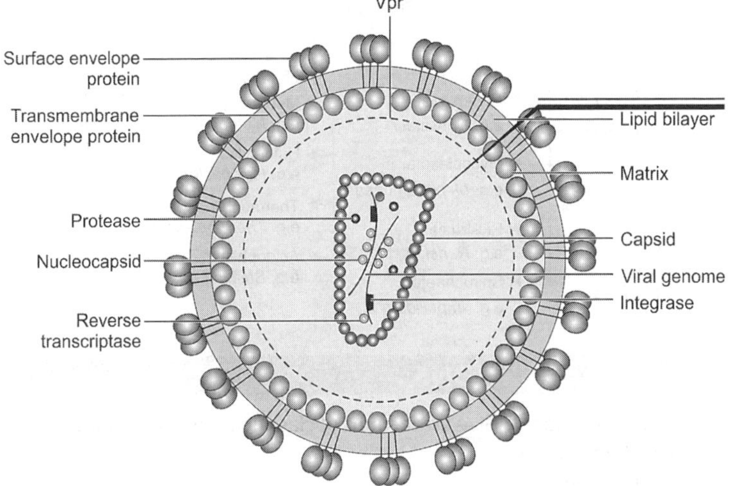

Figure 2.1.11: HIV, causal agent of AIDS.

Prions

- Are infectious particles associated with diseases of the central nervous system.
- Are made of proteins only.
- Diseases caused by prions are:
  - Scrapie disease in sheep and goats
  - Bovine spongiform encephalopathy ('mad cow disease') in cows
  - Kuru disease in humans (cannibals)
  - Creutzfeldt-Jakob disease in humans.

Viroids

- Are not cells and not visible with light microscope.
- Are obligate intracellular parasites.

- Are single-stranded, covalently closed, circular RNA molecules that exist as base-paired, rod like structures.
- Cause plant diseases but have not been proven to cause human disease, although the RNA of Hepatitis D virus (HDV) is viroid-like.

Flowchart 2.1.1: Classification of microorganisms.

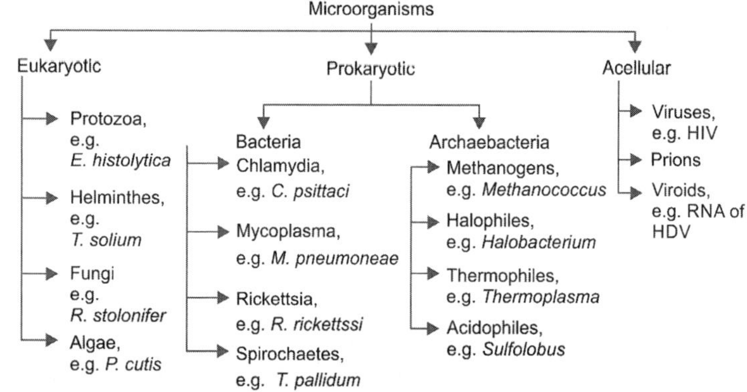

POSSIBLE QUESTIONS

1. What is taxonomy? Give an account of classification of microorganisms.
2. Write Short Notes:
   a. Parasites
   b. Tapeworm
   c. Protozoa
   d. Viruses
   e. Prions
   f. Extremophiles
   g. Lichens
   h. Viroids
   i. Rocky Mountain spotted fever
   j. Mycoplasma
   k. Spirochaete
   l. Rickettsia
   m. Saprophytes

MULTIPLE CHOICE QUESTIONS

1. Eukaryotic microorganisms have ribosome_______________.
   a. 80s b. 60s
   c. 40s d. 50s
2. Free-floating protozoa of oceans are called as__________.
   a. Phytoplankton b. Zooplankton
   c. Phagocytes d. None of the above
3. Amoebiasis is caused by ___________.
   a. *Entamoeba histolytica* b. *Ascaris lubrieoides*
   c. *Histoplasma capsulatum* d. *Prototheca cutis*
4. The wall that separates cylindrical hyphae into cells in fungi are called as ___________.
   a. Septa b. Fragments
   c. Lipopolysaccharides d. Flagella
5. Histoplasmosis in humans is caused by ___________.
   a. *H. capsulatum* b. *P. cutis*
   c. *V. cholerae* d. *R. prowazekii*
6. Chlamydia is ________ bacteria.
   a. Gram (+) b. Gram (-)
   c. Flagellated d. Both b and c
7. The word pleomorphic mean ___________.
   a. Occurs in various form b. Occurs only in one form
   c. Omnipresent d. Multicellular
8. Prokaryotic cell wall is made up of _________.
   a. Peptidoglycan b. Lipopolysaccharides
   c. Both a and b d. Cellulose
9. Trachoma is caused by ______________.
   a. *C. pneumoniae* b. *C. psittaci*
   c. *C. trachomatis* d. Both a and b
10. Siprochaetes reproduce through__________.
    a. Binary fission b. Budding
    c. Transverse fission d. Fragmentation

Answers

1. a	2. b	3. a	4. a	5. a
6. d	7. a	8. a	9. c	10. c

Structure of Microorganisms

WHAT ARE BACTERIA?

Bacteria (sing: bacterium) are the most well known microorganisms. These are microscopic, prokaryotic, unicellular organisms found everywhere.

DISTRIBUTION OF BACTERIA

Bacteria are found in every habitat starting from soil to volcanic zone. They are present in invisible form in the objects we touch, the food we eat, air we breathe, water we drink and from soil to volcanoes. They are found in plants, animals including human beings. The human mouth itself contains 500 species of bacteria. It has been estimated that a single teaspoon of fertile top soil contains more than a billion bacteria.

SIZE

Bacterial cells are extremely small. They vary in length and width. The size of bacteria is scientifically measured in the unit 'micron'. Bacteria range in size from 0.2–2 microns in width and 1–10 microns in length. It is important to know that bacteria have high surface: volume ratio.

Biggest Bacteria

Thiomargrita namibiensis: 100–300 µm

Smallest Bacteria

Mycoplasma: 0.2–0.3 µm

SHAPE

There are three basic shapes of bacteria, viz. Coccus, Bacillus and Spiral.

Table 2.2.1: Types of bacteria on the basis of their shape.

Coccus (Pleural—Cocci): They may be oval or flattened on one side. They can be of following types:			
Diplococci	Cocci that remain in pair	*Diplococcus pneumoniae*	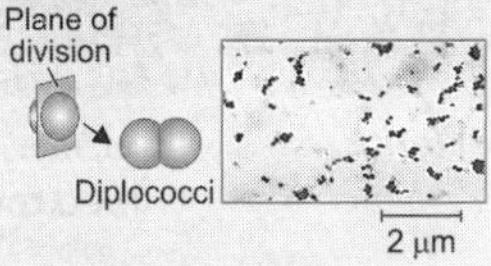
Streptococci	Cocci that remain in chain	*Streptococcus pneumoniae*	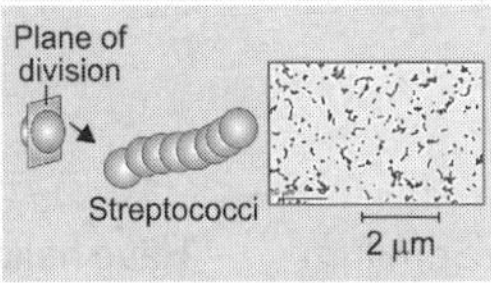
Tetrad	Cocci that remain in a group of 4	*Tessaracoccus bendigoensis*	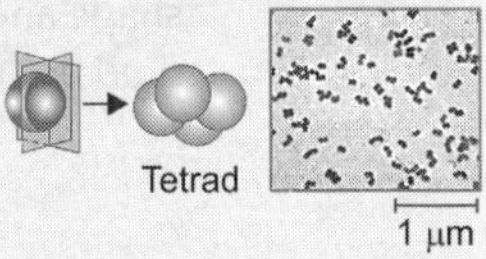
Sarcinae	Cocci that remain in group of 8 to form a cube like structure	*Sarcina ventriculi*	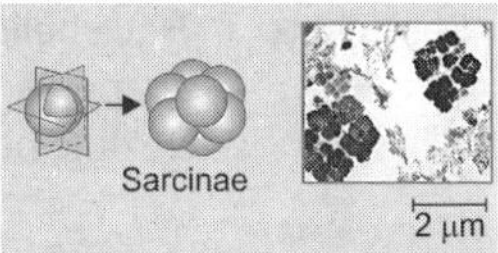
Staphylo-cocci	Cocci that remain in clusters	*Staphylococcus aureus*	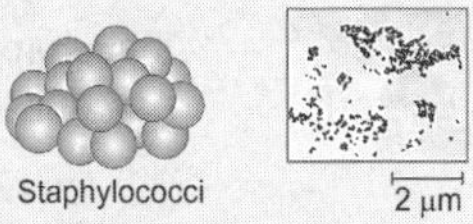
Bacillus (Pleural- Bacilli)			
These are of following types:			
Diplobacilli	Bacilli appearing in pair	*Diplobacillus* species	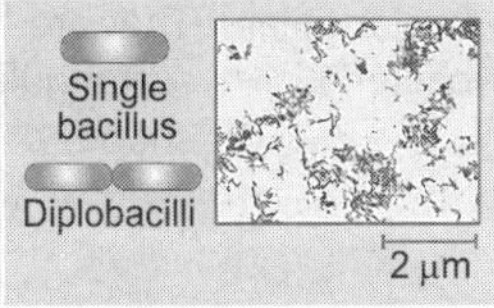
Streptobacilli	Bacilli that appear in chain	*Streptobacillus moniliformis*	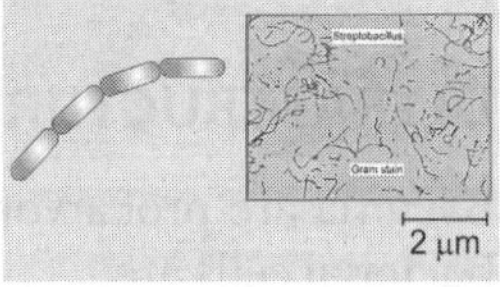

Contd...

Contd...

Cocco-bacilli	Bacilli which are short fat and look like cocci	*Acetobacter*	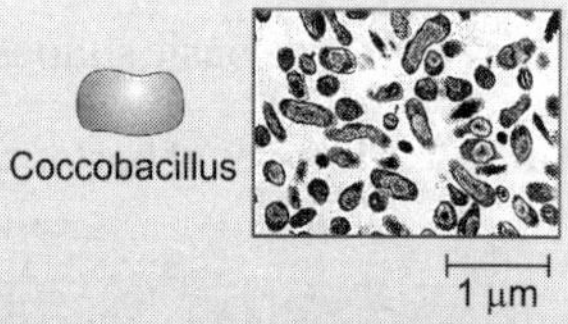 Coccobacillus 1 µm
Spiral bacteria These are spiral in shape and are of following types:			
Vibrio	Look like curved rods	*Vibrio*	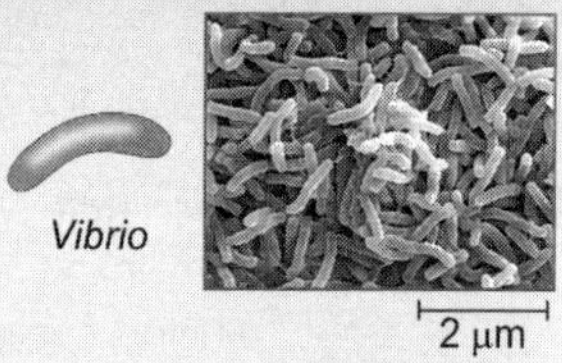 *Vibrio* 2 µm
Spirillum	Have helical shape and rigid body	*Borrelia*	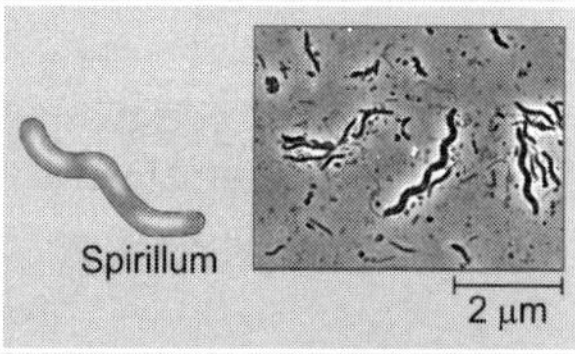 Spirillum 2 µm
Spirochete	Have helical shape and flexible body	*Leptospira*	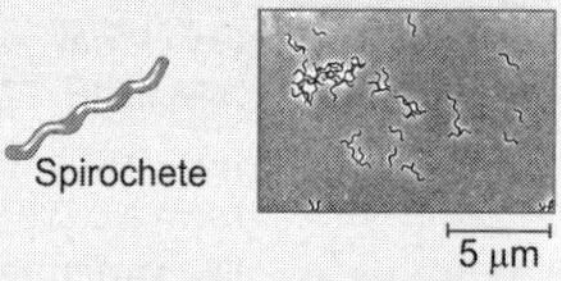 Spirochete 5 µm
Other shapes			
Stellar bacteria	Star shaped bacteria	*Simonsiella*	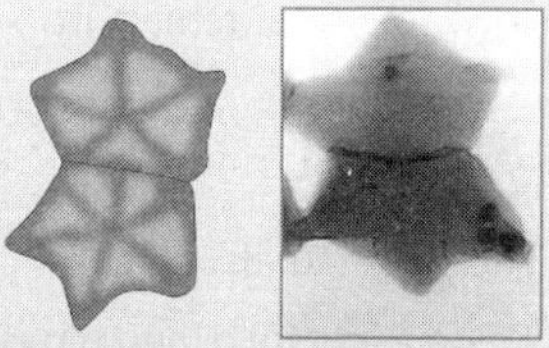
Rectangular bacteria	They are rectangular in shape	*Haloarcula* species	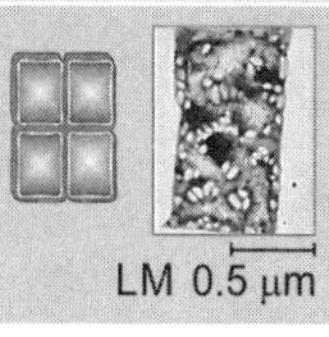 LM 0.5 µm

ULTRASTRUCTURE OF BACTERIAL CELL

Bacteria are prokaryotic by their cellular constitution. The parts of bacterial cells are:

a. Capsule and Slime layer
b. Cell wall
c. Cell membrane
d. Cytoplasm
e. Chromosome
f. Plasmids
g. Ribosomes
h. Locomotory organs
i. Inclusion bodies
j. Pili and fimbriae
k. Endospore

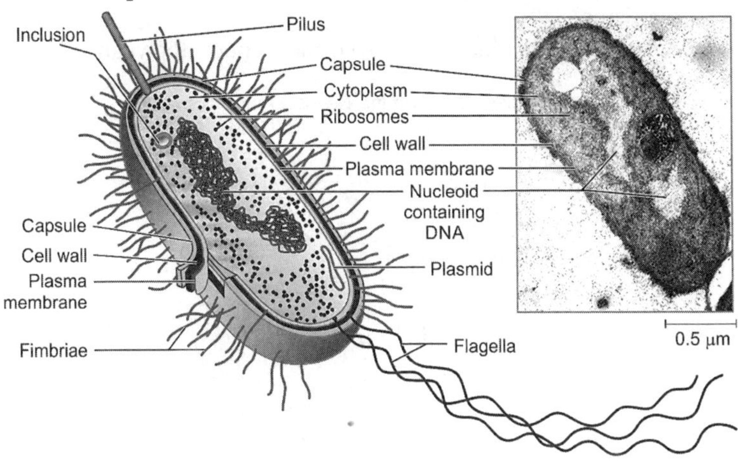

Figure 2.2.1: Ultrastructure of bacterial cell.

Capsule and Slime Layer

Location: A loose coating called Slime layer is usually deposited around the bacterial cell wall. In some bacteria Slime layers become thick and forms capsule.

Structure and composition: It is made-up of polysaccharides, lipids and proteins.

Function: It helps bacteria to attach on a particular surface. In some pathogenic bacteria (diseases causing bacteria), capsule protects bacterial cell from immune system of the host.

Cell Wall

Location: It is present next to capsule. In some bacterial cells where capsule is absent, cell wall acts as the outermost covering.

Thickness: Gram-positive bacteria - 20–80 nm

Gram-negative bacteria - 2–3 nm

Structure and composition: It is made-up of peptidoglycan which differs in two groups of bacteria, namely Gram-negative and Gram-positive. The properties of peptidoglycan are:

- **Polysaccharide backbone:** Consists of two alternating repeating sugars: NAG (N-Acetyl Glucosamine) and NAMA (N-Acety Imuramic Acid).
- **Tetra-peptide:** It is hung from polysaccharide backbone having Amino acids such as L-Alanine, D-Glutamic acid, D-Lysine and D-Alanine. (Note: D type Amino acids are very rare in living organisms).
- **Peptide cross bridge:** This link connects peptidoglycan subunits together.

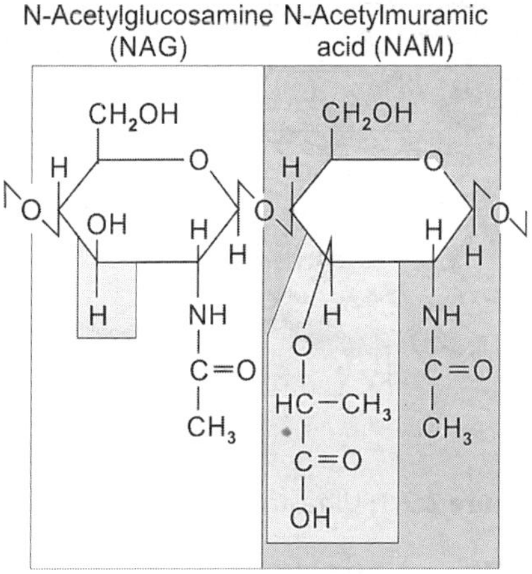

Figure 2.2.2: Peptidoglycan subunit comprising of N-acetylglucosamine (NAG) and N-acetylmuramic acid (NAM).

Function: It protects the cell from Osmotic shock and physical damage. It also provides rigidity and shape to bacterial cells.

Table 2.2.2: Difference between Gram-positive and Gram-negative bacteria.

Characteristic	Gram-positive	Gram-negative
Gram reaction	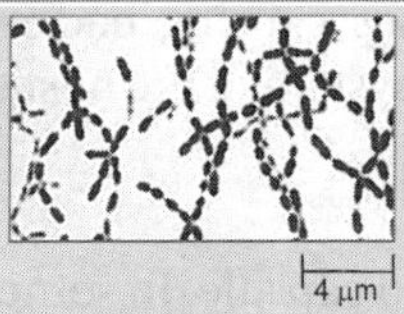 4 µm Retain crystal violet dye and stain blue or purple	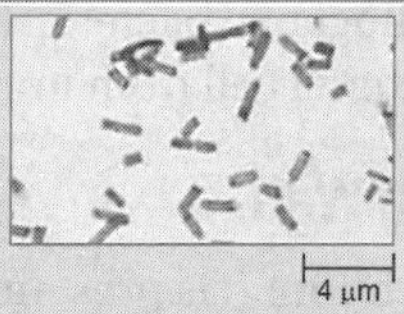 4 µm Can be decolorized to accept counterstain (safranin) and stain pink or red
Peptidoglycan layer	Thick (multilayered)	Thin (single-layered)
Teichoic acids	Present in many	Absent
Periplasmic space	Absent	Present
Outer membrane	Absent	Present

Contd...

Contd...

Characteristic	Gram-positive	Gram-negative
Lipopolysaccharide (LPS) content	Visually none	High
Lipid and lipoprotein content	Low (acid-fast bacteria have lipids linked to peptidoglycan)	High (because of presence of outer membrane)
Flagellar structure	2 rings in basal body	4 rings in basal body
Toxins produced	Exotoxins	Endotoxins and exotoxins
Resistance to physical disruption	High	Low
Cell Wall disruption by lysozyme	High	Low (acid-fast bacteria have lipids linked to Peptidoglycan)
Susceptibility to penicillin and sulfonamide	High	Low
Susceptibility to streptomycin, chloramphenicol, and tetracycline	High	High
Inhibition by basic dyes	High	Low
Susceptibility to anionic detergents	High	Low
Resistance to sodium salt	High	Low
Resistance to drying	High	Low

Cell Membrane

It is also called as cytoplasmic membrane or plasma membrane.

Location: It is present next to the cell wall and encloses cytoplasm.

Structure and composition: The cell membrane is made up of Phospholipid bilayer (two layers of phospholipid molecules) having thickness of 6–8 nm. A phospholipid molecule consists of one hydrophilic (water loving) phosphate group and two hydrophobic (water hating) fatty acid chains. Hydrophilic heads are exposed to external environment or cytoplasm. The fatty acid chains direct inwards, facing each other due to hydrophobic effects (staying away from water).

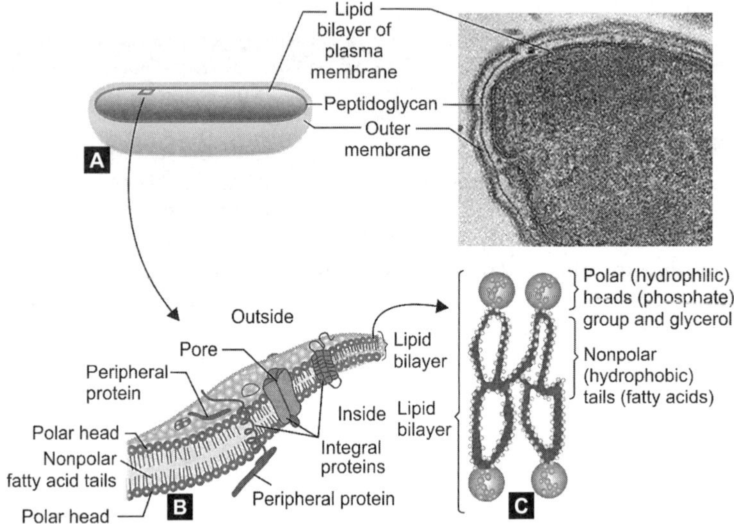

Figures 2.2.3A to C: (A) Plasma membrane of cell; (B) Lipid bilayer of plasma membrane; (C) Phospholipid molecules in lipid bilayer.

Apart from phospholipids following types of proteins are present in the cell membrane.

- Integral proteins firmly inserted in the membrane. These are mainly involved in transportation and are of three types—uniport, symport and antiport.
- Outer surface proteins usually present in Gram-negative bacteria. These interact with periplasmic proteins for the transport of large molecules in the cell.
- Inner surface proteins interact with other proteins in energy producing reactions and other important cellular functions.
- Mesosome: These are infoldings formed by the plasma membrane. These are commonly found in Gram-positive bacteria and play important roles in cell division and replication.

Function: Regulates the specific transport of substances between the cells and outer environment.

Cytoplasm

Location: It is present next to the cell membrane and fills entire inner space of the cell.

Composition: It is a semifluid substance enclosed by the cell membrane. It appears granular due to the presence of large number of ribosomes. Different structures such as chromosomes, plasmids as well as cytoplasmic organelles are found in the cytoplasm.

Note: Membrane bound cell organelles like mitochondria, chloroplasts, lysosomes, Golgi complex, vacuoles and endoplasmic reticulum are absent in bacterial cell.

Function: It is the site for various biochemical reactions and contains genetic material of the cell.

Chromosome

The space where the chromosome resides is called as **nucleoid.**

Location: Since the bacterial cell is prokaryotic, a membrane bound nucleus is absent. Bacterial chromosome is found to float freely in the cytoplasm.

Number: One chromosome in each cell.

Size: In ***E. coli*** the size of chromosome is 4640 kilo base pairs (kbp).

Structure and composition: It is made up of circular DNA attached at a point to the plasma membrane. The DNA in bacterial cell is not associated with histone protein. The DNA molecule is composed of nitrogen bases (Adenine, Guanine, Cytosine, Thymine), deoxyribose sugar and phosphate molecules.

Function: It is the storehouse of genetic information.

Plasmid

Apart from chromosomes, certain bacterial cells contain additional DNA molecule called as **plasmid.**

Location: Bacterial plasmid is found to float freely in the cytoplasm.

Number: Present from one to several in number.

Size: Plasmids are much smaller than chromosomes.

Structure and composition: It is a circular DNA molecule without histones. The plasmid DNA replicates independently.

Function: It contains some special genes such as Fertility factor (F-factor), Resistance factor (R-factor), Nitrogen fixing genes (Nif genes). Due to the presence of plasmid bacterial cells get special characteristics.

Note: Some plasmids may temporarily become associated with Nucleoid DNA and are called as Episomes.

Ribosomes

Location: These are evenly distributed in the cytoplasm.

Structure and composition: Bacteria contain 70S Ribosome and is made up of ribosomal RNA (rRNA) and proteins. 70S Ribosome has two subunits:

- 30S subunit: It has 21 proteins and 16S rRNA.
- 50S subunit: It has 34 proteins, 23S rRNA and 5S rRNA.

Note: "S" stands for Svedburg unit, which represents how rapidly particles or molecules sediment in an ultracentrifuge.

Function: These are involved in bacterial protein synthesis.

Locomotory Organs (Flagella and Cilia)

There are two types of locomotory organs in bacteria—the bigger one are called as flagella and the smaller one are called as cilia. Locomotory organs help in the movement or locomotion of bacterial cells. Depending on the presence or absence of locomotory organs bacteria are of two types:

1. **Motile:** Bacteria that can move, e.g., *Vibrio cholerae*
2. **Non-Motile:** Bacteria that cannot move, e.g., *Staphylococcus aureus.*

Location: It is present in outer surface of the cell.

Monotrichous	A single flagellum present at one pole of the bacterial cell	*Vibrio*	
Amphitrichous	Each pole of bacteria having one single flagellum		
Cephalotrichous	Each pole having a bunch of flagellae		
Lophotrichous	Bunch of flagellae present at one pole in bacterium	*Thiospirillum*	
Peritrichous	Flagella evenly distributed throughout the surface of the bacterial cell	*Salmonella typhii*	
Atrichous	Flagella is totally absent in such bacteria	*Staphylococcus*	

Structure and Composition

Flagella are made up of protein called as flagellin. The structure of flagella is divided into three parts:

1. **Filament:** Consists of flagellin protein.
2. **Hook:** Single type of protein that connects filament to basal body.
3. **Basal body:** Supports the filament at the base.

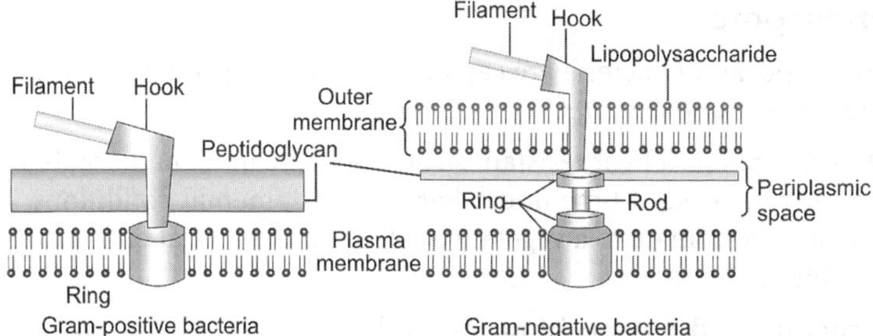

Figure 2.2.4: Flagella structure in Gram-positive and Gram-negative bacteria.

Function: The primary function of flagella is to make bacteria move. There are three types of movement seen:

Chemotaxis: Movement of bacteria towards or away from chemical stimuli.

Magnetotaxis: Movement along the earth's magnetic field.

Phototaxis: Movement of bacteria towards light of different intensities.

Inclusion Bodies

Location: Distributed in the cytoplasm.

These are non-living components present in the cell which do not possess metabolic activity. The most common inclusion bodies are glycogen, lipid droplets, crystals, pigments, volutin granules and metachromatic granules.

Pili and Fimbriae

Location: Distributed outside the cell surface.

Structure and Composition

Pili	Fimbriae
Pili are short, thin, straight, hair-like projections composed of protein pilin, carbohydrate and phosphates	Similar to pili but more in number

Function

Pili	Fimbriae
Surface adhesion	Surface adhesion
Sex pili participate in genetic material exchange between mating bacterial cells	Formation of biofilm

Endospore

Some species of bacteria are capable of producing endospores, e.g., *Clostridium* and *Bacillus.*

Definition: It is a heat resistant structure that can retain its viability over long period of time under harsh environmental conditions. It can later germinate to a vegetative cell upon the arrival of favorable conditions.

Structure and composition: An endospore has several coatings which are as follows:

- **Exosporium:** Outermost layer consisting of proteins
- **Spore coat:** Several layers of spore specific proteins
- **Cortex:** Loosely crossing peptidoglycan
- **Core:** Consists of core wall, cell membrane, cytoplasm, nucleoid, ribosomes and other cellular components.

Function: It helps bacteria to survive during unfavorable environmental conditions.

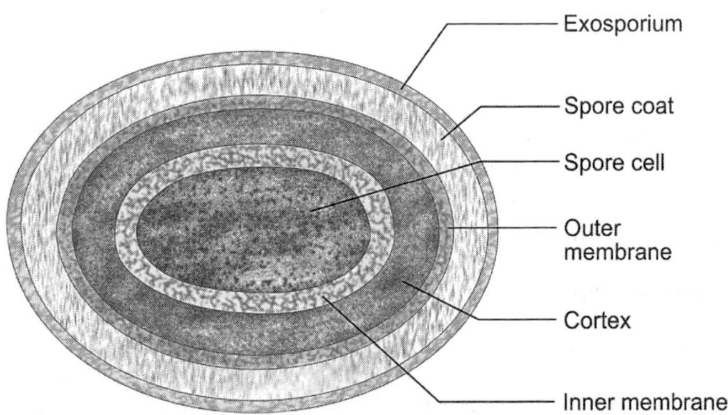

Figure 2.2.5: Bacterial endospore.

POSSIBLE QUESTIONS

1. Define bacteria. Give a detail account of the ultrastructure of a bacterial cell.
2. Write Short Notes:
   a. Shape of bacteria
   b. Endospore
   c. Peptidoglycan
   d. Inclusion bodies
   e. Nucleoid
   f. Plasmid
   g. Motility
   h. Membrane protein
3. Differentiate between the following:
   a. Gram-negative and Gram-positive bacteria
   b. Capsule and slime layer
   c. Pili and fimbriae
   d. Flagella and cilia
   e. Plasmid and chromosome

MULTIPLE CHOICE QUESTIONS

1. Name the biggest bacteria___________.
   a. Thiomargarita namibiensis
   b. *Streptococcus pneumoniae*
   c. Thiobacillus
   d. *E. coli*
2. Mycoplasma ranges from ___________.
   a. 100–200 μ
   b. 0.2–0.3 μ
   c. 5–6 μ
   d. None of the above
3. Bacilli that looks like curved rods are called as______.
   a. Streptobacilli
   b. *Vibrio*
   c. Spirillum
   d. Diplobacilli
4. The thickened slime layer is called as______.
   a. Capsule
   b. Cell wall
   c. Plasmid
   d. Endospore
5. Bacterial cell wall is made up of _____________.
   a. Peptidoglycan
   b. Cellulose
   c. Lignin
   d. Suberin
6. Peptidoglycan consists of____________.
   a. NAG and NAMA
   b. D-Glutamic acid
   c. L-amino acids
   d. None of the above
7. Gram-positive bacteria have ____________ cell wall
   a. Thick
   b. Thin
   c. Absent
   d. None of the above

8. Gram-negative bacteria have ____________ flagellar structure.
   a. 2
   b. 4
   c. 3
   d. 7
9. Outer layer of endosperm is called as ________.
   a. Cortex
   b. Core
   c. Exosporium
   d. Coat
10. Which of the following is not an inclusion body?
   a. Crystals
   b. Droplets
   c. Metachromatin
   d. None of the above

Answers

1. a	2. b	3. b	4. a	5. a
6. a	7. a	8. b	9. c	10. d

Viruses: Structure and Life Cycle

MEANING AND HISTORY OF VIRUSES

Viruses (Latin Venum-poisonous fluid) are simplest forms of life. They are not cells, but their study has provided a great deal of information about cells. Study of viruses is a branch of biology called virology. Viruses are cellular parasites. They are smaller than bacteria and have a much more simplified organization.

Properties of Virus

Some general properties of virus are as follows:

- **Size:**
  - The size of virus ranges from (20–300) nm in diameter.
  - Parvovirus is the smallest virus with size 20 nm whereas Poxvirus is largest being 400 nm.
- **Shape:**
  - The overall shape of virus varies in different groups of virus.
  - Most of animal viruses are spherical shape, Poxvirus is rectangular shape, TMV is rod shape, Poliovirus is bullet shape, etc.
  - Some virus are irregular and pleomorphic in shape.
- **Symmetry:**
  - Morphological protein subunits of capsid are arranged together to from a symmetrical structure of the virus.
  - Two basic symmetry are recognized in virus, they are helical symmetry and icosahedral symmetry.
  - In some virus, symmetry is more complex, which is other than helical or icosahedral.

- **Structure and chemical composition:**
  - *Genome:*
    - Viral genome or nucleic acid contains either DNA or RNA but not both.
    - The genome can be either ds DNA or ss DNA or ds RNA or ss RNA
    - The genome can exist as single piece or segmented, e.g., influenza virus contains 8 segments of ss RNA genome.
    - The genome may be linear or circular. Most virus possess linear genome except Papova virus which contains circular ss DNA.
    - Genome helps replication of virus in host cell.
  - *Capsid:*
    - Capsid is the outer shell of a virus.
    - It is chemically a viral protein.
    - Capsid is composed of capsomere.
    - Structure of capsid gives the symmetry of virus.
    - Capsid protects the nucleic acid and also helps in attachments on host cell surface during infection.
  - *Envelope:*
    - Some virus contains phospholipid bilayer known as envelope.
    - Virus lacking envelope is called naked virus.
    - Envelope is a lipid bilayer which is acquired from host cell membrane.
  - *Glycoprotein spike:*
    - Envelope of some virus contains viral coded spike projected outside the envelope called glycoprotein spike or peplomers.
    - Glycoprotein spike are viral coded protein with carbohydrate head.
    - Glycoprotein spikes is an important antigenic structure.
    - Neuraminidase and Hemagglutinin are glycoprotein spikes which helps in virus attachment to cellular receptor on host cell to establish infection.
  - *Enzymes:*
    - Some virus possess their own enzymes.
    - Retrovirus possess reverse transcriptase.

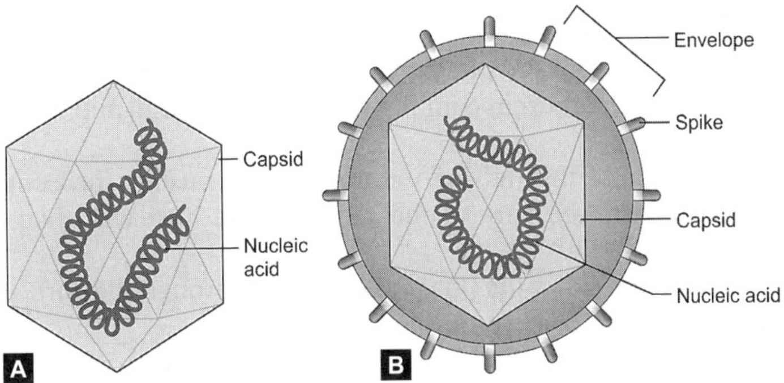

Figures 2.3.1A and B: Structure of virus: (A) Naked nucleocapsid virus; (B) Enveloped virus.

VIRAL REPLICATION

Replication of virus takes place by lytic and lysogenic cycle.

Replication of Virus by Lytic Cycle

This type of cycle is seen in T-even phages (T_2, T_4 etc.) which attack *Escherichia coli.*

The lytic cycle consists of five steps:

1. Adsorption
2. Infection
3. Synthesis of phage components in host cell
4. Formation of new phage particle
5. Liberation of phages from the host cell.

Adsorption

- The interaction between the phage specific organelle — the tail and the receptor site of the host cell is called the adsorption.
- The adsorption is facilitated by the negatively charged carboxyl groups on the host surface and the positively charged amino group of protein present at the tip of the phage tail.
- In T-even phages, the tip of the tail fiber first attaches to the cell surface. The tail fiber then bends and allows the tail pins to attach on the host surface that makes an irreversible attachment.

Infection

- After adsorption, the phage particle secretes an enzyme which hydrolyses the murein complex of the host cell wall and forms a pore.
- The sheath of the tail then contracts and pushes the central tubular part, i.e., core of the tail, into the host wall, like an injection needle.
- The nucleic acid of the phage then passes through the core and enters the host bacterium.
- The empty protein shell of the phage is called ghost, which may remain attached even after release of nucleic acid.
- Once the bacterial cell receives the nucleic acid of a phage, it becomes resistant to the other phages.

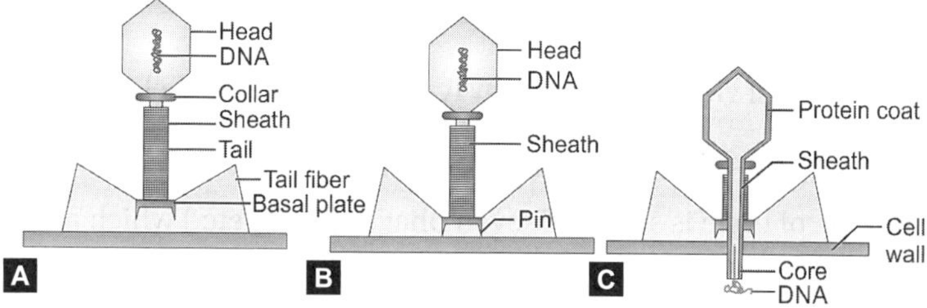

Figures 2.3.2A to C: Mechanism of DNA introduction by T-even phage into a host cell: (A) Attachment of phage on the host surface by tail fiber; (B) Attachment of pins of basal plate on host surface; (C) Contraction of sheath, pushing of core and releasing of DNA inside the host.

Synthesis of Phage Components in Host Cell

- Once the phage nucleic acid takes the entry inside the bacterial cell, it suppresses the synthesis of bacterial protein and directs to synthesize the proteins of the phage particle.
- The DNA of phage replicates following the semi-conservative process.
- Majority of the DNA acts as a template for its own synthesis and the rest is used as template for the synthesis of viral specific m-RNA by utilizing the RNA-polymerase of the host.

Formation of New Phage Particle

The new phage particles are formed by the assemblage of nucleic acid and protein. This process is called maturation, which is controlled by viral genome. In this process, initially the condensation of nucleic acid molecule takes place.

Liberation of Phages from the Host Cell

In a cycle of phage development, about 200 phages are formed which take about 30-90 minutes. In the host cell, the phage DNA secretes lysozyme (an enzyme) which causes the lysis of host cell wall. As a result of lysis, the phage particles are liberated.

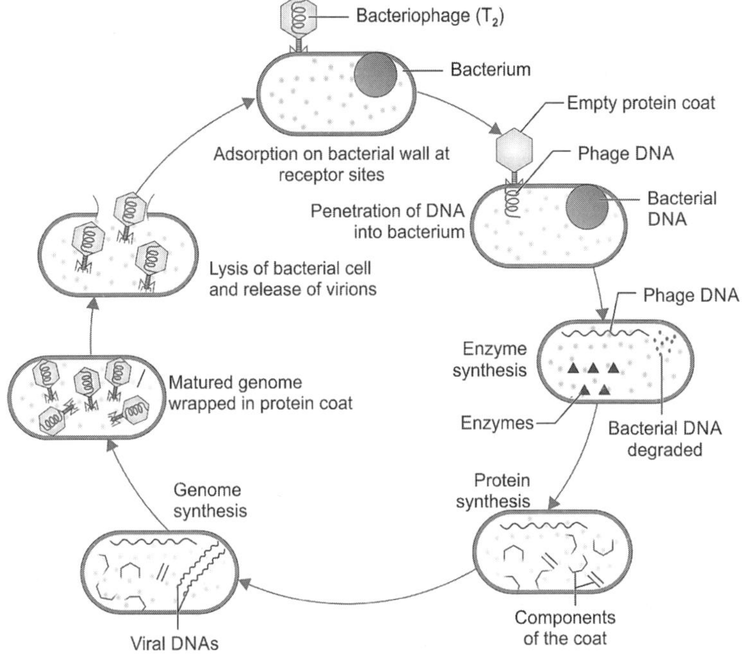

Figure 2.3.3: Lytic life-cycle of bacteriophage (T_2).

Replication of Virus by Lysogenic Cycle

- Lwoff (1953) discovered this type of cycle in Lambda (bacteriophages that attack, *E. coli*). The phage involved in this cycle is called temperate phage, the bacterium is the lysogenic strain and the entire process is called lysogeny.
- At first, the phage is adsorbed on the wall of the host bacterium and its DNA becomes injected into the host cell.
- Here the phage DNA, like the lytic cycle, does not take over the protein synthesis machinery of the host cell, instead, it becomes integrated with the nucleoid of the host genome.
- This integrated phage DNA is called a prophage. Thus the new composite genome replicates as one unit. The composite genome

then multiplies for indefinite number of times and produces daughter lysogenic bacteria.

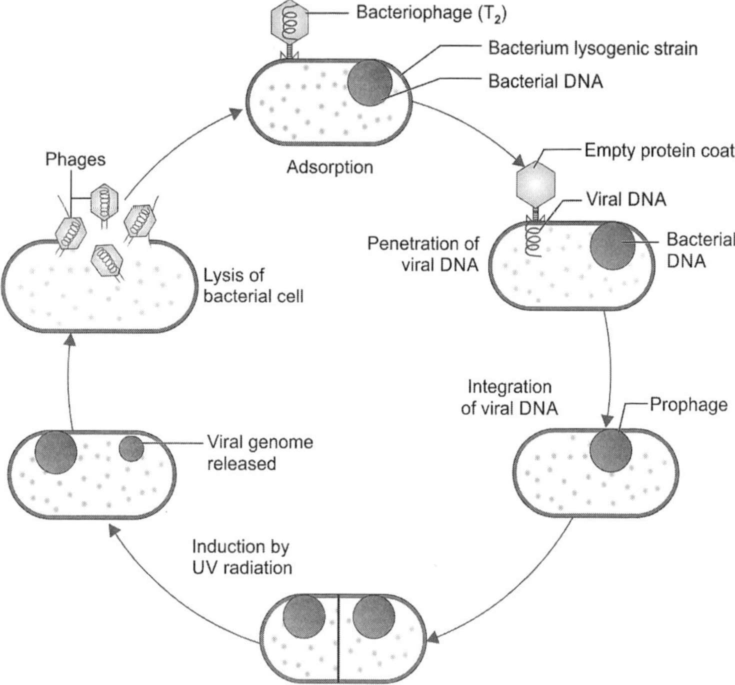

Figure 2.3.4: Lysogenic life-cycle of bacteriophage (λ-phage).

Table 2.3.1: Lytic vs lysogenic cycle.

Lytic cycle	Lysogenic cycle
The DNA of the virus doesn't integrate into the host DNA	The DNA of the virus integrates into the host DNA
Host DNA hydrolyzed	Host DNA not hydrolyzed
Absence of prophage stage	Presence of prophage stage
DNA replication of virus takes place independently from the host DNA replication	DNA replication of the virus takes place along with the host DNA replication
Occurs within a short period of time	Takes time
Symptoms of viral replication are evident	Symptoms of viral replication not evident
Genetic recombination in the host bacterium not allowed	Genetic recombination in the host bacterium allowed

Contd...

Contd...

Lytic cycle	Lysogenic cycle
The cellular mechanism of the host cell is totally undertaken by the viral genome	The cellular mechanism of the host cell is somewhat disturbed by the viral genome

- After a number of generations the viral genome gets detached from the composite genome and releases in the cytoplasm. This dissociation is called induction . The viral genome then enters the lytic cycle and forms temperate phages that are released by lysis of wall of the host bacterium.

DIAGNOSIS OF VIRUS

There are two broad approaches to detecting and diagnosing a viral infection in the laboratory: **viral detection** and **host response.**

Viral Detection

Cell Culture

- Viruses must be cultured in medium that contains living cells such as monkey kidney.
- Viral growth can be identified by observing:
  - **Cytopathic effect:** A characteristic cellular change due to viral growth (e.g., respiratory syncytial virus (RSV) culture leads to multinucleated giant cells).
  - **Hemadsorption:** The envelope protein hemagglutinin (HA) causes added red blood cells to attach to the viral infected cell. Examples include influenza and mumps virus.
  - **Viral antibody:** A positive response to the addition of viral antibody is detected by a range of methods, including enzyme-linked immunosorbent assay (ELISA) and immunofluorescence.

Microscopic Techniques

Light microscopy—detects inclusion bodies (collections of viral particles) within the infected cell. Some have a characteristic appearance such as Negri bodies with rabies infection.

Electron microscopy—detects viruses and viral particles.

Viral Antigen Detection

ELISA and immunofluorescence.

Viral Nucleic Acid

- The sequencing of viral nucleic acids has enabled the creation of highly sensitive diagnostic tests.
- A complementary DNA or RNA probe to the viral nucleic acid labelled with a marker will identify viral nucleic acid.
- Polymerase chain reaction (PCR) can amplify small amounts of nucleic acid.

Host Response

Antibody Detection

- **Interpretation**
  - **Immunoglobulin (Ig) M**—levels rise early and suggest recent or current infection.
  - **IgG**—must rise fourfold over a 2 week period to be diagnostic of a recent or current infection. Can also suggest previous infection.
- **ELISA**
- **Western Blot**
  - Electrophoresis is used to separate viral proteins in a gel solution.
  - These proteins are subsequently transferred (blotted) onto filter paper.
  - The sample serum is added to the paper; if viral antibodies are present, they will bind to the antigen.
  - This complex can be detected by adding a labelled antibody to human IgG and visualized in a similar manner to ELISA or immunofluorescence.

Table 2.3.2: Important human viral diseases.

Disease	Pathogen		Genome	Vector/Epidemiology
Polio	Entero-virus		(+) Single-stranded RNA	Acute viral infection of the CNS that can lead to paralysis and is often fatal. Prior to the development of Salk's vaccine in 1954, 60,000 people a year contracted the disease in the US alone

Contd...

Contd...

Disease	Pathogen		Genome	Vector/Epidemiology
Yellow fever	Flavivirus		(+) Single-stranded RNA	Spread from individual-to-individual by mosquito bites; a notable cause of death during the construction of the Panama Canal. If untreated, this disease has a peak mortality rate of 60%
Ebola	Filoviruses		(–) Single-stranded RNA	Acute hemorrhagic fever; virus attacks connective tissue, leading to massive hemorrhaging and death. Peak mortality is 50–90% if untreated. Outbreaks confined to local regions of central Africa
Influenza	Influenza viruses		(–) Single-stranded RNA	Historically a major killer (22 million died in 18 months in 1918-19); wild Asian ducks, chickens, and pigs are major reservoirs. The ducks are not affected by the flu virus, which shuffles its antigen genes while multiplying within them, leading to new flu strains
Measles	Paramyxo-viruses		(–) Single-stranded RNA	Extremely contagious through contact with infected individuals. Vaccine available. Usually contracted in childhood, when it is not serious; more dangerous to adults

Contd...

Contd...

Disease	Pathogen		Genome	Vector/Epidemiology
SARS	Corona-virus		(–) Single-stranded RNA	Acute respiratory infection; an emerging disease, can be fatal, especially in the elderly
Pneumonia	Influenza virus		(–) Single-stranded RNA	Acute infection of the lungs; often fatal without treatment
Rabies	Rhabdo-virus		(–) Single-stranded RNA	An acute viral encephalomyelitis transmitted by the bite of an infected animal. Fatal if untreated

MULTIPLE CHOICE QUESTIONS

1. Which of the following task is not performed of nurses?
   a. Assessment b. Diagnosis
   c. Evaluation d. Eradication
2. Microorganism which causes diseases are known as ________.
   a. Pathogens b. Microbes
   c. Phagocytes d. None of the above
3. Microbiology is the study of ________.
   a. Virus b. Bacteria
   c. Algae d. All of the above
4. A person who study microbiology is called as ________.
   a. Microcyst b. Micrologist
   c. Microbiologist d. All of the above
5. Microbiology is based on the principles of ________.
   a. Personal b. Community hygiene
   c. Both a and b d. Virus
6. Microbes that do not cause disease are known as ________.
   a. Pathogens b. Non-pathogens
   c. *Neisseria* d. *Salmonella*
7. Which system helps multicellular organism to resist harmful microorganisms?
   a. Digestive system b. Nervous system
   c. Immune system d. Reproductive system
8. A medicine or other substance that has a physiological effect on body when ingested is________.
   a. Drugs b. Alcohol
   c. Tobacco d. All of the above

9. Which of the following combinations are used to sterilize surgical knives, needles, etc.?
   a. Water and pesticides
   b. Hot water and antiseptics
   c. Antiseptics and drugs
   d. None of the above
10. Which is not a communicable disease?
   a. Hepatitis B
   b. HIV
   c. Influenza
   d. Diabetes
11. Tuberculosis is detected by the test_________.
   a. CT scan
   b. MRI
   c. Mantoux
   d. X-ray
12. Nurses should be _______ with the patients.
   a. Familiar
   b. Rude
   c. Strict
   d. Intolerant
13. Nursing don't include:
   a. Promotion of health
   b. Prevention of ill
   c. Taking care of ill and disabled people
   d. To become rude and unkind to patients
14. Which of the following sentence is correct about the responsibilities of nurses?
   a. Recording medical history and symptoms
   b. Administering medications and treatments
   c. Collaborating with teams for patient care
   d. All of the above
15. Microbiology in nursing refers to:
   a. Understand the concepts of reproduction, morphology, biochemical nature of microbes
   b. Learn the process of spread of infection
   c. Collect and handle specimen for examination
   d. All of the above
16. What is medical microbiology ?
   a. Study on pathogens
   b. Study on non-pathogens
   c. Study on microorganisms
   d. Both a and c

Answers

1. d	2. a	3. d	4. c	5. c
6. b	7. c	8. a	9. b	10. d
11. c	12. a	13. d	14. a	15. d
16. d				

CHAPTER

2.4

Growth and Nutrition of Microorganisms

WHAT IS GROWTH IN MICROORGANISMS?

Growth is an essential characteristic of living organisms. For example a human baby grows to become an adult, a small plant grows to become a huge tree, etc. But how do microorganisms grow? They are always microscopic after all. Growth of microorganisms always means increase in their population (i.e. cell number). In bacteria, this happens by the process of binary fission.

CLASSIFICATION OF MICROORGANISMS ON NUTRITION BASIS

All living organisms require a source of energy. Depending on this, the microbes can be classified as:

- Phototrophs: Organisms that use radiant energy (light) are called phototrophs. Example: Cyanobacteria.
- Chemotrophs: Microorganisms that obtain energy by Oxidation of electron donors in their environment. These molecules can be organic or inorganic. Example: *Nitrobacter*.
- Lithotrophs: Organisms that oxidize inorganic compounds are called lithotrophs. Example: Purple sulfur bacteria.

The carbon requirements of organisms must be met by organic carbon (a chemical compound with a carbon-hydrogen bond) or by CO_2.

- Heterotrophs: Organisms that use organic carbon are called as heterotrophs. Example: *E. coli.*
- Autotrophs: Organisms that use CO_2 as a sole source of carbon for growth are called **autotrophs**. Example: Green bacteria.

Table 2.4.1: Major nutritional types of prokaryotes.

Nutritional type	Energy source	Carbon source	Examples
Photoautotrophs	Light	CO_2	Cyanobacteria, some purple and green bacteria
Photoheterotrophs	Light	Organic compounds	Some purple and green bacteria
Chemoautotrophs or Lithotrophs (Lithoautotrophs)	Inorganic compounds, e.g. H_2, NH_3, NO_2, H_2S	CO_2	A few bacteria and many Archaea
Chemoheterotrophs or heterotrophs	Organic compounds	Organic compounds	Most bacteria, some Archaea

FACTORS AFFECTING MICROBIAL GROWTH

Nutrition

- Nutrients that are acquired from the environment are used for growth by microorganisms.
- These nutrients are classified as macro-and microelements.

The Macroelements

- Macroelements consist of C, H, O, N, S, P, K, Mg, Fe, Ca, Mn, Zn, Co, Cu, and Mo. These elements are found in the form of water, inorganic ions, small molecules and macromolecules which serve either a structural or functional role in cells.

Table 2.4.2: Major elements, their sources and functions in bacterial cells.

Elements	% of dry weight	Sources	Functions
Carbon	50	Organic compounds or CO_2	Main constituent of cellular material
Oxygen	20	H_2O, organic compounds, CO_2, and O_2	Constituent of cell material and cell water; O_2 is electron acceptor in aerobic respiration
Nitrogen	14	NH_3, NO_3, organic compounds, N_2	Constituent of amino acids, nucleic acids, nucleotides and coenzymes

Contd...

Contd...

Elements	% of dry weight	Sources	Functions
Hydrogen	8	H_2O, organic compounds, H_2	Main constituent of organic compounds and cell water
Phosphorus	3	Inorganic phosphates (PO_4)	Constituent of nucleic acids, nucleotides, phospholipids, LPS, teichoic acids
Sulphur	1	SO_4, H_2S, SO, organic sulphur compounds	Constituent of cysteine, methionine, glutathione, several coenzymes
Potassium	1	Potassium salts	Main cellular inorganic cation and cofactor for certain enzymes
Magnesium	0.5	Magnesium salts	Inorganic cellular cation, cofactor for certain enzymatic reactions
Calcium	0.5	Calcium salts	Inorganic cellular cation, cofactor for certain enzymes and a component of endospores
Iron	0.2	Iron salts	Component of cytochromes and certain nonheme iron-proteins and a cofactor for some enzymatic reactions

Microelements

Microelements or trace elements are metal ions required by certain cells in small amounts. Example: Mn, Co, Zn, Cu and Mo.

Oxygen Requirement

Microorganisms can be classified on the basis of oxygen requirement:

- Aerobes: They need oxygen for growth. Example: Streptococci, *Staphylococcus.*
- Anaerobe: They do not need oxygen for growth. Example: *Clostridium.*
- Obligate aerobes: They absolutely require O_2 for growth. Example: *Mycobacterium tuberculosis* and *Nocardia asteroides.*
- Obligate anaerobes (occasionally called aerophobes): They do not need O_2 at all. In fact, O_2 is poisonous to them. Example: Actinomyces, Bacteroides, Fusobacterium.

- Facultative anaerobes: They can switch between aerobic and anaerobic states. Example: *Escherichia coli (E. coli).*
- Aerotolerant anaerobes: They are insensitive to the presence of O_2. Example: *Clostridium intestinale.*
- Microaerophilic: They need little amount of oxygen for growth. Example: *Campylobacter jejuni.*

Table 2.4.3: Terms used to describe O_2 relations of microorganisms.

Organism	Obligate aerobe	Facultative anaerobe	Obligate anaerobe	Aeroto-lerant anaerobe	Microae-rophile
Effort of oxygen on oxygen	Oxygen required. Only can survive in aerobic conditions. Dies if oxygen is absent.	Growth in presence of oxygen, both aerobic and anaerobic.	Oxygen not required, only can survive in anaerobic conditions. Dies if oxygen is present.	Do not care if oxygen is present or absent. Just do not use the oxygen present.	Low oxygen concent-ration allowed for growth only.
Examples	*Mycoba-cterium*	*Strepto-coccus, Staphylo-coccus,* Entero-bacteriaceae	*Clostri-dium*	*Lacto-bacillus*	*Neisseria gonorrhoeae*

pH

- The pH is the hydrogen ion concentration $[H^+]$ of a liquid. It varies from 0.5–10.5 and above. If a liquid has a pH in the range 0.5–6 then it is considered as acidic, 7 is neutral (neither acidic nor alkaline) and 7 above is considered as alkaline or basic.

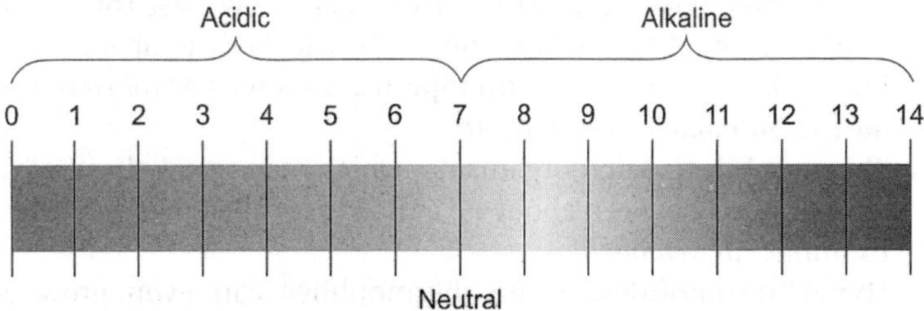

Figure 2.4.1: The pH scale.

- The range of pH over which a microorganism grows is defined by **three cardinal points: minimum pH** below which organisms cannot grow, maximum pH, above which organisms cannot grow and **optimum pH** at which the organism grows the best.
- Depending on the optimum pH requirement, microorganisms can be classified as:
- **Acidophiles:** Microorganisms which grow at an optimum pH well between 0.5-6 are called **acidophiles**. Example: *Thiobacillus, Sulfolobus.*
- **Neutrophiles:** Those which grow the best at neutral pH (pH 7) are called neutrophiles. Example: Soil bacteria and yeasts.
- **Alkaliphiles:** Those that grow best under alkaline conditions (pH above 7) are called alkaliphiles. Example: *Clostridium, Bacillus.*

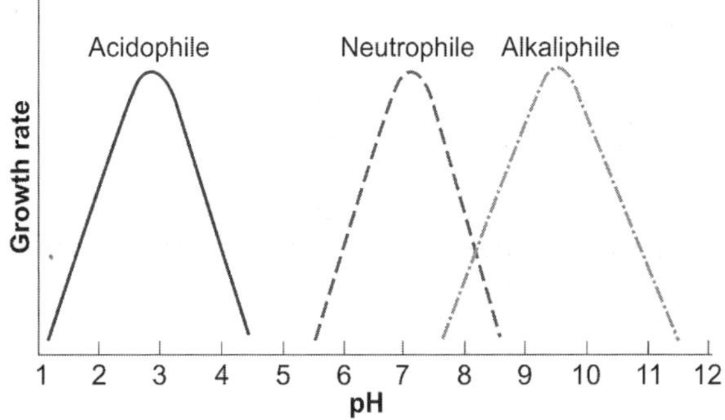

Figure 2.4.2: Growth rate vs pH for three environmental classes of microorganisms.

Temperature

Depending upon the temperature requirement, microorganisms can be categorized as:

- **Mesophile:** Microorganisms which can grow best (optimum temperature) at temperature near 37°C (the body temperature of human beings) are called **mesophiles**. Example: *Staphylococcus aureus, Salmonella, Listeria,* etc.
- **Thermophiles:** Microorganisms which can grow best at a temperature between about 45° and 70° are called **thermophiles**. Example: *Alicyclobacillus.*
- **Hyperthermophiles:** Some thermophiles can even grow at a temperature of 80°C or as high as 115°C. They are called as **hyperthermophiles**. Example: *Methanopyrus.*

- **Psychrophiles:** The cold-loving microorganisms are **psychrophiles**. They have the ability to grow at 0°C. Example: *Psychrobacter.*

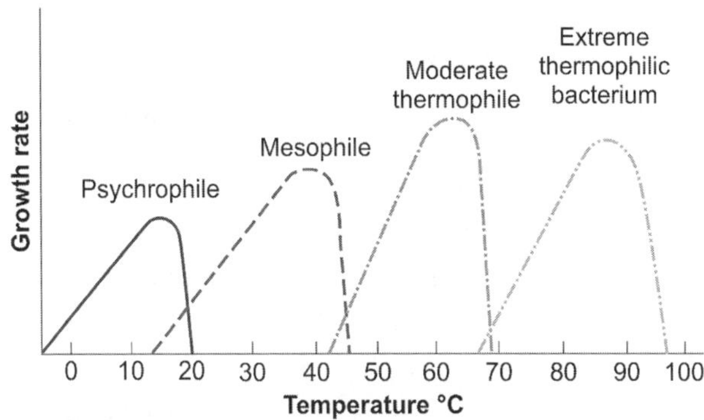

Figure 2.4.3: Microbial growth rate vs temperature.

Solute and Water Availability

For microorganisms solute can be salt (NaCl) or sugar. Depending on salt and water availability, the microorganisms could be categorized as follows:

- **Halophiles:** These are microorganisms that require sodium chloride (NaCl), the common salt, for growth. Example: Halobacteria. They are of following types;
  - **Mild halophiles** require 1-6% salt.
  - **Moderate halophiles** require 6-15% salt.
  - **Extreme halophiles** that require 15-30% salt.
- **Halotolerant:** These are microorganisms that are able to grow at moderate salt concentrations even though they grow best in absence of NaCl. Example: *Cyanobacteria.*
- **Osmophiles:** Microorganisms that are able to live in environments high in sugar. Example: *Enterobacter aerogenes, Micrococcus.*
- **Xerophiles:** Microorganisms which live in dry environment (made dry by lack of water). Example: *Trichosporonoides.*

CALCULATION OF MICROBIAL GROWTH

- Bacteria can increase their number by carrying out the process of binary fission. Suppose there is one bacterial cell. It takes 2 minutes to divide into two daughter cells through binary fission. So when one bacterial cell divides to form two we say one generation is over. The time taken by the bacterial cell to double its number is called as its generation time. For example, like in the above case the generation time is 2 minutes.

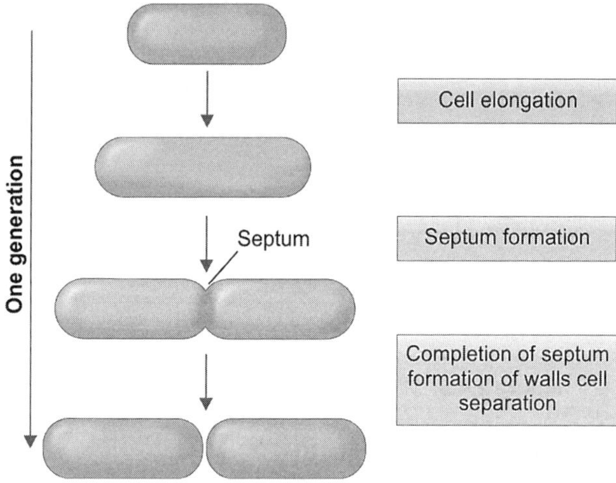

Figure 2.4.4: Formation of one generation in bacteria.

- The generation time can mathematically be expressed as:

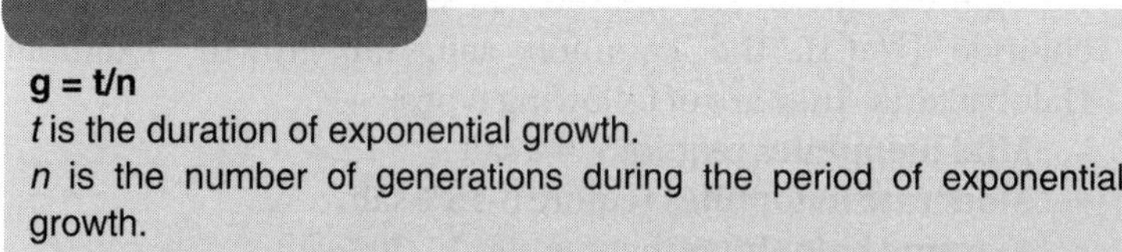

g = t/n

t is the duration of exponential growth.

n is the number of generations during the period of exponential growth.

Table 2.4.4: Generation times for some common bacteria.

Bacterium	Generation time (minutes)
Escherichia coli	17
Bacillus megaterium	25
Streptococcus lactis	26
Streptococcus lactis	48
Staphylococcus aureus	27–30
Lactobacillus acidophilus	66–87
Bhizobium japonicum	344–461
Mycobacterium tuberculosis	792–932
Treponema pallidum	1980

The growth pattern of bacteria is exponential in nature. This means under favorable conditions, a growing bacterial population doubles at regular intervals. Growth is by geometric progression: 1, 2, 4, 8, etc. or 20, 21, 22, 23.........2n (where n = the number of generations). This is called **exponential growth**.

A relationship exists between the initial and final number of bacterial cell present. This can be presented as follows:

$N = N_0 2^n$

N is the final cell number.

N_0 is the initial cell number.

n is the number of generations during the period of exponential growth.

MICROBIAL GROWTH CYCLE

The entire series of events that include birth, maturation and death of microorganisms could be put together to form the microbial growth cycle.

The microbial growth cycle is represented by microbial growth curve on a graph sheet. This has following phases:

- **Lag phase:** The population of microorganisms remains the same as bacteria become accustomed to their new environment.
- **Logarithmic phase (log phase):** Bacterial growth occurs at its optimal level and the population doubles rapidly.
- **Stationary phase:** The reproduction of bacterial cells is offset by their death and the population reaches a plateau. The reasons for bacterial death include accumulation of waste, lack of nutrients and unfavorable environmental conditions that may have developed.
- **Decline phase (Death phase):** If the conditions are not changed, the population will enter its decline or death phase. The bacteria die off rapidly, the curve turns downward and the last cell in the population soon dies.

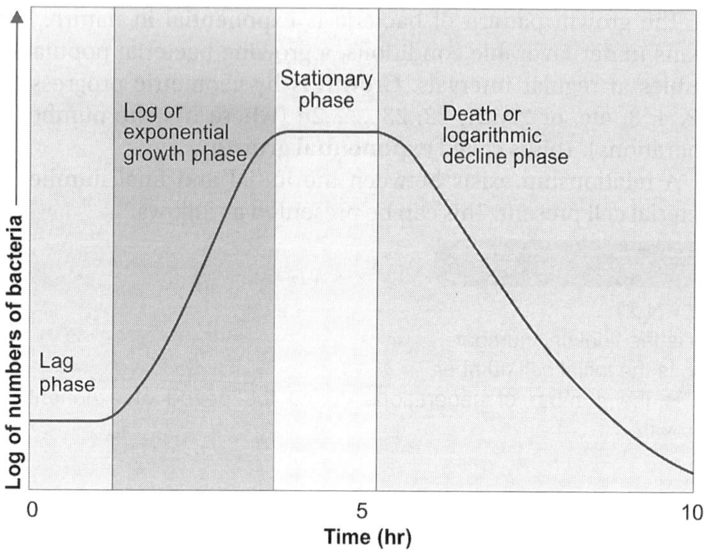

Figure 2.4.5: Growth curve of bacteria.

POSSIBLE QUESTIONS

1. What is microbial growth? What are the factors affecting the bacterial growth?
2. Discuss in detail about different phases of microbial growth curve.
3. Write Short Notes:
   a. Phototroph
   b. Chemotroph
   c. Lithotroph
   d. Macronutrients and Micronutrients
   e. Psychrophiles
   f. Mesophiles
   g. Thermophiles
   h. Halophiles
   i. Aerobe and anaerobe
   j. Microbial growth curve

MULTIPLE CHOICE QUESTIONS

1. The organism that use radiant energy for nutrition are called as ________.
   a. Phototrophs b. Chemotrophs
   c. Lithotrophs d. Heterotrophs
2. Which of the following bacteria oxidize inorganic compounds?
   a. Nitrobacteria b. Cyanobacteria
   c. Purple sulphur bacteria d. *E. coli*
3. Which of the following is not a microelements?
   a. Carbon b. Manganese
   c. Zinc d. Copper
4. The microorganisms which are insensitive to the presence of O_2 ___________.
   a. Aerotolerant anaerobes b. Aerobes
   c. Obligate anaerobes d. Facultative anaerobes
5. Microorganism that grow in an optimum pH well between 0.5–6 are called as ________.
   a. Acidophiles b. Alkaliphiles
   c. Mesophiles d. None of the above
6. The cold-loving microorganisms are called as___________.
   a. Psychrophiles b. Thermophiles
   c. Neutrophiles d. Mesophiles
7. Microorganisms that are able to grow in environments high in sugar are called as____________.
   a. Halophytes b. Osmophiles
   c. Halotolerant d. Xerophiles
8. In which phase population of microorganisms remain same as bacteria become accustomed to environment?
   a. Log phase b. Lag phase
   c. Decline phase d. Stationary phase
9. Bacteria can reproduce through______.
   a. Binary fission b. Conjugation
   c. Transformation d. All of the above
10. The relationship between the initial and final number of bacterial cell is ______.
   a. $N=N_0 2^n$ b. G=t/n
   c. $N/N_{0=}2^n$ d. Both a & b

Answers

1. a	2. c	3. a	4. a	5. a
6. a	7. b	8. b	9. d	10. d

Microbial Reproduction

WHAT IS REPRODUCTION?

All living things have the ability to reproduce. Reproduction is the process of generating offsprings. Microorganisms also reproduce by various methods in order to increase population. There are two main types of reproduction: Sexual reproduction and asexual reproduction. Some living organisms reproduce by only one method and others can reproduce using either method. Microorganisms can reproduce sexually and asexually. Microbes have an enormous population because they can reproduce quickly and in so many different ways.

TYPES OF REPRODUCTION IN MICROORGANISMS

Asexual Reproduction

It is a type of reproduction where cells from only one parent are used. Only genetically identical organisms are produced by this type of reproduction.

In this Type of Reproduction

- Donor (one which gives DNA) and recipient (one which receives DNA) cells are absent
- Exchange of genetic material (DNA) does not take place
- The offsprings are exact copies of Mother cell

Types of Asexual Reproduction

Budding

In this type of reproduction a small projection, called bud, develops at one end of the cell and one copy of the genetic material gets into the bud. Then the bud enlarges to form a new cell and gets separated from the parent cell.

It takes place in following steps:

- Parent cell gives rise to a lateral outgrowth called as bud.
- The chromosome of parent cell is duplicated and passes into the daughter cell.
- The bud grows in size while being attached to the parent body.
- It then gets separated from the parent by the formation of a wall.
- Thereafter the bud falls off and germinates into new individual.
- Thus budding results in formation of daughter cells of unequal size that later grow to adult bodies.

Example: Budding is found in Planctomyces and Yeasts.

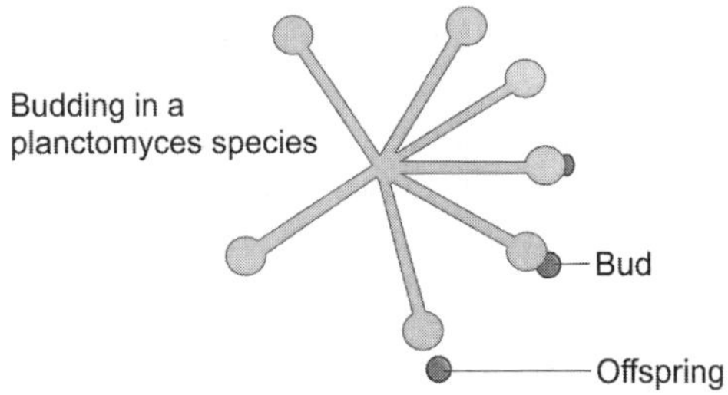

Figure 2.5.1: Binary fission.

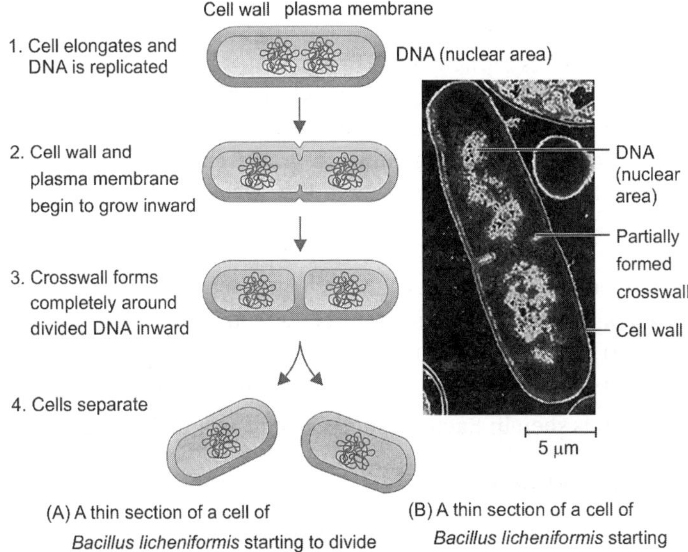

(A) A thin section of a cell of *Bacillus licheniformis* starting to divide

(B) A thin section of a cell of *Bacillus licheniformis* starting to divide

Figures 2.5.2A and B: Endospore formation.

Binary Fission

Binary fission generally takes place in bacteria. It is a simple process where the cell increases in size and a double wall develops across the midline of enlarged cell. The enlarged cell then gets separated to form two new cells. Each cell is able to function independently. The process of this type of multiplication in microorganisms is quite rapid. *E. coli* bacterium can double in every 20 minutes at favorable environmental conditions.

It occurs through following steps:
- Parental cell enlarges and duplicates its chromosome
- Septum formation (midline wall formation) divides the cell into two separate chambers
- The duplicated chromosome moves to newly formed chamber
- Complete division results in two identical cells
- Each new cell has an identical copy of DNA
- Example, mostly seen in Bacteria

Spore Formation or Sporulation

The process of endospore formation in bacteria is called sporulation. During unfavorable condition bacteria produce endospores through following steps:
- **Step 1:** DNA is replicated.
- **Step 2:** DNA aligns along the cell's long axis.
- **Step 3:** Cytoplasmic membrane invaginates to form forespore.
- **Step 4:** Cytoplasmic membrane grows and engulfs forespore within a second membrane. The DNA of vegetative cells disintegrates.
- **Step 5:** A cortex of Calcium and Dipicolinic acid is deposited between the membranes.
- **Step 6:** Spore coat forms around endospore.
- **Step 7:** Endospore matures.
- **Step 8:** Endospore releases from the Original cell.

Example: It is seen in Bacteria such as *Bacillus* and *Clostridium.*

Conidia Formation

It takes place in some bacterial and fungal cells. Mostly during unfavorable conditions, bacterial protoplasm divides into small compartments and then gets fragmentized forming minute bodies called as conidia. When the favorable condition arrives, each conidium develops itself into a new bacterium. Each conidium gets a copy of the genetic material.

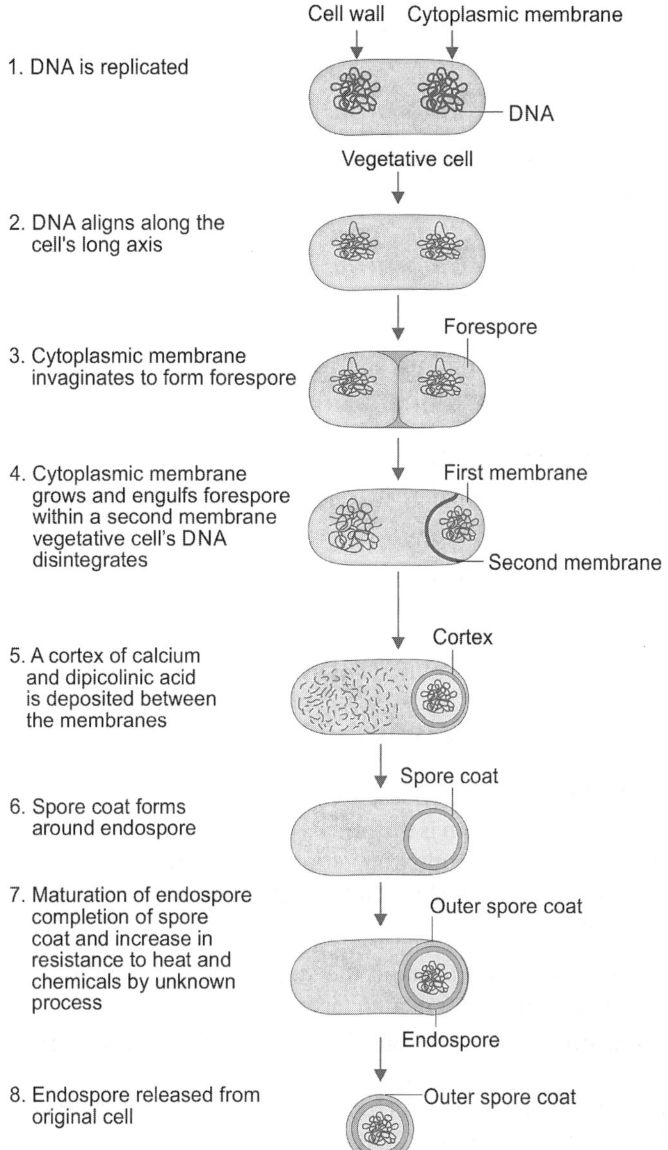

Figure 2.5.3: Endospore formation by bacteria.

Zoospores

This is a common method of asexual reproduction in *Rhizobium* which produces flagellated zoospores.

Cyst

In some bacteria, thick walled spores, similar to endospores are formed. These are called as cysts.

Example: *Azotobacter*

Fragmentation

It is mostly seen in fungi. In this process the mycelium (fungal filament) breaks into two or more similar fragments either accidentally or due to some external force and each fragment grows into a new fungal filament.

Sexual Reproduction

During sexual reproduction, two cells, one from each parent, fuse to form a new organism.

In this type of reproduction

- Donor (one which gives DNA) and recipient (one which receives DNA) cells are present
- Exchange of genetic material (DNA) takes place.

Types of Sexual Reproduction

Conjugation

Definition: Conjugation is the process of direct transfer of DNA from one bacterial cell to another bacterial cell. The transferred DNA is a plasmid, i.e., a circle of DNA that is distinct from the main bacterial chromosome.

Basic concept: To understand the steps of conjugation in bacteria one must know different related terms like:

- **F-plasmid:** It is a special plasmid called as Fertility. Plasmid present in some bacterial cell.
- **Donor:** The bacteria which contain the F-plasmid are called as F^+ cells or donor cells.
- **Recipient:** The bacteria which lack the F-plasmid are called as F^- cells or recipient cells.

- **Sex pilus:** This is a specialized thread-like structure present on the outer most surface of donor cells (F^+cells).

Steps of Conjugation

- **Step 1:** Donor cell is attached to a recipient cell with its pilus. The pilus draws the cell together.
- **Step 2:** The cells contact with one another.
- **Step 3:** One strand of F-plasmid DNA is transferred to the recipient
- **Step 4:** The recipient which was F^- before, becomes F^+ after getting the F-plasmid.

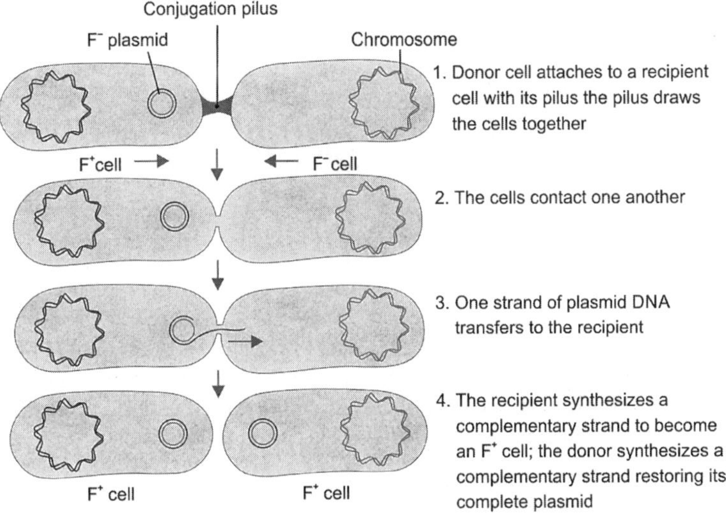

Figure 2.5.4: Conjugation between F^+ and F^- bacterial cell.

Transduction

Definition: Transduction is the process of DNA transfer from one bacterium (donor) to another (recipient) mediated by a virus called as bacteriophage. The recipient cell of a transduction process is called as transductant.

Basic concept: To understand the steps of conjugation in bacteria one needs to know following terms:

- **Bacteriophage:** It is a virus that attacks bacteria, multiplies inside it and finally kills it. Bacteriophage, like all other viruses, are made-up of nucleic acid and protein. The structure of a bacteriophage is as below:
  - **Nucleic acid:** The Nucleic acid present in bacteriophage is Deoxyribo Nucleic Acid (DNA). It carries all information

(genetic information) which are necessary to carry out the lytic cycle.

- **Protein Part:** Apart from DNA, all other parts of bacteriophage such as capsid head, collar, sheath, baseplate, spikes and tail fibers are made-up of proteins.

Example of a bacteriophage is a T4 phage.

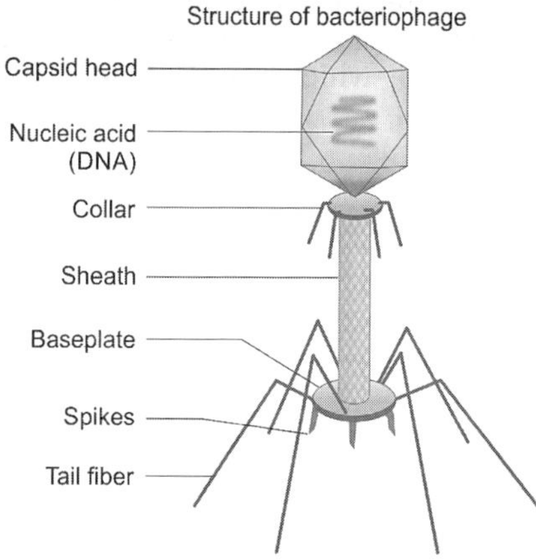

Figure 2.5.5: Bacteriophage.

- **Lytic cycle:** The process by which a bacteriophage attacks, multiplies and kills a bacterial cell is called as lytic cycle. The bacterial cell which is attacked is called as host cell.

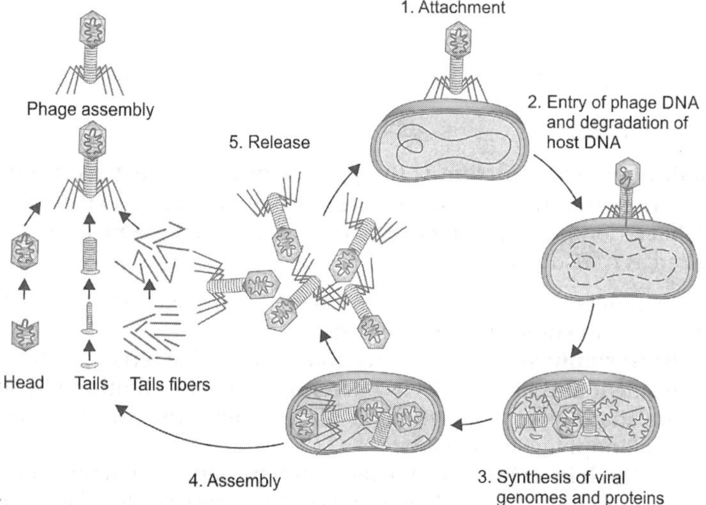

Figure 2.5.6: Steps of transduction.

Steps of Transduction

- **Step 1:** The bacteriophage attacks the host bacterial cell (called as donor cell) and injects its DNA.
- **Step 2:** The bacteriophage DNA then makes a special type of enzyme that degrades (or break down) the host DNA.
- **Step 3:** New bacteriophage particles are synthesized each having bacteriophage DNA (usual bacteriophage) and few with host's (or donor's) DNA (unusual bacteriophage). Such unusual bacteriophage is called as a transducing phage.
- **Step 4:** The transducing phage attacks another bacterial cell (also called as recipient cell) and injects donor's DNA.
- **Step 5:** Donor's DNA is then incorporated into recipient's chromosome by recombination. After this the recipient cell is called as transduced cell.

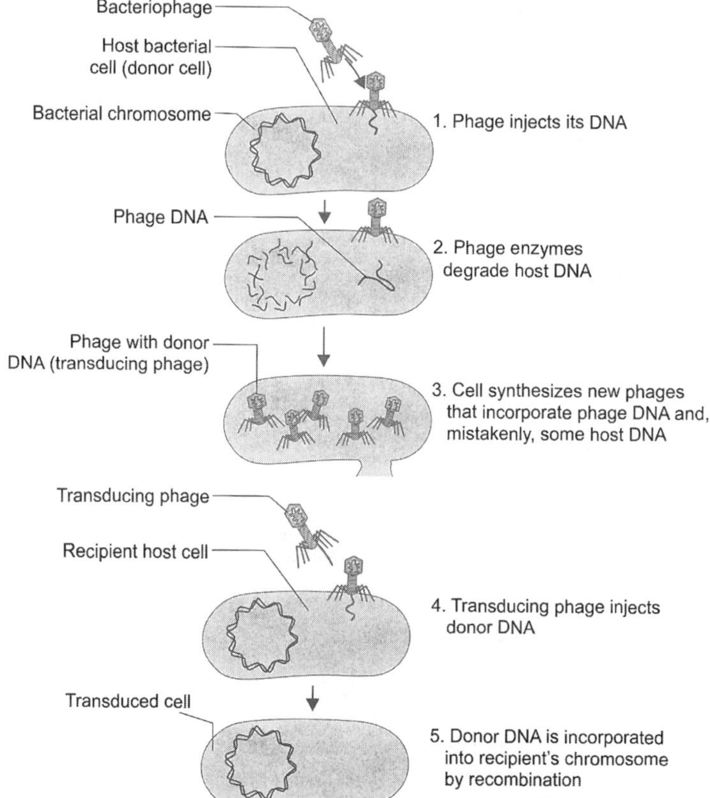

Figure 2.5.7: The process of transduction.

Transformation

Definition: Transformation is a process in which bacteria take-up DNA from the outside environment and integrates into its chromosome.

Steps of Transformation

- Naked DNA fragments from one bacterium (donor) released during cell lysis (when cell bursts) bind to the cell wall of another bacterium (recipient).
- The recipient bacterium must be competent which means that it has structures on its cell wall that can bind DNA and take it up into it.
- The DNA that has been brought in can then incorporate itself into the recipient.
- After this process, the recipient cell is called as transformed cell.

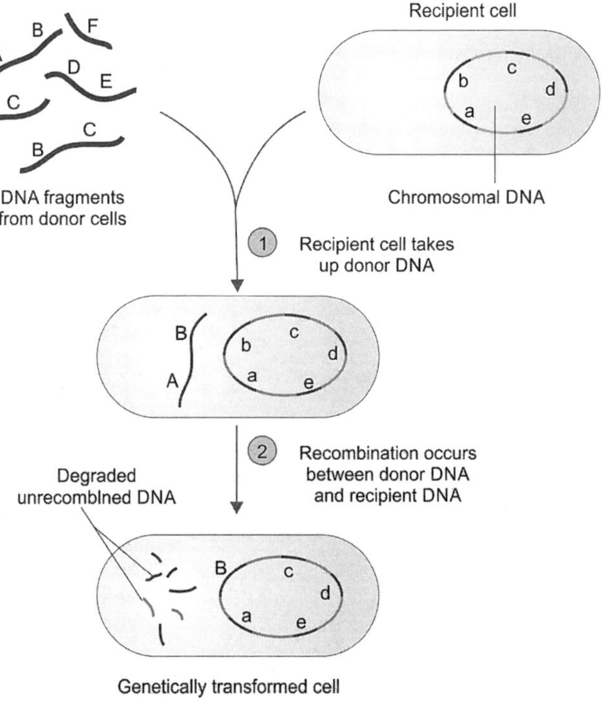

Figure 2.5.8: Transformation in bacteria.

POSSIBLE QUESTIONS

1. What is reproduction? Discuss various types of Asexual reproduction carried out by microorganisms.
2. Write an essay on various types of Sexual reproduction seen in Microorganisms.
3. What is sexual reproduction? How is it different from asexual reproduction? Write a short note on transduction.
4. Write Short Notes:
   a. Binary fission
   b. Budding
   c. Conidia
   d. Cyst
   e. Sporulation
   f. Endospore
   g. Bacteriophage
   h. Lytic cycle
   i. Transduction
   j. Conjugation
   k. Transformation
   l. Zoospores

MULTIPLE CHOICE QUESTIONS

1. Asexual reproduction involves______.
   a. Uniparental b. Biparental
   c. No parents required d. None of the above
2. Budding found in __________.
   a. Yeast b. Planctomyces
   c. Clostridium d. Both a and b
3. Sporulation is the process of formation of ______.
   a. Spores b. Endospores
   c. Exospores d. Both a and c
4. Rhizobium reproduces through _____________.
   a. Zoospores b. Aplanospores
   c. Conidia d. Chlamydospores
5. Azatobacter reproduces by ____________.
   a. Cyst b. Conidia
   c. Fragmentation d. Budding
6. The bacteria that contains F-plasmid are called as ____________.
   a. Recipient b. Donor
   c. F^+ cells d. Both b and c
7. Bacteriophage contains ___________.
   a. Nucleic acid b. Protein
   c. Both a and b d. Only protein

8. The process by which bacteriophage attacks, multiplies, and kills the bacterial cell is called as ____________.
   a. Lysogenic
   b. Lytic
   c. Transformation
   d. None of the above
9. The process by which a virus transfers genetic material from one bacterium to another is called as ____________.
   a. Transduction
   b. Sporulation
   c. Both a and b
   d. None of the above
10. Zoospores are ____________.
   a. Flagellated
   b. Non-flagellated
   c. Motile
   d. Both a and c

Answers

1. a	2. d	3. b	4. a	5. a
6. d	7. c	8. b	9. a	10. d

CHAPTER 2.6

Bacterial Culture and Isolation Techniques

WHAT IS CULTURE MEDIA?

The media is a source of nutrients to support the growth of the microorganisms in vitro. The media helps in the growth and counting of microbial cells, selection of microorganisms, and survival of microorganisms. The culture medium can be liquid or gel.

Common Ingredients of Culture Media

- **Peptone:** Source of carbon and nitrogen.
- **Beef extract:** Source of amino acid, vitamins and minerals.
- **Yeast extract:** Source of vitamin, carbon and nitrogen.
- **Distilled water**
- **Agar:** Solidifying agent.

HOW TO PREPARE CULTURE MEDIA?

- Weigh the amount of ingredients powder on weighing machine.
- Dissolve the ingredients in distilled water.
- Adjust PH of the medium if needed.
- Add agar and boiled it to dissolve.
- Pour the media into flask.
- Autoclave the media when ingredients fully dissolve.
- Sterilization is done in autoclave to prevent from contamination, at 121°C for 15 minutes at 15 lbs.
- After the autoclave place the media flask in laminar air flow.
- Sterilize the laminar air flow with 70% alcohol.
- A bit cools down the media and pours into sterile Petri plates for solidification.
- Then sample is ready to spread (spreader)/streak (inoculation loop) on the medium for identification or isolation of microbes.
- Sealed the Petri plates with paraffin, label them.
- Keep them inverted in incubator at 37°C for 24 hours.

- Observe the result next day colonies formation is visible on the media.

What is a Defined Medium?

A defined medium has a known quantity of all ingredients, like carbon source (glucose or glycerol) and nitrogen source (ammonium salt or nitrate as inorganic nitrogen). The medium needs in metabolic, nutritional, and physiological growth experiments.

What is an Undefined Medium?

This medium has different complex ingredients in unknown quantities, for example, yeast extract, beef, various salts, and enzymatic protein.

What is Complex Media?

This media is other than basal media; it has added ingredients to bring the characteristics of microorganisms with unique nutrients.

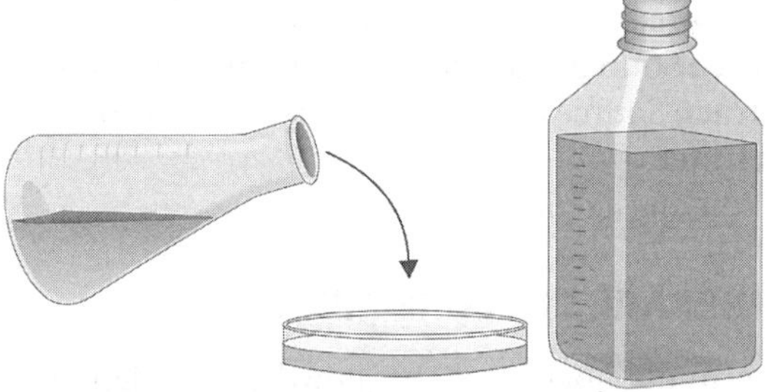

Figure 2.6.1: Types of culture media.

TYPES OF CULTURE MEDIA BASED ON CONSISTENCY/PHYSICAL STATE

1. Solid medium
2. Semi-solid medium
3. Liquid medium

Solid Media

Principle of Solid Media

It is for the isolation of bacteria as a pure culture on a solid medium. Robert Koch realized the use of solid media.

Agar is used to hardening the media at 1.5- 2.0% concentration. Solid media allows the growth of bacteria as colonies by streaking on the medium. It solidified at 37°C.

Agar is an un-branched polysaccharide extracted from red algae species like *Gelidium*. Colonies identification is done on this medium.

Examples of Solid Media

- Nutrient agar, MacConkey agar, Blood agar, Chocolate agar.
- Growth of bacteria on solid medium appear as smooth, rough, mucoid, round, irregular, filamentous, punctiform.

Semi-solid Media

Principle of Semi-solid Media

This media shows the motility of bacteria and the cultivation of microaerophilic bacteria. This media has agar at a concentration of 0.5% or less. It has a jelly consistency.

Examples of Semi-solid Media

Stuart's and Amies media, Hugh and Leifson's oxidation fermentation medium, and Mannitol motility media.
The growth of bacteria in semi-solid appears as a thick line in the medium.

Liquid Media

Principle of Liquid Media

- This media shows the growth of a large number of bacteria.
- It is called Broth that allows bacteria to grow uniformly with turbidity. The growth occurs at 37°C in an incubator for 24 hours.
- Liquid media don't have the addition of agar; it is for fermentation studies.

Examples of Liquid Media

- Nutrient broth, Tryptic soy broth, MR-VP broth, phenol red carbohydrate broth.
- Growth of bacteria in liquid media—turbidity is seen at the end of the broth.

TYPES OF CULTURE MEDIA BASED ON CHEMICAL COMPOSITION/APPLICATION

There are seven routine laboratory media.

1. Basal media
2. Enriched media
3. Selective media
4. Enrichment media
5. Indicator media or differential media
6. Transport media
7. Storage media

Basal Media

This media is simple as it enhances the growth of many microorganisms. It's a routinely used medium in the lab, having carbon and nitrogen. This media allows the growth; of non- fastidious bacteria without any enrichment source; used for sub-culturing. It's a non-selective medium.

Staphylococcus and *Enterobacteriaceae* grow in this media.

Examples of Basal Media

Nutrient agar, Peptone water.

Enriched Media

This media requires the addition of other substances like blood, egg, or serum. An enriched media allows the growth of devised microorganisms but inhibits other and fastidious microbes grow as they require nutrients like vitamins and growth-promoting substances.

Example of Enriched Media

Blood agar, chocolate agar, LSS, Monsor's taurocholate, Lowenstein-Jensen media. Blood agar identifies hemolytic bacteria, chocolate media for *N. gonorrhoeae.*

Selective Media

As by name, we can tell, this media shows the growth of selective; microbes or desired microorganisms and inhibits the growth of unwanted microbes. The inhibition occurs by adding bile salts, antibiotics, dyes, PH adjustments. Media is agar-based; any media is possible to transform into selective by adding inhibitory agar.

Examples of Selective Media

S. No.	Media	Bacteria
1.	**Mannitol agar:** It has 7% of sodium chloride that inhibits the growth of other microbes and promotes the growth of *Staphylococci. It has phenol red dye that produces acid Staphylococcus used the mannitol for the acid production and the* color of phenol red changes from red to yellow	Selective for *Staphylococcus aureus*
2.	Salmonella-Shigella agar deoxycholate agar	It is used for the isolation of *Salmonella* bacteria that causes typhoid Selective for *Shigella*
3.	**MacConkey agar:** It has bile salts that inhibit the growth of gram-positive bacteria	Selective isolation for *Enterobacteriaceae*
4.	**TCBS agar:** Light green translucent media bile salt inhibits the growth of unwanted bacteria	Selective for *Vibrio cholera. V. cholera* produces acid by fermentation of sucrose that acts as indicator called bromothymol blue and yellow colonies appears
5.	**Lowenstein Jensen media:** It is made selective by adding malachite green and stops the unwanted growth of pathogens	Selective *for M. tuberculosis*

Enrichment Media

It is a liquid medium, which also permits the growth of desired bacteria at a low density. The media provides an environment and conditions as selective media and inhibits unwanted bacteria from growing. It is for the isolation of the soil and fecal microorganisms.

Examples of Enrichment Media

Selenite F-broth does the isolation of *Salmonella* Typhi from a fecal sample. Selenium allows the growth of desired organisms and, detection levels increase for intestinal flora.

Indicator or Differential Media

This media shows visible changes due to the presence of an indicator. It differentiates bacteria based on colony color growing on the same plate; biochemical characteristics show organism's growth with chemical indicators like neutral red, phenol red, methylene blue.

Examples of Indicator or Differential Media

Mannitol salt agar (mannitol fermentation shows yellow color colonies); blood agar is used to differentiate between hemolytic and non-hemolytic. MacConkey agar produces pink colonies due to lactose utilization and, non-lactose shows pale color colonies.

Transport Media

The media transport specimens after collection to control the overgrowth of organisms. For the cultivation, this media act as temporary storage. It also maintains the viability of pathogens in the specimen and prevents them from drying.

Examples of Transport Media

Stuart's transport medium (lacks carbon, nitrogen, growth factors). Cary Blair's transport media and VR are used to transport feces samples from cholera patients. Pikes medium helps to transport streptococci from throat patients.

Storage Media

It maintains the longevity of bacterial culture.
Examples are cooked meat broth, NA egg saline.

TYPES OF CULTURE MEDIA BASED ON OXYGEN REQUIREMENT

Microorganisms have different requirements for growth depending on oxygen requirements.

Aerobic Media

In this media, it is easy to cultivate microbes, on solid media, the growth occurs by keeping the culture in the incubator. It shows the growth; of non-fastidious microorganisms.

Examples of aerobic media are liquid media, solid media

Peptone water—1% peptone + 0.5% Nacl +100 mL water.

Nutrient agar- nutrient broth + 2% agar.

Anaerobic Media

The media cultivates anaerobic bacteria at low oxygen, reducing oxidation-reduction potential. Anaerobic media contains extra nutrients like vitamin K, hemin, and oxygen that get reduced by a physical or chemical process. The addition of glucose (1%), thioglycollate (0.1%), ascorbic acid (0.1%), cysteine (0.05%), or iron fillings added to cause the medium to reduce. The medium is boiled in a water bath to force out dissolved oxygen and packed with sterile paraffin.

Examples of Anaerobic Media

RCM (Robertson cooked meat) isolation for *Clostridium* sp.
Thioglycolate broth: Thioglycollate has sodium glycolate that maintains low oxygen.

TYPES OF SPECIAL PURPOSE CULTURE MEDIA

Assay Media

The media assay vitamins, amino acids, and antibiotics. For example, antibiotic sensitivity test the media used is Muller-Hinton agar has 1.7% agar for better diffusion of antibiotics. It also contains starch, which absorbs toxins released by bacteria. In this media plate, zone of inhibition is seen around antibiotics.

Minimal Media

Principle of Minimal Media

Minimal media is a defined medium with different compositions depending on microorganisms cultured. It contains a carbon source like sugar/succinate and inorganic salts like magnesium, nitrogen, sulfur, phosphorus. Carbon is a source of energy; magnesium and ammonium salts are the sources of ions for metabolism stimulation. Phosphate is a buffering agent.

The growth comparison of microbe culture and mutant forms—minimal media and supplementary-minimal media—allow the differentiation of wild-type and mutant cells.

Use: The selection of recombinants, for the growth of wild-type microorganisms.

Fermentation Media

The media is for optimum microorganisms. Fermentation media produce high yields of the product; media provide energy and nutrients for growth, and medium gives the substrate for the synthesis of products in the fermentation.
Fermentation media contains major and minor components.

Major components—carbon and nitrogen for energy.

Minor components—this contains inorganic salts, growth factors, vitamins, buffer, anti-foaming agents, dissolved oxygen, gases, growth inhibitors, enzymes.

The nutrients in fermentation media depend on the organism and type of fermentation process.

Growth Media

It has low nutrients and creates raw material for further fermentation.

Fermentation Media

It has high nutrients and creates end products.

Example: The yeast requires 1% carbon, but the fermentation of alcohol, demands 12-13% carbon in the medium.

Resuscitation Culture Media

The resuscitation method is for the stressed bacterial recovery; this is a specialized medium that allows the growth of microbes that have lost the ability to produce because of the environmental harness. The culture provides nutrients and recovers their metabolism.

For example, bacteria require histamine for growth, and the medium lacks this component. Then it inhibits growth. The same bacterium is put in a medium having histamine, then it starts to grow again, and this medium acts as resuscitation media.

For example, tryptic Soy Agar.

Application of Culture Media

- To culture microbes.
- To identify the cause of infection.
- To identify characteristics of microorganisms.
- To isolate pure culture.
- To store the culture stock.
- To observe biochemical reactions.
- To test microbial contamination in any sample.
- To check antimicrobial agents and preservatives effect.
- To observe microbe colony type, its color, shape, cause.
- To differentiate between different colonies.
- To create antigens for laboratory use.
- To estimate viable count.
- To test antibiotic sensitivity.

Limitations of Culture Media

- Risk of cross-contamination.
- High skill required for optimal results.
- Increased drying out of media can occur.

METHODS OF ISOLATION OF BACTERIA

Methods of isolation of bacteria can be broadly classified into two:

- Culture methods
  - On solid media
  - On liquid media
  - Automated systems
- Non-culture methods

Culture Methods

The specimens received in the laboratory are plated on the culture media. The appropriate culture media is selected depending upon the bacteria suspected. The following precautions need to be taken into consideration when the culture methods are processed:

- Optimal atmospheric conditions
- Optimal temperature
- Growth requirement of the bacteria

Atmospheric conditions: Colonies of bacteria are usually large enough to identify after 18–24 hours of incubation (usually at 37°C), but for some bacteria longer incubation times are required (from

2 days to several weeks). Culture plates are incubated (1) in air, (2) in air with added carbon dioxide (5%), (3) anaerobically (without oxygen), or (4) micro-aerophilically (a trace of oxygen) according to the requirements of the different types of bacteria that may be present in specimens.

In case of mycobacteria especially the scotochromogen the culture bottles are placed in dark or the bottles are covered with black paper and kept for incubation at 37°C.

Temperature: Most of the bacteria requires a temperature of 37°C for optimal growth. This temperature is provided placing the inoculated culture plates in the incubator set at 37°C temperature.

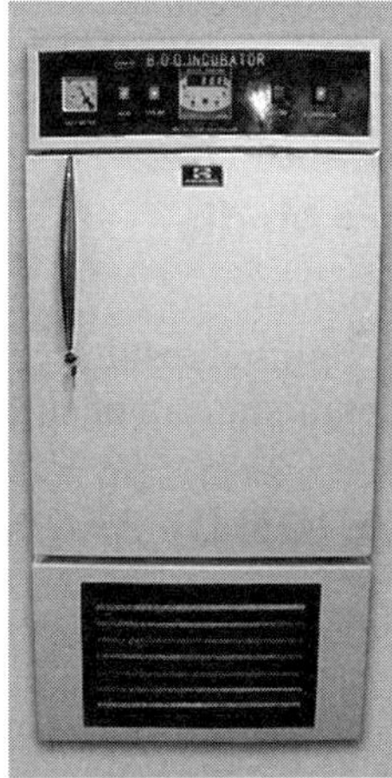

Figure. 2.6.2: Incubator.

Growth requirement of the bacteria: Different bacteria have different growth requirements. For example, *streptococcus pneumoniae* requires factor V and factor X for its growth, which are found in chocolate agar. Thus for sample suspected of *S. pneumoniae* the samples are plated on chocolate agar. Similarly depending upon the growth requirements the appropriate culture media are used.

Culture on Solid Media

The principal method for the detection of bacteria from clinical specimens is by culture on solid culture media. Bacteria grow on the surface of culture media to produce distinct colonies.

Different bacteria produce different but characteristic colonies, allowing for early presumptive identification and easy identification of mixed cultures. There are many different types of culture media. Agar is used as the gelling agent to which is added a variety of nutrients (e.g., blood, peptone and sugars) and other factors (e.g., buffers, salts and indicators).

Some culture media are non-selective (e.g., blood agar, nutrient agar) and these will grow a wide variety of bacteria. While some, e.g., MacConkey agar are more selective (in this case through the addition of bile salts selecting for the 'bile- tolerant' bacteria found in the large intestine, such as *Escherichia coli* and *Enterococcus faecalis*). MacConkey agar also contains lactose and an indicator system that identifies lactose-fermenting coliforms (e.g., *Escherichia coli, Klebsiella*) from lactose non-fermenting coliforms (e.g., *Morganella, Salmonella*). Media can be made even more selective by the addition of antibiotics or other inhibitory substances, and sophisticated indicator systems can allow for the easy detection of defined bacteria from mixed populations.

Method of Inoculating the Solid Culture Media

Method used for inoculating the solid media depends upon the purpose of inoculation- whether to have isolated colonies or to know the bacterial load of the sample (quantitative analysis).

For obtaining the isolated colonies streaking method is used, the most common method of inoculating an agar plate is streaking.

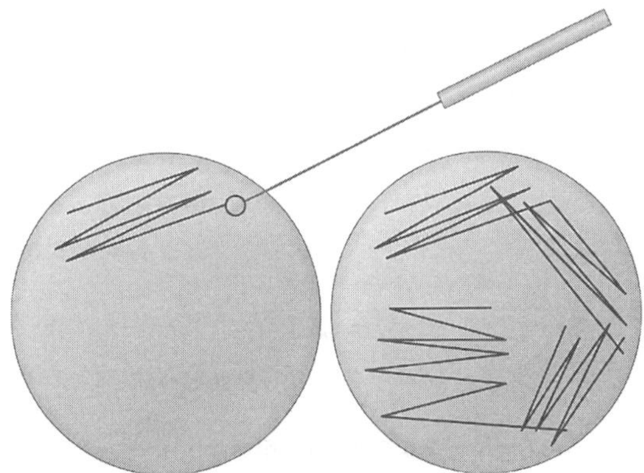

Figure. 2.6.3: Streaking method.

Streak Plates

- A small amount of sample is placed on the side of the agar plate (either with a swab, or as a drop from an inoculating loop).
- A sterile loop is then used to spread the bacteria out in one direction from the initial site of inoculation. This is done by moving the loop from side to side, passing through the initial site.
- The loop is then sterilized (by flaming) again and the first streaks are then spread out themselves.
- This is repeated 2-3 times, moving around the agar plate as shown in the figure.

In this method, single bacterial cells get isolated by the streaking, and when the plate is incubated, forming discrete colonies that will have started from just one bacterium each.

For quantitative analysis or semi quantitative analysis of the sample, for example, in case of urinary tract infection. In fact, *E. coli* is implicated as the causative organism in urinary tract infection only if there are >10^5Colony forming units per millilitre of urine. The method of inoculating the solid culture media is as shown in the figure.

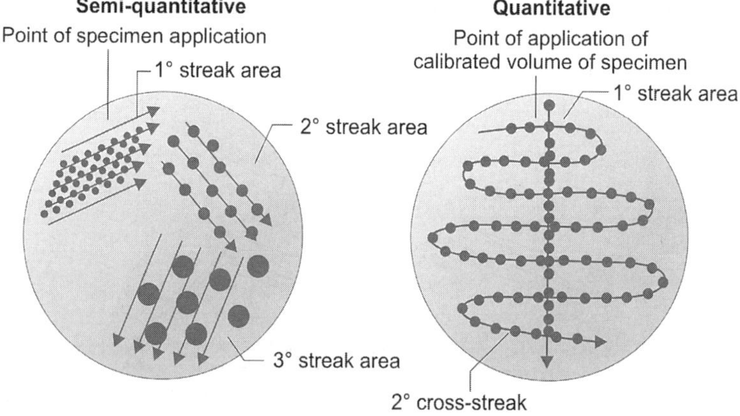

Figure. 2.6.4: Inoculation methods.

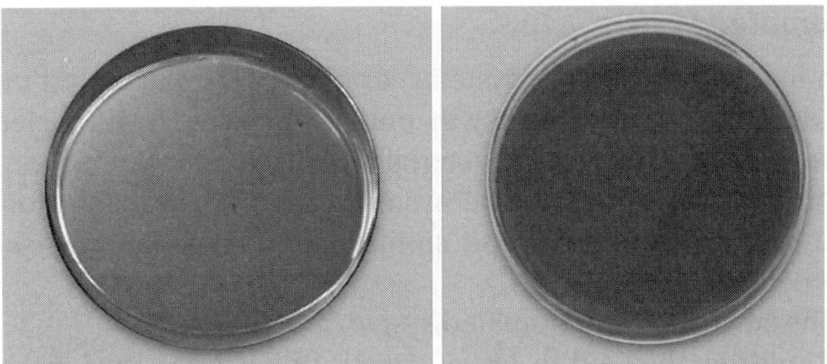

Figure. 2.6.5: Uninoculated MacConkey agar and blood agar plate.

Culture in Liquid Media

Bacteria can also be grown in liquid media (broth). Like agar plates, broth cultures may be non-selective or selective. Bacterial growth is easy to detect as the clear liquid turns turbid, usually within 24–48 hour, but incubation may need to be extended to 14 days or more.

The advantage of broth culture is that it is significantly more sensitive than direct culture on agar. The disadvantage is that, by itself, it is not easy to determine the type of bacteria present or whether a mixed growth has occurred, and in most cases, the broth must be subcultured onto solid agar plates. This causes an additional delay in culture results. Broth cultures are also prone to contamination.

Broth enrichment media are used when high sensitivity is required, e.g., for detection of bacteria from CSF, or to detect small numbers of *Salmonella* in a stool sample containing many millions of other bacteria.

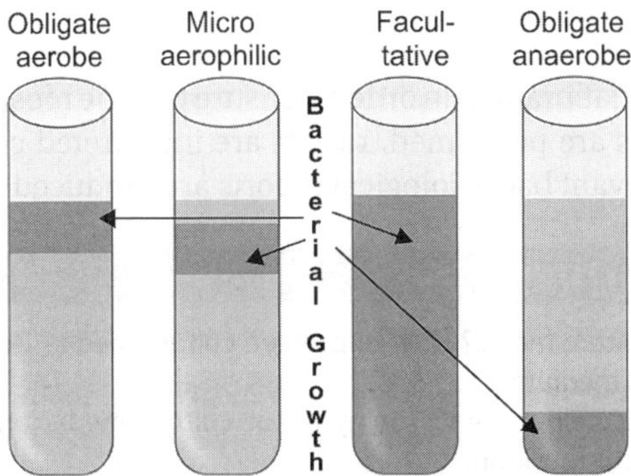

Figure. 2.6.6: Liquid media.

Automated System

Automated blood culture systems, e.g., BACTEC, BacteAlert utilize liquid culture. Bacterial growth may be detected by a variety of methods (e.g., detection of bacterial CO_2 production).

Automated liquid culture systems are also available for the culture of mycobacteria, and similar technology can be used to automate sensitivity.

The advantage of automated system are:

Rapidity: They aid in faster growth of bacteria. Thus less time consuming. The incidence of contamination during the processing of sample are minimized real time monitoring of the growth.

One of the main limitations is the commercial viability.

Non-culture Methods

Isolation of bacteria can also be carried out by non-culture methods. In particular, the more advanced amplification techniques like polymerase chain reaction (PCR), ligase chain reaction (LCR), strand displacement amplification (SDA), and nucleic acid sequence based amplification (NASBA) are being used in clinical laboratories for isolation and identification of bacteria.

The following are some of the factors that are considered in interpreting bacteriological culture results:

- Type of specimen
- Any delays in processing
- Types of bacteria recovered
- Knowledge of the normal human flora at different sites
- Clinical information provided on the request form
- Details of recent antibiotic therapy

There must be good liaison between healthcare workers and the microbiology laboratory, in order to ensure that the most appropriate investigations are performed, results are interpreted correctly, and clinically relevant bacteriological reports are produced.

POSSIBLE QUESTIONS

1. What is culture media? How to prepare culture media? Define solid and semi-solid medium.
2. Give an account details on types of culture media on the basis of chemical composition.
3. Describe methods of isolation of bacteria.

SHORT NOTES

1. Application of culture media.
2. Fermentation media.
3. Culture of bacteria in liquid medium.
4. Define medium and undefined medium.

MULTIPLE CHOICE QUESTIONS

1. Peptone is a source of ____________.
   a. Carbon b. Sulphur
   c. Oxygen d. Hydrogen
2. Agar is extracted from ___________.
   a. Red algae b. Blue algae
   c. Green algae d. None of the above
3. Lowenstein Jensen Media is made by adding _______________ to the culture media.
   a. Malachite green b. TCBS agar
   c. Deoxycholate agar d. None of the above
4. The optimal temperature for bacterial growth _____________.
   a. 37°C b. 34°C
   c. 32°C d. 38°C
5. *Streptococcus pneumoniae* requires which factor for its growth?
   a. V and X factor b. V and S factor
   c. X and S factor d. None of the above
6. Which is not a ingredient of culture media?
   a. Peptone b. Agar
   c. Beef extract d. Cellulose
7. Who discovered solid media?
   a. Robert Koch b. Robert brown
   c. Robert hook d. None of the above
8. Lowenstein Jensen Media is selective for which bacteria?
   a. *V. cholera* b. *M. tuberculosis*
   c. *Salmonella* d. Enterobacteriaceae
9. Which media maintains the longevity of bacterial culture?
   a. Transport media b. Enrichment media
   c. Storage media d. None of the above
10. Which media has high nutrients?
    a. Growth media b. Formation media
    c. Aerobic media d. Anaerobic media

Answers

1. a	2. a	3. a	4. a	5. a
6. d	7. a	8. b	9. c	10. b

The Normal Flora of Human Body

WHAT IS NORMAL FLORA?

- The normal flora are microorganisms (mostly bacteria) which are found in or on our body without causing any disease. There are more bacteria living in or on our bodies, than that of our cells. A human body contains around 10^{13} cells and is home to around 10^{14} bacteria. One fourth of fecal weight is made up of bacteria!
- The skin and mucous membranes carry a variety of microorganisms that can be arranged into two groups:
  - The resident flora consists of permanent microorganisms which are regularly found in a given area at a given age.
  - The transient flora consists of nonpathogenic or pathogenic microorganisms that stay on the skin or mucous membranes for hours, days, or weeks. They come from the environment, do not produce disease and do not stay permanently on the surface.

DISTRIBUTION OF NORMAL FLORA IN THE BODY

The most common sites of body inhabited by normal flora are the skin, eye, mouth, upper respiratory, gastrointestinal and urogenital tracts.

BENEFICIAL FUNCTIONS OF NORMAL FLORA

- **The normal flora synthesize and excrete vitamins** in excess of their own needs which can be absorbed as nutrients by their host. For example, in humans, enteric bacteria secrete vitamin K and vitamin B_{12}, and lactic acid bacteria produce certain B-vitamins.
- **The normal flora prevent spreading of pathogens by competing for** attachment sites or for getting essential nutrients.

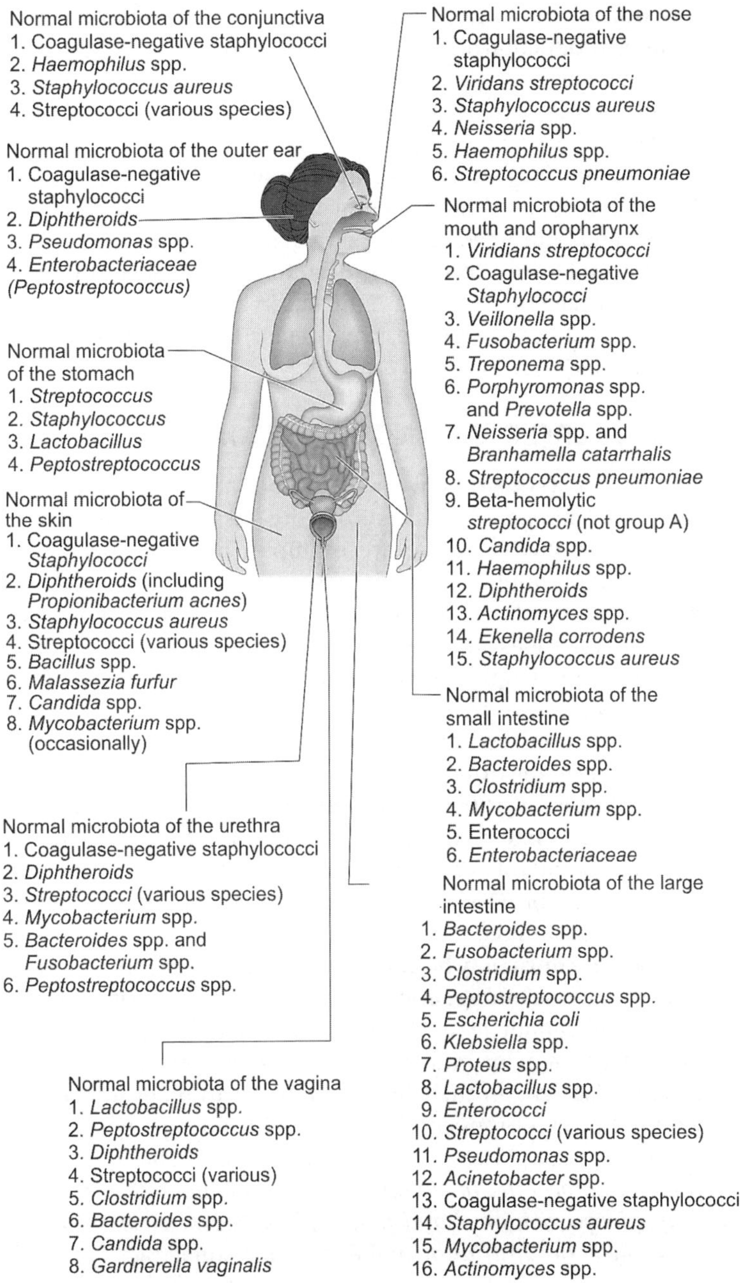

Figure 2.7.1: Normal flora of human body.

- **The normal flora may antagonize (act against) other bacteria** through production of substances which inhibit or kill pathogenic bacteria. For example, the intestinal bacteria produce a variety of substances such as bacteriocins, which inhibit or kill other bacteria.
- **The normal flora stimulates development of certain tissues.** For example, the caecum of germ-free animals is enlarged, thin-walled and fluid-filled compared to that in other animals.
- **The normal flora stimulates production of natural antibodies.** Since normal flora behave as antigens in an animal, they induce an immunological response, in particular, an antibody-mediated immune (AMI) response.

HARMFUL EFFECTS OF NORMAL FLORA

- **Bacterial synergism** between a member of normal flora and a potential pathogen. This means one organism is helping another to grow or survive. There are examples of a member of the normal flora supplying vitamin or some other growth factor that a pathogen needs in order to grow. This is called **cross-feeding** between microbes. Another example of synergism occurs during treatment of **"staph-protected infections"** when a penicillin-resistant *Staphylococcus* that is a component of the normal flora shares its drug resistance with pathogens that are otherwise susceptible to the drug.
- **Competition for nutrients** Bacteria in the gastrointestinal tract must absorb some of the host's nutrients for their own needs.
- Minute amounts of bacterial toxins (e.g. endotoxin) may be found in the circulation. Of course, it is these small amounts of bacterial antigen that stimulate the formation of natural antibodies.
- **The normal flora may be agents of disease.** Members of normal flora may cause **endogenous disease** if they reach a site or tissue where they cannot be restricted or tolerated by the host defenses.
- Some pathogens of humans that are members of normal flora may also rely on their host for transfer to other individuals where they can produce disease. This includes pathogens that colonize the upper respiratory tract such as *Neisseria meningitidis, Streptococcus pneumoniae, Haemophilus influenzae and Staphylococcus aureus and potential pathogens such as E. coli, Salmonella or Clostridium* in the gastrointestinal tract.

POSSIBLE QUESTIONS

1. Write an essay on the normal flora of human body.
2. Explain about normal flora of human body. What are its benefits and harmful effects?

MULTIPLE CHOICE QUESTIONS

1. A human body consists __________ numbers of cell.
   a. 10^{13} b. 10^{12}
   c. 10^{16} d. 10^{14}
2. Which of the following is not a function of Normal Flora?
   a. Synthesizes and excrete vitamins
   b. Prevent spreading of pathogens
   c. Stimulates production of natural antibiotics
   d. Prevent development of certain tissue
3. A phenomenon in which aerobic and anaerobic bacteria help each other's growth is called as __________.
   a. Bacterial synergism b. Bacterial transportation
   c. Bacterial communication d. None of the above
4. Enteric bacteria secretes which vitamins?
   a. Vit-K b. Vit-B_{12}
   c. Vit-C d. Both a and b
5. Lactic acid bacteria produces __________ vitamins.
   a. Vit-B b. Vit-D
   c. Vit-K d. Vit-E
6. Human body contains how many numbers of bacteria?
   a. 10^{12} b. 10^{13}
   c. 10^{14} d. 10^{15}
7. Bacteriocins are produced by __________.
   a. Intestinal bacteria b. Conjunctiva bacteria
   c. Oropharynx bacteria d. Both b and c

Answers

1. a 2. d 3. a 4. d 5. a
6. c 7. a

Pathogenic Microorganisms

INTRODUCTION

- Microorganisms can be found at every place and in close association with every type of multicellular organism. They grow on healthy human body by billions as harmless normal flora. All microoraganisms do not cause disease. Those relatively few species of microorganisms that are harmful to humans by causing diseases are called as pathogens.
- Most infectious disease started by colonization (the establishment of multiplying microorganisms on the skin or mucous membranes). Microbial colonization may result in: Elimination (or removal) of microorganism without affecting the host
- Infection in which the organisms multiply and cause the host to react
- A short period or prolonged carrier state.

Infectious disease occurs when an organism causes tissue damage and affecting body function.

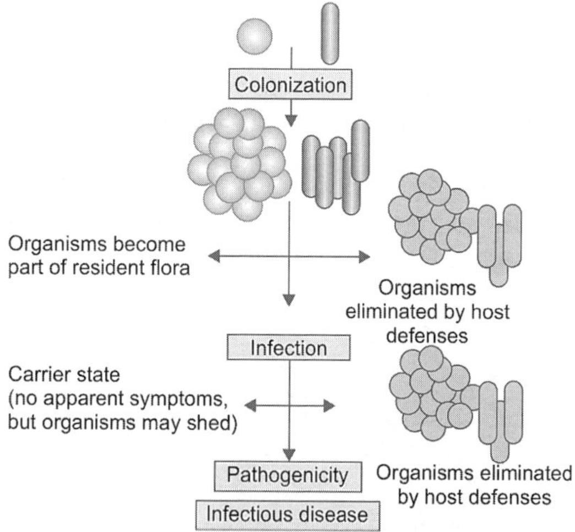

Figure 2.8.1: Some possible outcomes following exposure of microorganisms.

PATHOGENIC AND NON-PATHOGENIC MICROORGANISMS

Any organism or agent that produces a disease is called as a pathogen (Greek *patho,* disease, and *gennan,* to produce). Its ability to cause disease is called pathogenicity. Microorganisms which do not cause any disease are called as non-pathogenic microorganisms. Followings are types of pathogen:

- **Primary pathogen** is any organism that causes disease in a healthy host by direct interaction.
- **Opportunistic pathogen** is an organism that is either normally free-living or a part of the host's normal flora but which may adopt a pathogenic role under certain circumstances such as when the immune system is weak.
- Host is a living organism on which the pathogen grow and cause disease. Followings are the types of hosts:
  - **Final host:** The host on or in which the parasitic organism either attains sexual maturity or reproduces.
  - **Intermediate host:** A host that serves as a temporary but essential environment for some stages of development.
  - **Transfer host:** This is not necessary for completion of the organism's life cycle but is used as a vehicle for reaching a final host.
  - **Reservoir host:** A host infected with a parasitic organism that also can infect humans.

Table 2.8.1: Categorization of parasitic organisms and agents by size.

Discipline		Parasitic group		Approximate size
Virology		Prions		350 k Da
		Viroids	} 25–400 nm	130 k Da
		Viruses		
Bacteriology		Chlamydia		0.2–1.5 mm
		Mycoplasmas		0.3–0.8 mm
		Rickettsias		0.5–2 mm
		Other bacteria		

Contd...

Contd...

Discipline		Parasitic group		Approximate size
			Micro-organisms (Microbiota)	
Mycology		Fungi		3-15 mm diameter (hyphae)
Protozoology		Protozoa		1-150 mm
Helminthology	} Parasitology	Nematodes Platyhelminthes (cestodes, trematodes)	} Parasites	3 mm – 30 cm 1 mm – 10 m
Entomology		Ticks and miles		15 mm
Zoology		Horsehair worms Mesozoa Leeches	} Ectoparasites	10-20 cm Up to 100 cm 1-5 cm

HOST-PARASITE RELATIONSHIP

- If an organism either harms or lives at the expense of another organism (the host) then the former an organism is called as a parasitic organism and the relationship is called parasitism. The parasitic organism is usually smaller and is dependent on the host. There are many parasitic agents or organisms among the viruses, bacteria, fungi, plants and animals.
- There are two types of parasites which are:
  1. Ectoparasite: If an organism lives on the surface of its host.
  2. Endoparasite: If it lives internally inside the body of the host.

When a parasite is growing and multiplying within or on a host, the host is said to have an infection. An infection may or may not result in disease. An infectious disease is any change from a state of health in which part or all of the host body is not capable of carrying on its normal functions due to the presence of an organism or its products.

- The term virulence refers to the degree or intensity of pathogenicity of pathogen. It is determined by three characteristics of the pathogen:
  - Invasiveness: The ability of an organism to spread to adjacent or other tissues.
  - Infectivity: The ability of an organism to establish a point of infection.
  - Pathogenic potential: This refers to the degree that the pathogen causes damage. A major aspect of pathogenic potential is toxigenicity.
- Toxigenicity is pathogen's ability to produce toxins. Toxins are chemical substances that will damage the host and produce disease.

The outcome of most host-parasite relationships is dependent on three main factors:

1. The number of organisms present in or on the host
2. The virulence of an organism
3. The host's defenses or degree of resistance.

Table 2.8.2: Terms used to describe infection.

Type	Definition
Abscess	A localize infection with collection of pus surrounded by an inflamed area
Acute	Short but severe course
Bacteremia	Presence of viable bacteria in the blood
Chronic	Persists over a long time
Covert	Subclinical, no symptoms
Cross	Transmitted between hots infected with different organisms
Focal	Exists in circumscribed areas
Fulminating	Infectious agent multiplies with great intensity
Latrogenic	Caused as a result of health care
Latent	Persists in tissues for long periods, during most of which there are no symptoms
Localized	Restricted to a limited region or to none or more anatomical areas
Mixed	More than one organism present simultaneously

Contd...

Contd...

Type	Definition
Nosocomial	Develops during a stay at a hospital or other clinical care facility
Oppo-rtunistic	Due to an agent that does not harm a healthy host but takes advantage of an unhealthy one
Overt	Symptomatic
Phytogenic	Caused by plant pathogens
Primary	First infection that often allows other organisms to appear on the scene
Pyogenic	Result in pus formation
Secondary	Caused by an organism following an initial or primary infection
Sepsis	The condition resulting from the presence of bacteria or their toxins in blood or tissues; the presence of pathogens or their toxins in the blood or other tissues
	Systemic response to infection; this systemic response is manifested by two or more of the following conditions as a result of infection: temperature, >38°C or <36°C; heart rate, >90 beats per min; respiratory rate, >20 breaths per min, or pCO_2, <32 mm Hg; leukocyte count, > 12000 cells per mL^3. Or >10% immature (band) forms
Septicemia	Blood poisoning associated with persistence of pathogenic organisms or their toxins in the blood
Septic shock	Sepsis with hypotension despite adequate fluid resuscitation, along with the presence of perfusion abnormalities that may include but are not limited to, lactic acidosis, oliguria, or an acute alteration in mental status
Severe sepsis	Sepsis is associated with organ dysfunction, hypoperfusion, or hypotension; hypoperfusion and perfusion abnormalities that may include; but are not limited to, lactic acidosis, oliguria, or an acute alteration in mental status
Sporadic	Occurs occasionally
Subclinical (inapparent or convert)	No detectable symptoms or manifestations
Toxemia	Condition arising from toxins in the blood
Zoonosis	Caused by a parasitic organism that is normally found in animals orther than humans

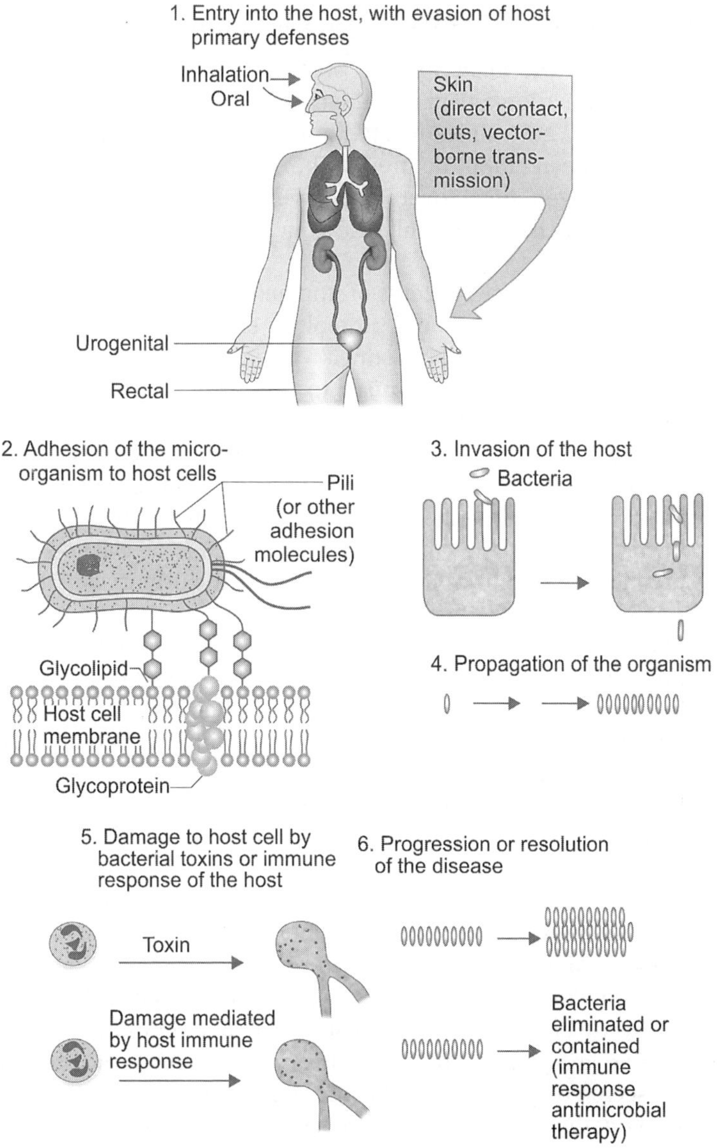

1. Entry into the host, with evasion of host primary defenses

Inhalation
Oral
Skin (direct contact, cuts, vector-borne transmission)
Urogenital
Rectal

2. Adhesion of the micro-organism to host cells

Pili (or other adhesion molecules)
Glycolipid
Host cell membrane
Glycoprotein

3. Invasion of the host

Bacteria

4. Propagation of the organism

5. Damage to host cell by bacterial toxins or immune response of the host

Toxin
Damage mediated by host immune response

6. Progression or resolution of the disease

Bacteria eliminated or contained (immune response antimicrobial therapy)

Figure 2.8.2: Mechanism of infectious process.

MECHANISM OF INFECTIOUS PROCESS

- **Entry into the host:** The first step of infectious process is the entry of microorganism into the host by one of several ports: via respiratory, gastrointestinal (GI), urogenital tract or through skin that has been cut, punctured, or burnt. Once entry is achieved, the pathogen must overcome diverse host immune system before it can establish itself. These include:
  - Phagocytosis
  - The acidic environments of stomach and urogenital tract
  - Various hydrolytic and proteolytic enzymes found in saliva, stomach and small intestine.
- **Adherence of microorganism to host cells:** Various bacteria follow different mechanisms to adhere (attach) to the surface of host cells. For example, *Escherichia coli* use pili whereas Group A *Streptococci* uses its fimbriae to adhere to the surface of the host cells. In each case, adherence enhances virulence by preventing bacteria from being carried away by mucous or washed from organs with significant fluid flow, such as the urinary and the GI tracts.
- **Invasion of the host:** Invasive bacteria are those that can enter host cells or penetrate mucsal surfaces, spreading from the initial site of infection. Invasiveness is facilitated by several bacterial enzymes, the most notable of which are collagenase and hyaluronidase.
- **Propagation of the microorganism:** Once the pathogen has entered the host it will start to propagate (or multiply) very fast in order to increase its number.
- **Damage to host cell:** While propagating itself in the host cell, microorganisms can damage the host cell by producing toxins. They are of two types:
  - *Exotoxins:* These are toxins which are produced and released by the pathogenic bacteria at the site of their multiplication. For example, diphtheria toxin. Exotoxins are proteins secreted by both Gram-positive and Gram-negative bacteria.
  - *Endotoxins:* These are not released out but instead is part of the cell walls of Gram-negative bacteria. For example, LPS, layer of Gram-negative bacteria.

Table 2.8.3: Characteristics of bacterial endotoxins and classic exotoxin.

Property	Endotoxin	Exotoxin
Chemical nature	Lipopolysaccharide (mw = 10 kDa)	Protein (mw = 50–1000 kDa)
Relationship to cell	Part of outer membrane	Extracellular, diffusible
Denatured by boiling	No	Usually
Antigenic	Yes	Yes
Form toxoid	No	Yes
Potency	Relatively low (>100 μg)	Relatively high (1 μg)
Specificity	Low degree	High degree
Enzymatic activity	No	Often
Pyrogenicity	Yes	Occasionally

Damage of the host cell is also possible due to host immune response.

- **Progression or resolution of disease:** If the pathogen is not removed by immune system then the disease is established. If the pathogen fails to multiply then there is no disease.

POSSIBLE QUESTIONS

1. What are pathogenic microorganisms? How are they different from non-pathogenic microorganisms?
2. Write an essay on host-parasite relationship.
3. What is infection? Give a detailed account of the mechanism of infectious process.
4. Write Short Notes:
   a. Pathogen
   b. Parasite
   c. Pathogenicity
   d. Virulence
   e. Host
   f. Infection
   g. Invasiveness
   h. Endotoxins and Exotoxins
   i. Infectivity

MULTIPLE CHOICE QUESTIONS

1. Microorganisms that causes harmful disease to human beings are called as ______
   a. Pathogens b. Phagocytes
   c. Bacteriophage d. All of the above
2. What is parasitism?
   a. Relationship between two parasites for beneficial expense of the other
   b. One parasite kills other parasite
   c. Parasite that grow on host
   d. Parasite that kills host
3. If an organism lives on the surface of its host is called as ______
   a. Endoparasite b. Ectoparasite
   c. Phagosomes d. None of these
4. The degree of damage caused by the pathogens are called as______
   a. Infectivity b. Pathogenic potential
   c. Toxigenicity d. Invasiveness
5. The word Overt refers to ______
   a. Subclinical b. No symptoms
   c. Symptomatic d. Short but severe
6. The condition resulting from the presence of bacteria is known as ______
   a. Chronic b. Acute
   c. Sepsis d. Mixed
7. Zoonosis refers to ______
   a. No detectible symptoms
   b. Occurs occasionally
   c. Caused by parasite that present in animal
   d. Restricted to limited region
8. The chemical nature of Endotoxin is ______
   a. Protein b. Lipoprotein
   c. Lipopolysaccharide d. Water
9. Diphtheria toxins are ______
   a. Exotoxin b. Endotoxin
   c. No toxin is found d. Both a and c
10. Streptococci uses ______ for its adhere to the surface of the host cell.
    a. Pili b. Fimbriae
    c. Flagella d. Plasmids

Answers

1. a	2. a	3. b	4. b	5. c
6. c	7. c	8. c	9. a	10. b

Diseases Caused by Microorganisms

INTRODUCTION

A few harmful microbes, for example, less than 1% of bacteria, can invade our body (the host) and make us ill. They are called as pathogenic microorganisms.

Pathogens establish infection and damage tissues by any of three mechanisms:

1. They can contact or enter host cells and directly cause of death cells.
2. They may release toxins that kill cells at a distance, release enzymes that degrade tissue components or damage blood vessels.
3. They can induce host immune responses that although directed against the invader (pathogen), cause additional tissue damage.

COMMON DISEASES CAUSED BY BACTERIA

Millions of bacteria normally live on the skin, in the intestines and on genitalia. The vast majority of bacteria do not cause disease. Many bacteria are actually helpful and even necessary for good health.

These bacteria are sometimes referred to as "good bacteria" or "healthy bacteria."

Harmful bacteria that cause bacterial infections and diseases are called pathogenic bacteria. Bacterial diseases occur when pathogenic bacteria get into the body, begin to reproduce and crowd out healthy bacteria, or to grow in tissues that are normally sterile. Harmful bacteria may also emit toxins that damage the body. Common pathogenic bacteria and the types of bacterial diseases they cause include:

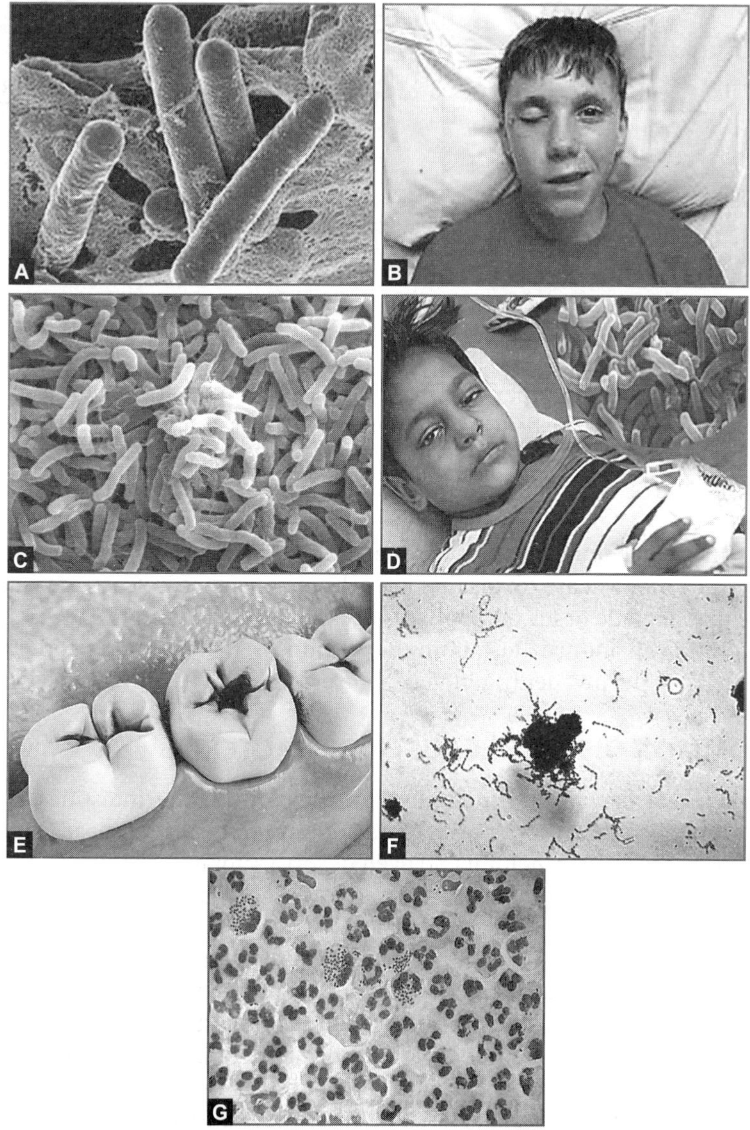

Figures 2.9.1A to G *(For color version see Plate 2)*

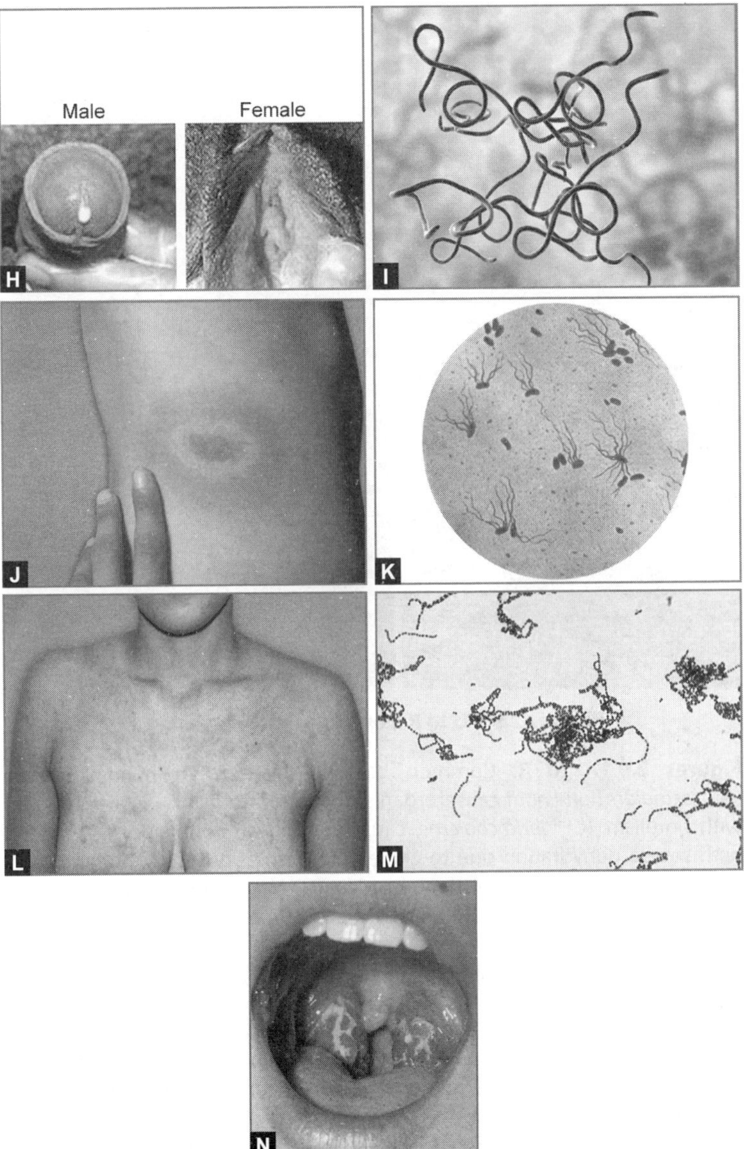

Figures 2.9.1H to N *(For color version see Plate 3)*

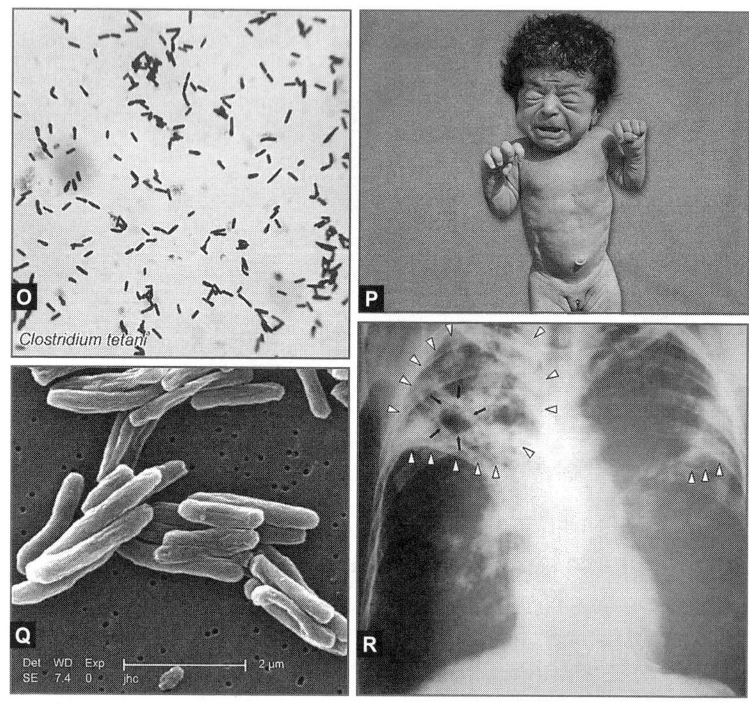

Figures 2.9.1 O to R *(For color version see Plate 4)*

Figures 2.9.1A to R: Common bacterial diseases of human beings. (A) *Clostridium botulinum*, causal organism of botulism; (B) A 14-year-old patient with botulism; (C) *Vibrio cholerae,* causal organism of cholera; (D) A person with severe dehydration due to cholera; (E) Dental caries; (F) *Streptococcus mutans*, causal organism of dental caries; (G) *Neisseria gonorrhoeae*, causal organism of gonorrhoeae; (H) Gonorrhoeae in male and female; (I) *Borrelia burgdorferi*, causal organism of lyme disease; (J) Classic bull's-eye appearance is also called erythema migrans; (K) *Salmonella typhi*, causal organism of typhoid; (L) Rose spots on the chest of a patient with typhoid fever due to the bacterium *Salmonella*; (M) *Streptococcus pyogenes,* causal organism of streptococcal pharyngitis; (N) Streptococcal pharyngitis; (O) *Clostridium tetani*, causal organism of tetanus; (P) A child suffering from tetanus; (Q) *Mycobacterium tuberculosis*, causal organism of tuberculosis; (R) Chest X-ray of a person with advanced tuberculosis: Infection in both lungs is marked by white arrow-heads and the formation of a cavity is marked by black arrows.

Table 2.9.1: Common bacterial diseases.

Diseases	Pathogenic agent	Transmission	Symptoms	Target body part	Treatment and prevention
Botulism	*Clostridium botulinum*	Improperly preserved foods	Difficulty swallowing/speaking dry mouth Facial weakness Burred vision Trouble breathing Nausea, abdominal cramps	Nerves	The Patient is kept on a ventilator for weeks/ months. Patient is treated with Antitoxin
Cholera	*Vibrio cholerae*	Contaminated water and food	Diarrhea, vomiting, dehydration (loss of water), headache, stomach ache	Intestine	Antibiotics, Vaccination, Replace fluids intravenously, drinking boiled water
Dental Caries	*Streptococcus mutants*	Enter the mouth from environment	Presence of a small pit, or hole, in the tooth, Sensitivity to hot and cold food and beverages, Bad breath (halitosis), Bitter taste in the mouth, Swelling of the gums, Facial swelling with enlarged glands in the neck	Teeth	Amalgam filling, Prevented by Brushing, flossing and reducing the intake of refined and processed sugars
Gonorrhea	*Neisseria gonorrhoeae*	By sexual contact	In Women-Greenish yellow or whitish discharge from the vagina, Lower abdominal or pelvic pain, Burning when urinating, Conjunctivitis (red, itchy eyes),	Female reproductive system—vagina, fallopian tubes, uterus, etc.	Effective antibiotic treatment is given prevention—practice safer sex or no sex

Contd...

Contd...

Diseases	Pathogenic agent	Transmission	Symptoms	Target body part	Treatment and prevention
			Bleeding between periods, Spotting after intercourse, Swelling of the vulva (vulvitis), Burning in the throat (due to oral sex), Swollen glands in the throat (due to oral sex) In Man-Greenish yellow or whitish discharge from the penis, Burning when urinating, Painful or swollen testicles,	Male reproductive and encretory organs—penis, urethra, urinary canal	untill antibiotic treatment is completed follow up test must be done to ensure clearance of infection
Lyme Disease	*Borrelia burgdorferi*	Tick bite	Fever, headache and fatigue. A rash occurs in 70– 80% of infected persons at the site of the tick bite after a delay of 3–30 days (average is about 7 days), and may or may not appear as the well-publicized bull's-eye	Skin, joints, heart	Oral administration of doxycycline. Protective clothing. Light-colored clothing makes the tick more easily visible before it attaches itself. People should use special care in handling and allowing outdoor pets inside homes because they can bring ticks into the house

Contd...

Contd...

Diseases	Pathogenic agent	Transmission	Symptoms	Target body part	Treatment and prevention
Salmonella Food Poisoning (Typhoid)	*Salmonella typhi*	Contaminated water and food	Rash, headache, fever, coughing, body ache, weakness	Intestine	Vaccination, Antibiotics, Drinking boiled water
Throat infection	*Streptococcus pyogenes*	Sneezing, coughs or direct person-to-person contact	Sore throat, fever of greater than 38°C (100 °F), tonsillar exudates (pus on the tonsils), and large cervical lymph nodes	Upper respiratory tract, blood, skin	Analgesics such as non-steroidal anti-inflammatory drugs (NSAIDs) and paracetamol (acetaminophen) help significantly in the management of pain associated with strep throat. To avoid getting strep throat, it is a good idea to avoid contact with anyone who has a strep infection. Wash hands when you meet someone with bacterial or viral illnesses. Do not share toothbrushes or eating and drinking utensils.

Contd...

Contd...

Diseases	Pathogenic agent	Transmission	Symptoms	Target body part	Treatment and prevention
Tetanus	*Clostridium tetani*	Contaminated wounds	Headache, Jaw cramping, Sudden, involuntary muscle tightening—often in the stomach (muscle spasms), Painful muscle stiffness all over the body, Trouble swallowing, Jerking or staring (seizures), Fever and sweating, High blood pressure and fast heart rate.	Nerves at synapses	Can be treated with; • Tetanus immunoglobulin, also called tetanus antibodies or tetanus antitoxin • Metronidazole IV for 10 days • Diazepam There are three different types of tetanus vaccines. Diphtheria, tetanus, and pertussis (DTaP), Tdap (tetanus, diphtheria, and pertussis), Td (tetanus and diphtheria) vaccine.

COMMON DISEASES CAUSED BY VIRUSES

Viral diseases are extremely widespread infections caused by viruses, a type of microorganism. There are many types of viruses that cause a wide variety of viral diseases. The most common type of viral disease is the common cold, which is caused by a viral infection of the upper respiratory tract (nose and throat). Other common viral diseases include:

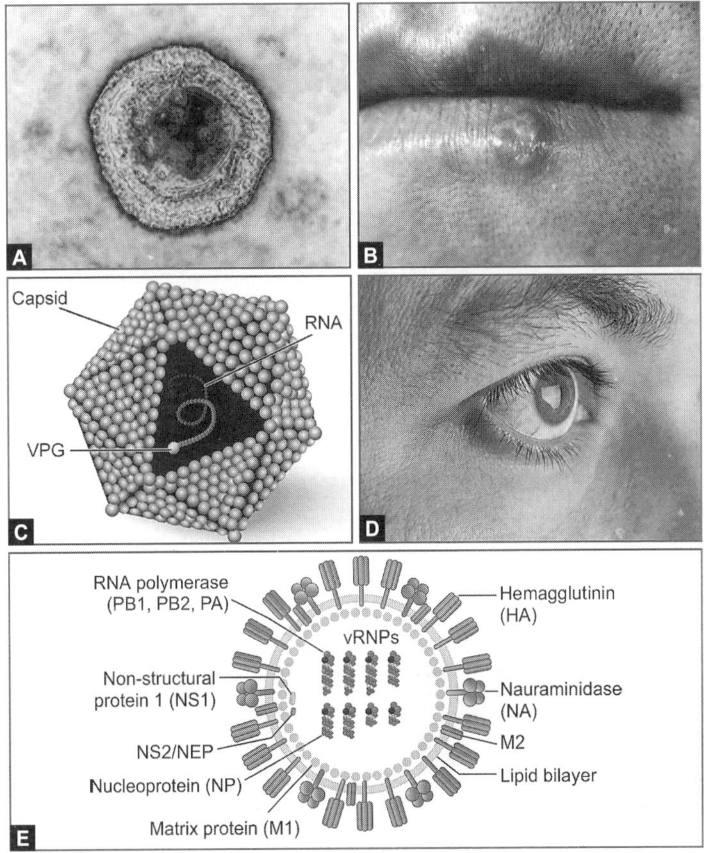

Figures 2.9.2A to E *(For color version see Plate 5)*

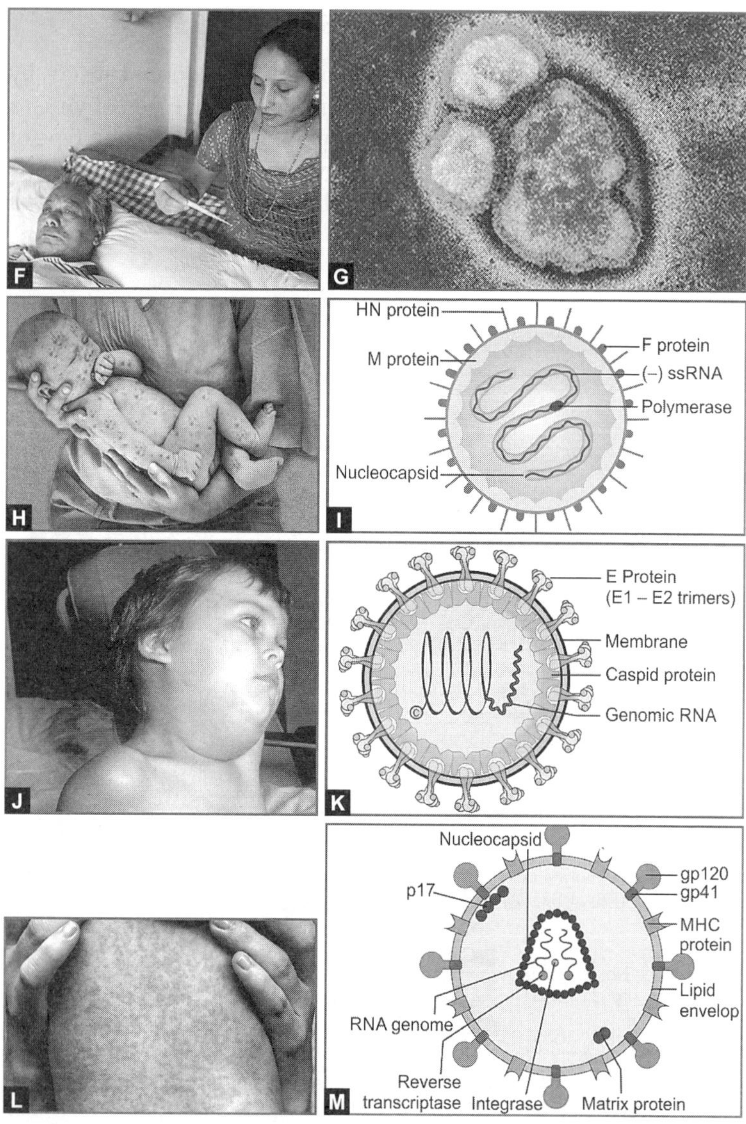

Figures 2.9.2F to M *(For color version see Plate 6)*

COMMON DISEASES CAUSED BY FUNGI

Clinical Categories of Fungal Infections

- **Superficial/Cutaneous:** Infection of outer layer of skin by lipophilic or keratinolytic fungi, e.g., pityriasis, dermatophytosis

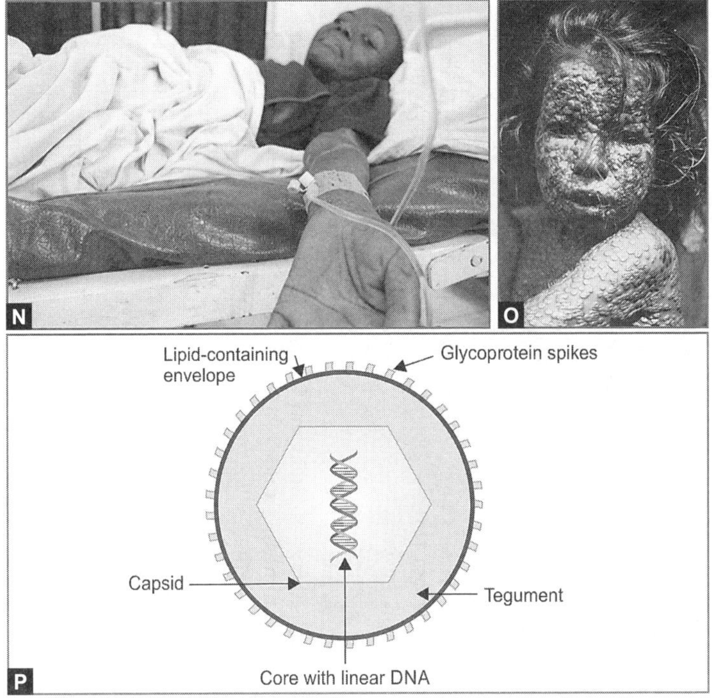

Figures 2.9.2N to P *(For color version see Plates 7).*

Figures 2.9.2A to P: Common viral diseases in human beings. (A) Herpes virus; (B) Herpes labialis (blister) of the lower lip in a herpes patient; (C) Hepatitis A virus; (D) A case of jaundice caused by hepatitis A; (E) Influenza viru; (F) A patient suffering from Influenza; (G) Measles virus; (H) A patient suffering from measles; (I) Mumps virus; (J) A patient suffering from mumps; (K) Rubella virus; (L) A patient suffering from Rubella (German fever); (M) Human immunodef iciency virus (HIV); (N) A patient suffering from acquired immunodeficiency syndrome (AIDS); (O) *Varicella zoster* virus; (P) A child suffering from smallpox.

- **Subcutaneous:** Infection of subcutaneous tissues from the painful implantation of the fungus into the skin, e.g., sporotrichosis
- **Systemic:**
  - **The true pathogenic fungi**—can cause disease even in immunocompetent hosts: histoplasmosis, coccidioidomycosis, blastomycosis
  - **The opportunistic fungi**—generally cause disease only in immunocompromised hosts: cryptococcosis, candidiasis, aspergillosis, mucormycosis

Table 2.9.2: Common viral diseases.

Diseases	Pathogenic agent	Transmission	Symptoms	Target body part	Treatment and prevention
Tuber-culosis	*Mycob-acterium tuberculosis*	Person-to-person by coughs	A bad cough that lasts 3 weeks or longer, Pain in the chest, Coughing up blood or sputum (phlegm from deep inside the lungs), Weakness or fatigue,Weight loss, No appetite, Chills, Fever.	Lung, bones, other organs	Antibiotics used in the treatment of tuber-culosis are !soniazid, Rifampin (Rifadin, Rimactane), Ethambutol (Myambutol) and Pyrazina-mide. Children are vaccinated with Bacille Calmette-Guerin (BCG) vaccine. For adults there is no vaccine.
Bacterial meningitis (Infection of sac around brain and spinal chord)	*Streptococcus pneumonia, Neisseria meningitides, Haemophilus influenzae* type b	Person-to-person through tiny drop-lets that are sent into the air during talking, laughing, coughing and sneezing. It can also spread by kiss-ing, sharing eating utensils, and hand-to-hand contact	Headache, sensitivity to light, neck stiffness, fever, loss of appetite, rashes, seizure, irritability in children and difficulty thinking clearly	Brain and Spinal Chord	Vaccination, Antibiotics such as ceftriaxone and vancomycin, Corticosteroids, drinking plenty of boiled water along with ample rest is advised. Prevention include—washing hands after contacting with patients

Contd...

Contd...

Diseases	Pathogenic agent	Transmission	Symptoms	Target body part	Treatment and prevention
Herpes Simplex	Herpes virus hominis	Infections through droplets or infectious smears. Human may be carrier without symptoms	Fever blisters, severe weakness	Microscopically by demonstration of intran-uclear inclusion bodies in cells from lesions	Aciclovir
Hepatitis A	Hepatitis A Virus (HAV), Hepatitis epidemica	Oral infection by feces, dirty hands or objects. Often transmitted by water, Active and passive vaccination in humans	Jaundice, fever, diarrhea, rejection of food, seizures, itching, weakness, green-brown urine, often fatal	Detection of HAV in feces; antibodies in serum	There is no specific treatment for hepatitis A. Sufferers are advised to rest, avoid fatty foods and alcohol (these may be poorly tolerated for some additional months during the recovery phase and cause minor relapses), eat a well-balanced diet, and stay hydrated
Influenza (Flu)	Influenza virus of humans; Coryza-Rhino viruses	Infection by humans (aerosol infection by sneezing) and in experiments	Sneezing, coughing, rhinitis, fever, headache, may affect respiratory organs	Viruses in respiratory tract	In case of secondary infections (pneumonia)

Contd...

Contd...

Diseases	Pathogenic agent	Transmission	Symptoms	Target body part	Treatment and prevention
Rabies	Rabies virus	Infection by bites, saliva of infected animals (carnivores, domestic animals) or by improper vaccination	Overexcitability, self-multilation, inability to drink water, paralysis	Viruses in saliva, tears	Vaccination
Measles	Measles virus	It is spread when an infected person coughs, sneezes, or shares food or drinks. The measles virus can travel through the air.	Runny nose, high temperature, sore, red eyes, white spots inside mouth, red blotchy rash—it actually starts on the head and neck and spreads down the body, fever	Detected by viral culture or blood test	The measles vaccine protects against the illness. This vaccine is part of the MMR (measles, mumps, and rubella)
Mumps	Mumps virus	Mumps is highly contagious. The virus is spread directly from one person to another via respiratory droplets, can also be transmitted via hand-to-mouth contact after touching infected pillows or bedsheets	Swollen and painful salivary glands, flu like symptoms, such as aches, pains and tiredness. Abdominal pain and headaches	Detected by clinical examination of parotid gland enlargement	The mumps vaccine protects against the illness. This vaccine is part of the MMR (measles, mumps, and rubella). Taking analgesics (acetaminophen, ibuprofen) and applying warm or cold packs to the swollen and inflamed salivary gland region may be helpful

Contd...

Contd...

Diseases	Pathogenic agent	Transmission	Symptoms	Target body part	Treatment and prevention
Rubella (German Measles)	Rubella virus	It can spread when an infected person coughs or sneezes, or it can spread by direct contact with an infected person's respiratory secretions, such as mucus. It can also be transmitted from a pregnant woman to her unborn child via the bloodstream	Rash that starts on face and spreads to the rest of the body, swollen glands behind ears and possibly in other parts of the body, mild fever, cold, cough, sore throat and red eye	Viral rashes are observed. Virus culture or a blood test can detect the presence of different types of rubella antibodies in your blood. These antibodies indicate whether the patient had a recent or past infection or a rubella vaccine	No treatment will shorten the course of rubella infection, and symptoms are so mild that treatment usually isn't necessary. The rubella vaccine protects against the illness. This vaccine is part of the MMR (measles, mumps, and rubella)
AIDS	Human Immuno-deficiency Virus (HIV)	From infected person via blood transfusion, semen (unprotected sex), use of infected needles, newborn may acquire HIV from infected mother also	Infected individuals have a flu-like illness within month or two after exposure to the virus, with fever, headache, tiredness, and enlarged lymph nodes (glands of the immune system).	By testing blood for the presence of antibodies (disease-fighting proteins) to HIV	Since there is no accurate medication for HIV combined antiviral drugs are given to the patients.

Contd...

Contd...

Diseases	Pathogenic agent	Transmission	Symptoms	Target body part	Treatment and prevention
			These symptoms usually disappear within a week to a month and are often mistaken for those of other viral infections. During this period, people are very infectious, and HIV is present in large quantities in blood, semen, and vaginal fluids. More severe HIV symptoms—such as profound and unexplained fatigue, rapid weight loss, frequent fevers, or profuse night sweats—may not appear for 10 years or more after HIV first enters the body in adults, or within two years in children born with HIV infection		Prevention: Because there is no cure or vaccine to prevent HIV, the only way people can prevent infection from the virus is to avoid high-risk behaviors putting them at risk of infection, such as having unprotected sex or sharing needles

Contd...

Contd...

Diseases	Pathogenic agent	Transmission	Symptoms	Target body part	Treatment and prevention
Viral Gastro-enteritis (Stomach Flu)	Rotavirus, Novovirus	Highly contagious, spreads through close contact with people who are infected, or through contaminated food or water	Nausea, vomiting, loss of appetite, and watery diarrhea, fever and body aches, chills, sweating, abdominal cramps and pain, etc.	A stool sample is tested for the type of virus or the doctor finds out illness is due to a parasitic or bacterial infection, if not then its viral.	The main focus of treatment is to prevent dehydration by drinking plenty of fluids and electrolytes. Proper rest and food should be taken in small amounts. In severe cases, hospitalization and intravenous fluids are necessary
Chicken Pox	*Varicella-Zoster Virus*	Virus can spread easily from one person to another. It most often spreads through the respiratory tract, such as mucus membranes of the mouth and nose. One can get chickenpox through the air from an infected person's sneezing or coughing	Fever, tired and sluggish, no appetite, headache, sore throat, itchy rash and red spots or blisters all over the body	Diagnosis is usually done based on the rash looks	Prevention: Chickenpox Vaccination

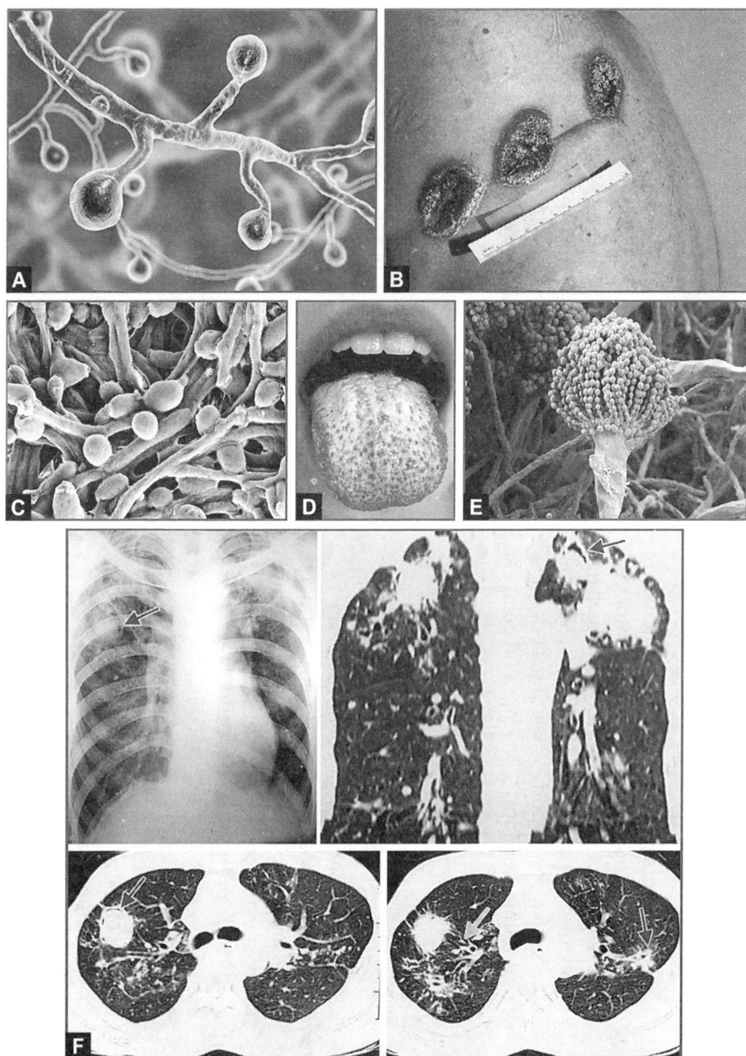

Figures 2.9.3A to F *(For color version see Plates 8)*

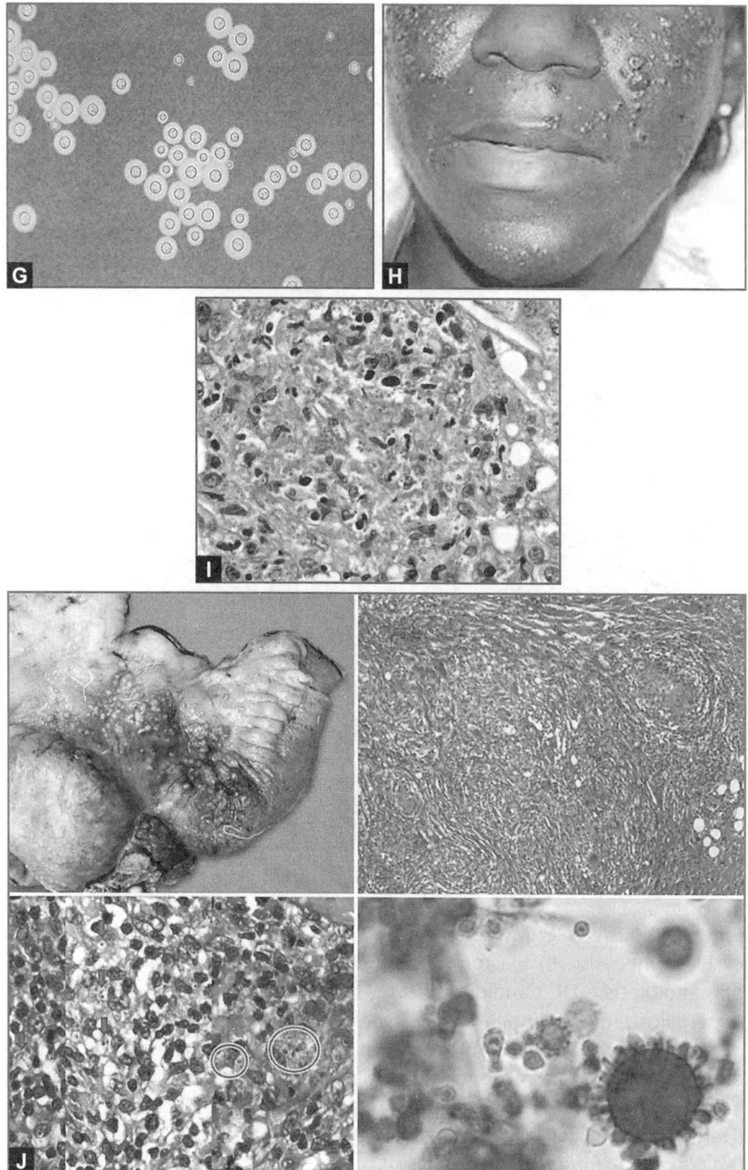

Figures 2.9.3G to J *(For color version see Plates 9)*

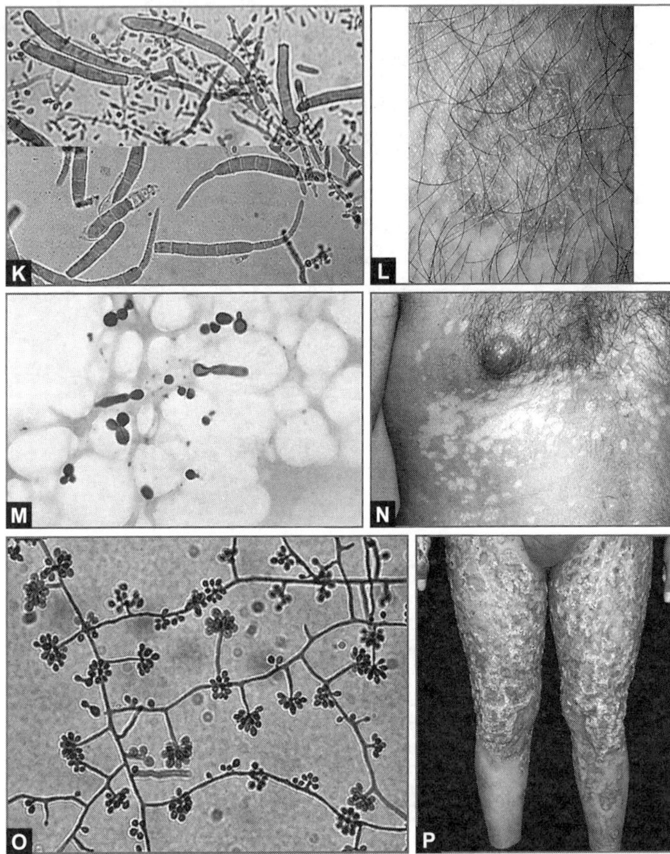

Figures 2.9.3K to P *(For color version see Plates 10)*

Figures 2.9.3A to P: Mycosis: (A) *Blastomyces dermatitidis*, causal organism of Blastomycosis; (B) Blastomycosis; (C) *Candida albicans*, causal organism of candidiasis; (D) Candidiasis; (E) *Aspergillus* spp., causal organism of Aspergillosis; (F) Aspergillosis; (G) *Cryptococcus neoformans*, causal organism of Cryptococcosis; (H) Cryptococcosis; (I) *Histoplasma capsulatum*, causal organism of Histoplasmosis; (J) Colony of *Histoplasma capsulatum* inside the lungs of the patient suffering from Histoplasmosis; (K) *Tricophyton rubrum* (Dermatophyte), causal organisms of Dermatophytosis; (L) Dermatophytosis; (M) *Malassezia furfur*, causal organisms of Tinea versicolor; (N) Tinea versicolor; (O) *Sporothrix schenckii*, causal organism of Sporotrichosis; (P) Sporotrichosis.

Table 2.9.3: Common fungal infections (Mycosis).

Disease	Pathogenic organisms	Pathogenesis	Symptoms	Diagnostic tests	Treatment
Superficial fungal infections					
Dermatophytosis	Dermatophytes (Members of genera *Trichophyton, Microsporum and Epidermophyton)*	Spores on shed skin or hairs adhere to stratum corneum, germinate, invade. Organisms confined to stratum corneum, with surrounding inflammation penetrating deeper layers of skin	Can affect the skin on almost any area of the body, such as the scalp, legs, arms, feet groin, and nails. These infections are usually itchy. Redness, scaling, cracking of the skin, or a ring-shaped rash may occur. If the infection involves the scalp or beard, hair may fall out. Infected nails become discolored, thick, and may possibly crumble. More serious infections may lead to an abscess or cellulitis	Characteristic appearance, smear and culture of specimen	Azoles (for surface treatment). Griseofulvin, azoles and allylamines (for internal treatment)
Pityriasis versicolor (a lipophilic yeast)	*Malassezia furfur*	Yeasts proliferate in settings of lipids and sweat. Rare in kids, appears in adolescence	Patches that may be white, pink, red, or brown and can be lighter or darker than the skin around them. Spots that do not tan the way the rest of your skin does. Spots that may occur anywhere on your body but are most commonly seen on your neck, chest, back, and arms	Characteristic appearance; UV light fluorescence	Selenium sulfide or azoles

Contd...

Contd...

Disease	Pathogenic organisms	Pathogenesis	Symptoms	Diagnostic tests	Treatment
Subcutaneous fungal infections					
Sporo-trichosis	*Sporothrix schenckii*	Thorny plants (roses) or splinters inoculate fungus into subcutaneous tissues. Infection spreads slowly along draining lymphatics. Tissue reaction mixed pyogenic and granulomatous	Once the mold spores move into the skin, the disease takes days-to-months to develop. The first symptom is a firm bump (nodule) on the skin that can range in color from pink to nearly purple	Culture of tissue or drainage (fungi rarely seen on smear or section). Skin test determines exposure but not disease	Ketoconazole, itraconazole, Amphotericin B
Pathogenic fungal infections					
Histoplasmosis	*Histoplasma capsulatum*	Spores inhaled from soil, transform to yeast in lungs, phagocytosed by macrophages. May resolve, resolve with scarring, remain active in lungs, or, especially in settings of immunocompromise, disseminate.	Symptoms are similar to those of pneumonia and include: fever, chest pains and a dry or non-productive cough. Some people may also experience joint pain. If the disease is not treated, it can disseminate (spread) from the lungs to other organs	Skin test confirms exposure, but not infection. Antibody titers are often unreliable, especially in immunocompromise.	Amphotericin B

Contd...

Contd...

Disease	Pathogenic organisms	Pathogenesis	Symptoms	Diagnostic tests	Treatment
		Moves through reticuloendothelial organs (liver, spleen, lymph nodes)		Organisms seen intracellularly in blood/bone marrow/ liver/ urine/tissue and/or grown in culture	
Coccidio-idomycosis (Valley Fever)	*Coccidioides immitis*	Inhaled spores swell into spherules in lung, burst releasing hundreds of endospores. Hematogenous dissemination of endospores to meninges, skin, bone, liver, spleen with lesions ranging from pyogenic abscesses to granulomas	Symptoms of valley fever include: Fatigue (tiredness), Cough, Fever, Short-ness of breath, Headache, Night sweats, Muscle aches or joint pain, Rash on upper body or legs. In extremely rare cases, the fungal spores can enter the skin through a cut, wound, or splinter and cause a skin infection	Coccidioidin skin test positive 1-3 weeks after infection but not reliable: anergy common in disseminated disease.Complement fixation antibody may be + in disseminated disease, but not helpful in immunocompromised hosts. Best: smear and culture of pus, tissue	Amphotericin B; fluconazole; itraconazole

Contd...

Contd...

Disease	Pathogenic organisms	Pathogenesis	Symptoms	Diagnostic tests	Treatment
Blastomycosis	*Blastomyces dermatitidis*	Conidia inhaled, convert to yeast form in lungs. Dissemination via infected macro-phages to skin, bone, urinary tract	Similar to flu symptoms and include fever, chills, cough, muscle aches, joint pain, and chest pain. In very serious cases of blastomycosis, the fungus can disseminate (spread) to other parts of the body, such as the skin and bones	No adequate skin test, antibody or antigen assays exist. Best option is smear or culture of affected site	Amphotericin B, Ketoconazole, Itraconazole
Opportunistic fungal infections					
Cryptococcosis	*Cryptococcus neoformans*	Aerosolized yeasts inhaled. Hematogenous dissemination to central nervous system	Pulmonary disease (nodular, miliary) may occur. Mucoid, cloudy meninges in central nervous system, intra-cerebral masses of yeasts may form (cryptococcomas)	India ink prepa-ration, culture of cerebrospi-nal fluid (or other body site). Polysaccharide capsule allows for easy crypto-coccal antigen assay in serum or cerebrospinal fluid – sensitive and specific when titers are high	Amphotericin B + 5- flucytosine Fluconazole

Contd...

Contd...

Disease	Pathogenic organisms	Pathogenesis	Symptoms	Diagnostic tests	Treatment
Candidiasis	*Candida albicans*	Dissemination occurs via defect in mucosa, or formation of biofilm on catheter, other foreign body	Vaginitis, dysuria, fever, chills, renal dysfunction, endophthalmitis, skin lesions	1. Pathognomonic appearance (thrush) 2. Smear/culture of usually sterile site 3. Pathologic confirmation: organism in tissue	Nystatin, Clotrimazole, Amphotericin B, Fluconazole, Voriconazole, Caspofungin
Aspergillosis	*Aspergillus fumigatus, A. flavus*	Airborne spores are inhaled	Symptoms of allergic bronchopulmonary aspergillosis (ABPA) may include: Wheezing, Coughing, Fever (in rare cases) Symptoms of invasive aspergillosis may include: Fever, Chest pain, Coughing, Shortness of breath, Aspergilloma, or "fungus ball"	Stain and culture of tissue biopsy specimen. (Positive culture of a secretion may represent contamination)	Corticosteroids, Amphotericin B, Itraconazole, Voriconazole, Caspofungin

COMMON DISEASES CAUSED BY PROTOZOA

Protozoa are one of the three main classes of parasites that cause diseases in humans. They are single-celled organisms and can only be seen under microscope. When they invade a human they are able to multiply easily which causes them to be at a great advantage and put humans at a disadvantage. This helps them to be survive in the human body and causes serious infection even with the arrival of a single protozoon.

Infections caused by protozoa are contagious. Those protozoa that have inhabited the human intestine can be transmitted from one human to the other via the fecal-oral route, such as through sharing food the infected person has touched and through direct person-to-person contact. Protozoa living in the blood or tissue can be transmitted through a third source such as mosquito. Infections are easily transmitted and persons carrying this parasite should avoid interactions with others, especially those with compromised and weakened immune systems.

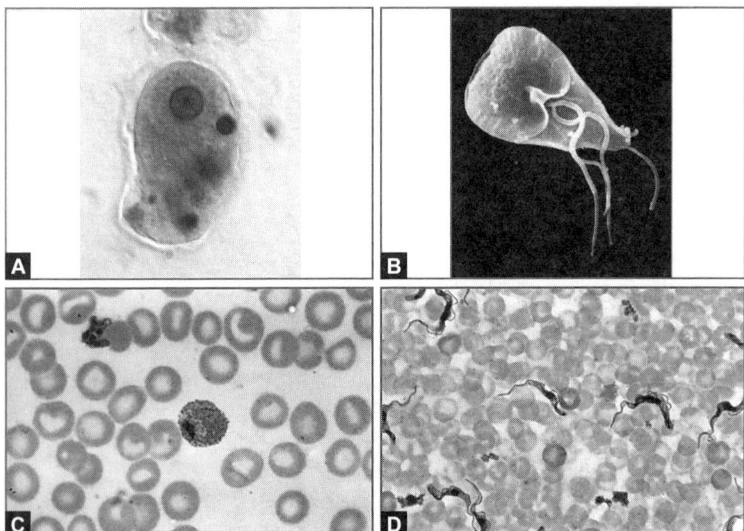

Figures 2.9.4A to D: Common protozoan parasites of human beings. (A) *Entamoeba histolytica*, causal organism of amoebiasis; (B) *Giardia lamblia*, causal organism of giardiasis; (C) *Plasmodium vivax*, causal organism of malaria; (D) *Trypanosoma brucei*, causal organism of African sleeping sickness. *(For color version see Plate 11)*

Table 2.9.4: Common protozoan diseases.

Disease	Pathogenic agent	Transmission	Symptoms	Diagnosis	Treatment
Amoebiasis	*Entamoeba histolytica*	Usually in feces, via water and contaminated salad and fruits	Dysentery, flatulence, loss of water, thirst, depression, gut ulceration, enlarged liver, if severe death can also occur within 4-weeks	Feces is microscopically examined, histology of gut content is studied	Metronidazol, Diiodo-hydroxyquin
Giardiasis	*Giardia lamblia*	Direct infection	Bloody diarrhea, vomiting	Feces examined	Metronidazol, Carnidazol
Malaria	*Plasmodium* species	It spreads when an infected Anopheles mosquito bites a person. This is the only type of mosquito that can spread malaria. The mosquito becomes infected by biting an infected person and drawing blood that contains the parasite. When that mosquito bites another person, that person becomes infected	Fever, Chills, Headache, Sweats, Fatigue, Nausea and vomiting, Back pain, Dry cough, etc.	Blood test is conducted for the presence of parasite	Common antimalarial drugs include: Chloroquine, Quinine sulfate, Hydroxy-chloroquine

Contd...

Contd...

Disease	Pathogenic agent	Transmission	Symptoms	Diagnosis	Treatment
Trypano-somiasis (African sleeping sickness)	Trypanosoma species	The disease is mostly transmitted through the bite of an infected tsetse fly, Mother-to-child infection, Mechanical transmission through other blood sucking insects is also possible	Fever, headaches, joint pains and itching, changes of behavior, confusion, sensory disturbances and poor coordination, Disturbance of the sleep cycle	Screening for potential infection: This involves using serological tests (only available for *T.b.gambiense*) and checking for clinical signs - generally swollen cervical glands	Pentamidine, Suramin, Melarsoprol, etc.

Table 2.9.5: Common diseases caused by mycoplasma.

Diseases	Causal agent	Transmission	Symptoms	Areas affected	Treatment and prevention
Mycoplasma Pneumonia	*Mycoplasma pneumonia*	*Mycoplasma* is spread through contact with droplets from the nose and throat of infected people especially when they cough and sneeze	Persistent fever, dry cough, bronchitis, sore throat, headache, tiredness. Infection may become dangerous and cause damage to heart and central nervous system	Respiratory tract and ears	Antibiotics, such as erythromycin azithromycin, tetracycline, quinolones, etc. Corticosteroids, Immunomodulatory therapy Prevention: 6-8 hours of sleep, balanced diet, washing hands before eating or after interacting with sick patients
M. haemophilis infection	*Mycoplasma haemophilis*	It is transmitted via blood sucking arthropod vectors including fleas, mosquitoes and ticks	Anemia (infection of erythrocytes), lethargy, fever and anorexia	Blood, spleen, liver, lungs, bone marrow	Antibiotics, such as Doxycyclin and Enrofloxacin are used for treatment
M. genitalium infection	*Mycoplasma genitalium*	Transmitted between partners during unprotected sexual intercourse	Urethritis (in men), discharge in both sexes, burning while urinating, arthritis, vaginal itching, pain during intercourse in women	Genitals of men and women	Antibiotics, such as Azythromycin, Erythromycin, Ofloxacin, Levofloxacin, Doxycyclin are used for treatment

COMMON DISEASES CAUSED BY CHLAMYDIA

Chlamydia is a sexually transmitted disease (STD) caused by the bacteria *Chlamydia trachomatis.* When transmitted through sexual contact, the bacteria can infect the urinary and reproductive organs. Two other types of Chlamydia species can also lead to illness:

1. *Chlamydia pneumoniae,* which can be spread through coughing and sneezing.
2. *Chlamydia psittaci,* which birds can pass to humans.

Symptoms

In many cases, Chlamydia causes only mild symptoms or no symptoms at all. So an infection can last for weeks or months before it is discovered.

Symptoms include:

- Burning feeling during urination
- Discharge from the penis or vagina
- Vaginal irritation
- Pain in the lower abdomen
- Painful sexual intercourse in women
- Pain in the testicles in men

Untreated Chlamydia in females can lead to pelvic inflammatory disease (PID), which can affect the vagina, cervix, uterus, fallopian tubes and ovaries. Sometimes, PID causes no symptoms; more often, it causes abdominal or lower back pain, painful urination, pain during intercourse, bleeding between menstrual periods, nausea, vomiting, fatigue, or fever. It can cause scarring of the fallopian tubes which can lead to serious health problems, such as chronic pelvic pain, infertility, or ectopic (tubal) pregnancy.

Untreated infections in males can lead to epididymitis, an inflammation of the coiled tubes in the back of the testicles. This can result in testicular swelling, pain and even infertility.

Transmission

Chlamydia is contagious. It can be transmitted through sexual contact via semen and vaginal secretions. Chlamydia does not spread through casual contact such as shaking hands or using the same toilet as someone who is infected.

Diagnosis

Tests can be done to find out if the bacteria that cause Chlamydia is in the body. A urine test will be taken. In case of females, the cervix can also be swabbed while the urethra, where urine flows from, may be swabbed in case of males. If there is a chance, the Chlamydia is in the rectum or throat, these areas may be swabbed as well.

Treatment

If detected early Chlamydia can easily be treated with antibiotics and the symptoms alleviated within 7 to 10 days. Azithromycin is an antibiotic usually prescribed in a single dose while doxycycline must be taken twice per day for about one week.

The sexual partners of anyone who has (or is thought to have) Chlamydia or any other STD should be examined and treated. Those diagnosed with an STD should inform their partners as soon as possible so that they too can be examined and treated to prevent complications and avoid spreading the infection.

Prevention

Because Chlamydia is spread through sexual contact, the best way to prevent it is to abstain from having sex. Sexual contact with more than one partner or with someone who has more than one partner increases the risk of contracting any STD.

In addition, when properly and consistently used, condoms decrease the risk of STDs, including Chlamydia.

COMMON DISEASES CAUSED BY RICKETTSIA

Rickettsial disease encompasses a group of diseases caused by the microorganism *Rickettsiae.*

The organisms cause disease by damaging blood vessels in various tissues and organs. In severe cases multiple tissues and organs are affected.

Table 2.9.6: Common diseases caused by *Rickettsia.*

Disease	Causative *Rickettsia*	Transmitting vector/Carrier
Rocky mountain spotted fever (RMSF)	*R. rickettsia*	Vector: Wood tick, dog tic and lone star tick Humans become incidental host after being bitten by infected adult tick

Contd...

Contd...

Disease	Causative *Rickettsia*	Transmitting vector/Carrier
Rickettsialpox	*R. akari*	Vector: House mouse is the natural host of the mouse mite transmitting rikettsialpox Distribution: Russia, South Africa, Korea
Boutonneuse fever	*R. conorii*	Vector: Various ticks including dog ticks
Louse-borne typhus	*R. prowazekii*	Vector: Lice pedicures
Brill-Zinsser disease	*R. prowazekii*	Vector: Lice Reactivation of the organism form a latent state up to decades after primary infection
Murine	*R. typhi and R. felis*	Transmitted between RATS by rat flea Humans accidentally infected by the feces of infected fleas
Tsutsugamushi disease	*O. tsutsug-amushi*	Vector: Larval trombiculid mites in soil and scrub
Q fever	*C. burnetii*	Vector: Airborne droplets from infected cattle, sheep goats, rodents and cats

Table 2.9.7: Symptoms of rickettsial diseases.

Rickettsial disease	Characteristic signs and symptoms
RMSF	• Onset gradual or abrupt, starting about 2–8 days after a tick bite • Fever, headache, confusion, aching muscles, gastrointestinal symptoms • Rash from day 2–3 consisting of small red blotches on wrist and ankles that become widespread and sometimes blister • 20% of cases do not develop rash (spotless RMSF)
Rickettsial-pox	• Irregular fluctuating fever occurs and lasts for <1 week • Headache, chills, aching muscles, runny nose, sore throat, nausea and vomiting • Red raised spot develops at the site of mites bite, later forming a dry scab (eschar) • Rash distributed on the face, neck, trunk and extremities, and is easily confused with rash of varicella (chickenpox)

Contd...

Contd...

Rickettsial disease	Characteristic signs and symptoms
Boutonneuse fever	• Fever, headache, malaise, aching muscles • Rash appears on days 35 of illness, spreading from the extremities to the trunk neck, face, palms and soles within 36 hours • Rash is spotty and blotchy and may persist for 2–3 weeks • In half the cases, a dry scab known as a tache noire (black spot) develops
Louse-borne typhus Brill-Zinsser disease	• Abrupt onset occurring 1–2 weeks after louse bite • Fever and intractable headache • On days 4–7 of illness, rash appears and soles are usually not affected • Rash initially splotchy, developing into raised red spots • Brill-Zinsser disease is usually milder
Murine	• Similar to louse-borne typhus but tends to have a milder and shorter course • Flea-bite does not have an eschar
Tsutsugamushi disease	• Generalized swelling of the lymph nodes is common • Fever and headache • Rash occur 1–3 weeks after a mite bite and is a dry scab-like lesion • Rash usually only around the trunk and has a short duration
Q-fever	• Onset is usually abrupt with fever, intractable headache, chills, muscle pain, cough and chest pain • Usually no rash appears • Pneumonitis (lung involvement) occurs in more than half of patients

Diagnosis

This is a blood test that detects the presence of antibodies to rickettsial antigens.

Treatment

- All rickettsial diseases should be treated with antibiotic therapy.
- Doxycycline is the drug of choice. Chloramphenicol may be used as an alternative.

COMMON DISEASES CAUSED BY SPIROCHETES

Table 2.9.8: Spirochetes and the human diseases they produce.

Organism	Disease
Borrelia burgdorferi	Lyme disease
Borrelia species	Relapsing fever
	Louse-borne
	Tick-borne
Treponema pallidum pallidum	Syphilis
Treponema pallidum pertenue	Yaws
Treponema pallidum endemicum	Bejel (endemic syphilis)
Treponema carateum	Pinta
Leptospirosis interrogans	Leptospira
	Anicteric
	Icteric

POSSIBLE QUESTIONS

1. Give a detail account of the diseases caused by bacteria.
2. Write an essay on common diseases caused by microorganisms.
3. What is AIDS? Give an account of its causal agent, symptoms, diagnosis, treatment and prevention.
4. Give a brief note on protozoa and discuss the diseases caused by them.
5. Discuss diseases caused by chlamydia in detail.
6. Write short notes:
   a. *Mycoplasma* and diseases caused
   b. Diseases caused by rickettsia
   c. RMSF
   d. Protozoan parasites

MULTIPLE CHOICE QUESTIONS

1. Pathogenic agent for Botulism is___________.
   a. *Borrelia burgdorferi* b. *C. botulinum*
   c. *S. mutants* d. *C. tetani*
2. Gonorrhea affects which body parts?
   a. Nerves b. Female reproductive system
   c. Intestine d. Upper respiratory tract

3. Lyme disease is caused by ____________.
   a. *Borrelia burgdorferi* b. *C. botulinum*
   c. *S. typhi* d. *N. gonorrhoeae*
4. Bacterial meningitis affects which body parts?
   a. Brain and spinal chord b. Lungs
   c. Bones d. Eyes
5. Acyclovir is an antibiotic for ____________.
   a. TB b. Hepatitis-A
   c. Rabies d. Herpes Simplex
6. The pathogenic agent of German measles is:
   a. Rubella virus b. Measles virus
   c. Mumps virus d. HIV
7. Chickenpox is caused by _________.
   a. Varicella-zoster virus b. Rotavirus
   c. Novovirus d. Rubella virus
8. Rickettsial disease is caused by ___________.
   a. Rickettsiae b. *S. typhi*
   c. *C. burnetii* d. None of the above
9. *Clostridium tetani* is the pathogenic agent for ___________.
   a. Tetanus b. Throat infection
   c. Murine d. Q-fever
10. *Rickettsia* can be treated by ___________.
    a. Doxycycline b. Chloramphenicol
    c. RMSF d. Both a and b

Answers

1. b	2. b	3. a	4. a	5. d
6. a	7. a	8. a	9. a	10. d

Coronavirus Disease 2019 (COVID-19)

In this study guide, learn all the important information about Coronavirus 2019 (COVID-19) including how it is transmitted, its symptoms, how it is diagnosed, its preventive measures, nursing management, and advice for the health workers.

Coronavirus Disease 2019 (COVID-19) identified as the cause of an outbreak first discovered at a local seafood/wild animal market in Wuhan, China. The COVID-19 has been declared by the World Health Organization (WHO) as a pandemic where it is reported that around 5,000,000 people are affected in more than 200 countries around the world.

WHAT IS CORONAVIRUS 2019 (COVID-19)?

Coronavirus 2019 (COVID-19) is a disease caused by a new strain of coronavirus called *severe acute respiratory syndrome coronavirus 2 (SARS-CoV-2)* that can cause symptoms from common cold to more severe disease such as pneumonia and eventually it may lead to death especially those in vulnerable groups such as the elderly, the very young, and people with an underlying chronic health condition.

- Limited information is available to characterize the spectrum of clinical illness associated with COVID-19.
- The CDC clinical criteria for a COVID-19 patient under investigation (PUI) have been developed based on what is known about MERS-CoV and SARS-CoV and are subject to change as additional information becomes available.
- Early on, many of the patients in the outbreak in Wuhan, China reportedly had some link to a large seafood and animal market, suggesting animal-to-person spread.
- However, a growing number of patients reportedly have not had exposure to animal markets, indicating person-to-person spread is occurring.

Pathophysiology

Coronaviruses are common in many different species of animals, including bats, camels, cats, and cattle.

- COVID-19 is a beta-coronavirus, like MERS and SARS, all of which have their origins in bats.
- The sequences from US patients are similar to the one that China initially posted, suggesting a likely single, recent emergence of this virus from an animal reservoir.
- When person-to-person spread has occurred with MERS and SARS, it is thought to have happened mainly via respiratory droplets produced when an infected person sneezes, similar to how influenza and other respiratory pathogens spread.
- Most coronaviruses infect animals, but not people; in the future, one or more of these other coronaviruses could potentially evolve and spread to humans, as has happened in the past.
- Many of the patients have direct or indirect contact with the Wuhan Huanan Seafood Wholesale Market that is believed to be the original place of the outbreak of COVID-19.
- However, the transmission of COVID-19 from fish to humans is unlikely.
- The COVID-19 and fish coronaviruses such as Beluga Whale CoV/SW1 belong to different genera and apparently have different host ranges.
- As the Wuhan market seafood market also sells other animals, the natural host of COVID-19 awaits to be identified.
- Due to the possibility of transmission from animal to human, CoVs in livestock and other animals including bats and wild animals sold on the market should be constantly monitored.
- In addition, more and more evidence indicates the new virus COVID-19 is spread via the route of human-to-human transmission because there are infections of people who did not visit Wuhan but had close contact with family members who had visited Wuhan and got infected.

Causes

Coronaviruses are named for the crown-like spikes on their surface.

- There are four main sub-groupings of coronaviruses, known as alpha, beta, gamma, and delta.
- Human coronaviruses were first identified in the mid-1960s.

- The seven coronaviruses that can infect people are 229E (alpha coronavirus), NL63 (alpha coronavirus), OC43 (beta coronavirus), and HKU1 (beta coronavirus).
- Other human coronaviruses are MERS-CoV, SARS-CoV, and COVID-19.

Statistics and Incidences

An outbreak of pneumonia of unknown etiology in Wuhan City was initially reported to WHO on December 31, 2019.

- Chinese health authorities have confirmed more than 40 infections with a novel coronavirus as the cause of the outbreak.
- Reportedly, most patients had epidemiological links to a large seafood and animal market; the market was closed on January 1, 2020.
- Globally, there are 5,030,914 confirmed cases and 326,182 deaths confirmed as of May 21, 2020.
- The United States has the highest number of coronavirus cases in the world with more than 1.5 million cases (New York City being the most affected).
- Most countries have declared nationwide lockdowns and have restricted travel.
- International conveyance cases identified on the Diamond Princess cruise ship currently in Japanese territorial waters have reached 712.

Clinical Manifestations

For confirmed COVID-19 infections, reported illnesses have ranged from people being mildly sick to people being severely ill and dying; these symptoms may appear in as few as 2 days or as long as 14 after exposure based on what has been seen previously as the incubation period of MERS viruses.

- Fever
- Dry cough
- Shortness of breath

Other symptoms may include:

- Sore throat
- Runny nose
- Diarrhea
- Fatigue/tiredness
- Difficulty of breathing (in severe cases)

Assessment and Diagnostic Findings

At this time, diagnostic testing for COVID-19 can be conducted only at CDC

- To increase the likelihood of detecting infection, CDC recommends collection of three specimen types: *lower respiratory, upper respiratory, and serum specimens* for testing.
- CDC has deployed multidisciplinary teams to Washington, Illinois, California, and Arizona to assist health departments with clinical management, contact tracing, and communications.
- CDC has developed a real-time Reverse Transcription-Polymerase Chain Reaction (rRT-PCR) test that can diagnose COVID-19 in respiratory serum samples from clinical specimens.
- Currently, testing for this virus must take place at CDC, but in the coming days and weeks, CDC will share these tests with domestic and international partners.
- CDC uploaded the entire genome of the virus from all five reported cases in the United States to GenBank.
- CDC is also growing the virus in cell culture, which is necessary for further studies, including for additional genetic characterization.

Medical Management

The best way to prevent infection is to avoid being exposed to this coronavirus.

- **Hand hygiene:** Wash hands often with soap and water for at least 20 seconds; if water and soap are not available, use an alcohol-based hand sanitizer.
- **Keep hands off your face:** Avoid touching the eyes, nose, and mouth with unwashed hands.
- **Maintain social distancing:** Avoid close contact with people at least 3 feet (1 meter) who are sick, and stay at home when you are sick.
- **Proper cough and sneeze etiquette:** Cover your cough or sneeze with a tissue, then throw the tissue in the trash.
- **Supportive care:** People infected with COVID-19 should receive supportive care to help relieve symptoms.
- **Severe cases:** For severe cases, treatment should include care to support vital organ functions.

For Healthcare Workers

Healthcare workers are the very people who will be working day-and-night to treat and assist coronavirus patients are among the most exposed population for becoming infected. The protection of vulnerable members is one of the priorities for the response to COVID-19 outbreaks. Occupational health services in healthcare facilities play a vital role in helping, supporting, and ensuring that workplaces are safe and healthy and addressing health problems when they arise. WHO emphasizes the rights and responsibilities of health workers, including explicit criteria required to preserve occupational safety and health.

Health worker rights include that employers and managers in health facilities:

- Assume overall responsibility to ensure that all necessary preventive and protective measures are taken to minimize occupational safety and health risks.
- Provide information, instruction, and training on occupational safety and health, including;
  - Refresher training on infection prevention and control (IPC)
  - Use, putting on, taking off and disposal of personal protective equipment (PPE).
- Provide adequate IPC and PPE supplies (masks, gloves, goggles, gowns, hand sanitizer, soap and water, cleaning supplies) in sufficient quantity to healthcare or other staff caring for suspected or confirmed COVID-19 patients, such that workers do not incur expenses for occupational safety and health requirements.
- Familiarize personnel with technical updates on COVID-19 and provide appropriate tools to assess, triage, test and treat patients and to share infection prevention and control information with patients and the public.
- As needed, provide appropriate security measures for personal safety.
- Provide a blame-free environment for workers to report on incidents, such as exposures to blood or bodily fluids from the respiratory system or to cases of violence, and to adopt measures for immediate follow-up, including support to victims.
- Advise workers on self-assessment, symptom reporting and staying home when ill.
- Maintain appropriate working hours with breaks.
- Consult with health workers on occupational safety and health aspects of their work and notify the labor inspectorate of cases of occupational diseases.

- Not be required to return to a work situation where there is continuing or serious danger to life or health, until the employer has taken any necessary remedial action.
- Allow workers to exercise the right to remove themselves from a work situation that they have reasonable justification to believe presents an imminent and serious danger to their life or health. When a health worker exercises this right, they shall be protected from any undue consequences.
- Honor the right to compensation, rehabilitation, and curative services if infected with COVID-19 following exposure in the workplace. This would be considered occupational exposure and resulting illness would be considered an occupational disease.
- Provide access to mental health and counseling resources.
- Enable co-operation between management and workers and/or their representatives.

Health workers should:

- Follow established occupational safety and health procedures, avoid exposing others to health and safety risks and participate in employer-provided occupational safety and health training.
- Use provided protocols to assess, triage and treat patients.
- Treat patients with respect, compassion, and dignity.
- Maintain patient confidentiality.
- Swiftly follow established public health reporting procedures of suspected and confirmed cases.
- Provide or reinforce accurate infection prevention and control and public health information, including to concerned people who have neither symptoms nor risk.
- Put on, use, take off and dispose of personal protective equipment properly.
- Self-monitor for signs of illness and self-isolate or report the illness to managers, if it occurs.
- Advise management if they are experiencing signs of undue stress or mental health challenges that require support interventions.
- Report to their immediate supervisor any situation which they have reasonable justification to believe presents an imminent and serious danger to life or health.

Pharmacologic Management

There is no specific antiviral medication yet is recommended for COVID-19 infection, and no current vaccine to prevent it.

NURSING MANAGEMENT

Nursing management for patients with COVID-19 infection include the following:

Nursing Assessment

Assessment of a patient suspected of COVID-19 should include:

- **Travel history:** Healthcare providers should obtain a detailed travel history for patients being evaluated with fever and acute respiratory illness.
- **Physical examination:** Patients who have fever, cough, and shortness of breath and who has traveled to Wuhan, China recently must be placed under isolation immediately.

Nursing Diagnosis

Based on the assessment data, the major nursing diagnosis for a patient with COVID-19 are:

- **Infection** related to failure to avoid pathogen secondary to exposure to COVID-19.
- **Deficient knowledge** related to unfamiliarity with disease transmission information.
- **Hyperthermia** related to increase in metabolic rate.
- **Impaired breathing pattern** related to shortness of breath.
- **Anxiety** related to unknown etiology of the disease.

Nursing Care Planning and Goals

The following are the major nursing care planning goals for COVID-19:

- Prevent the spread of infection.
- Learn more about the disease and its management.
- Improve body temperature levels.
- Restore breathing pattern back to normal.
- Reduce anxiety.

Nursing Interventions

Listed below are the nursing interventions for a patient diagnosed with COVID-19:

- **Monitor vital signs:** Monitor the patient's temperature; the infection usually begins with a high temperature; monitor the respiratory rate of the patient as shortness of breath is another common symptom.

- **Monitor O_2 saturation:** Monitor the patient's O_2 saturation because respiratory compromise results in hypoxia.
- **Maintain respiratory isolation:** Keep tissues at the patient's bedside; dispose secretions properly; instruct the patient to cover mouth when coughing or sneezing; use masks, and advise those entering the room to wear masks as well; place respiratory stickers on chart, linens, and so on.
- **Enforce strict hand hygiene:** Teach the patient and folks to wash hands after coughing to reduce or prevent the transmission of the virus.
- **Manage hyperthermia:** Use appropriate therapy for elevated temperature to maintain normothermia and reduce metabolic needs.
- **Educate the patient and folks:** Provide information on disease transmission, diagnostic testing, disease process, complications, and protection from the virus.

Evaluation

Nursing goals are met as evidenced by:

- Patient was able to prevent the spread of infection.
- Patient was able to learn more about the disease and its management.
- Patient was able to improve body temperature levels.
- Patient was able to restore breathing pattern back to normal.
- Patient was able to reduce anxiety.

Documentation Guidelines

Documentation guidelines for a patient with COVID-19 include the following:

- Individual findings, including factors affecting, interactions, nature of social exchanges, specifics of individual behavior.
- Cultural and religious beliefs, and expectations.
- Plan of care.
- Teaching plan.
- Responses to interventions, teaching, and actions performed.
- Attainment or progress toward the desired outcome.

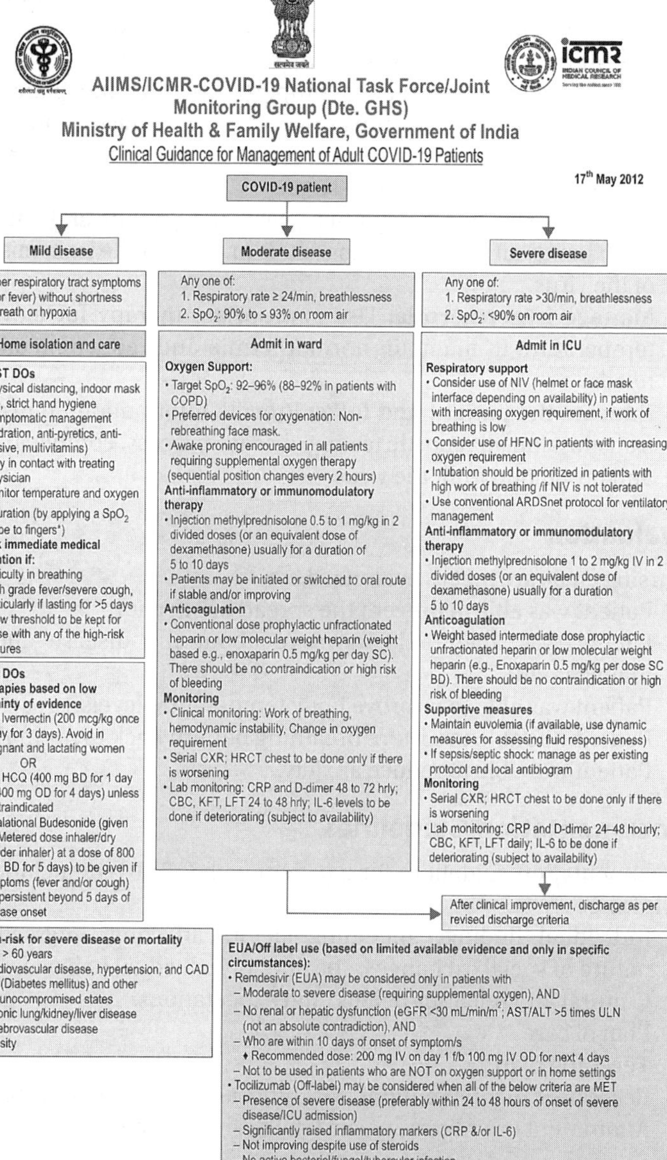

AIIMS/ICMR-COVID-19 National Task Force/Joint Monitoring Group (Dte. GHS)
Ministry of Health & Family Welfare, Government of India
Clinical Guidance for Management of Adult COVID-19 Patients

17th May 2012

COVID-19 patient

Mild disease

Upper respiratory tract symptoms (&/or fever) without shortness of breath or hypoxia

Home isolation and care

MUST DOs
- Physical distancing, indoor mask use, strict hand hygiene
- Symptomatic management (hydration, anti-pyretics, anti-tussive, multivitamins)
- Stay in contact with treating physician
- Monitor temperature and oxygen saturation (by applying a SpO_2 probe to fingers*)

Seek immediate medical attention if:
- Difficulty in breathing
- High grade fever/severe cough, particularly if lasting for >5 days
- A low threshold to be kept for those with any of the high-risk features

MAY DOs
Therapies based on low certainty of evidence
- Tab Ivermectin (200 mcg/kg once a day for 3 days). Avoid in pregnant and lactating women
  OR
- Tab HCQ (400 mg BD for 1 day f/b 400 mg OD for 4 days) unless contraindicated
- Inhalational Budesonide (given via Metered dose inhaler/dry powder inhaler) at a dose of 800 mcg BD for 5 days) to be given if symptoms (fever and/or cough) are persistent beyond 5 days of disease onset

Moderate disease

Any one of:
1. Respiratory rate ≥ 24/min, breathlessness
2. SpO_2: 90% to ≤ 93% on room air

Admit in ward

Oxygen Support:
- Target SpO_2: 92–96% (88–92% in patients with COPD)
- Preferred devices for oxygenation: Non-rebreathing face mask.
- Awake proning encouraged in all patients requiring supplemental oxygen therapy (sequential position changes every 2 hours)

Anti-inflammatory or immunomodulatory therapy
- Injection methylprednisolone 0.5 to 1 mg/kg in 2 divided doses (or an equivalent dose of dexamethasone) usually for a duration of 5 to 10 days
- Patients may be initiated or switched to oral route if stable and/or improving

Anticoagulation
- Conventional dose prophylactic unfractionated heparin or low molecular weight heparin (weight based e.g., enoxaparin 0.5 mg/kg per day SC). There should be no contraindication or high risk of bleeding

Monitoring
- Clinical monitoring: Work of breathing, hemodynamic instability, Change in oxygen requirement
- Serial CXR; HRCT chest to be done only if there is worsening
- Lab monitoring: CRP and D-dimer 48 to 72 hrly; CBC, KFT, LFT 24 to 48 hrly; IL-6 levels to be done if deteriorating (subject to availability)

Severe disease

Any one of:
1. Respiratory rate >30/min, breathlessness
2. SpO_2: <90% on room air

Admit in ICU

Respiratory support
- Consider use of NIV (helmet or face mask interface depending on availability) in patients with increasing oxygen requirement, if work of breathing is low
- Consider use of HFNC in patients with increasing oxygen requirement
- Intubation should be prioritized in patients with high work of breathing /if NIV is not tolerated
- Use conventional ARDSnet protocol for ventilatory management

Anti-inflammatory or immunomodulatory therapy
- Injection methylprednisolone 1 to 2 mg/kg IV in 2 divided doses (or an equivalent dose of dexamethasone) usually for a duration 5 to 10 days

Anticoagulation
- Weight based intermediate dose prophylactic unfractionated heparin or low molecular weight heparin (e.g., Enoxaparin 0.5 mg/kg per dose SC BD). There should be no contraindication or high risk of bleeding

Supportive measures
- Maintain euvolemia (if available, use dynamic measures for assessing fluid responsiveness)
- If sepsis/septic shock: manage as per existing protocol and local antibiogram

Monitoring
- Serial CXR; HRCT chest to be done only if there is worsening
- Lab monitoring: CRP and D-dimer 24–48 hourly; CBC, KFT, LFT daily; IL-6 to be done if deteriorating (subject to availability)

After clinical improvement, discharge as per revised discharge criteria

***High-risk for severe disease or mortality**
- Age > 60 years
- Cardiovascular disease, hypertension, and CAD
- DM (Diabetes mellitus) and other immunocompromised states
- Chronic lung/kidney/liver disease
- Cerebrovascular disease
- Obesity

EUA/Off label use (based on limited available evidence and only in specific circumstances):
- Remdesivir (EUA) may be considered only in patients with
  - Moderate to severe disease (requiring supplemental oxygen), AND
  - No renal or hepatic dysfunction (eGFR <30 mL/min/m^2; AST/ALT >5 times ULN (not an absolute contradiction), AND
  - Who are within 10 days of onset of symptom/s
    - ♦ Recommended dose: 200 mg IV on day 1 f/b 100 mg IV OD for next 4 days
  - Not to be used in patients who are NOT on oxygen support or in home settings
- Tocilizumab (Off-label) may be considered when all of the below criteria are MET
  - Presence of severe disease (preferably within 24 to 48 hours of onset of severe disease/ICU admission)
  - Significantly raised inflammatory markers (CRP &/or IL-6)
  - Not improving despite use of steroids
  - No active bacterial/fungal/tubercular infection
    - ♦ Recommended single dose: 4 to 6 mg/kg (400 mg in 60 kg adult) in 100 mL NS over 1 hour
- Convalescent plasma (off label) may be considered only when following criteria are MET
  - Early moderate disease (preferably within 7 days of symptom onset, no use after 7 days)
  - Availability of high titre donor plasma (signal to cut-off ratio (S/O) >3.5 or equivalent depending on the test kit being used)

Figure 2.10.1: Clinical guidelines for the management of COVID-19 patients.

POSSIBLE QUESTIONS

1. What is COVID-19? Describe its causes, symptoms, diagnostic and prevention.

SHORT NOTES

1. Pathophysiology
2. Clinical manifestation of COVID-19.

MULTIPLE CHOICE QUESTIONS

1. Corona virus was first found in ___________.
   a. China b. India
   c. Australia d. Brazil
2. COVID-19 is caused by:
   a. SARS-CoV-2 b. MERS-CoV
   c. Both a and b d. SRES-COV
3. Origin of SARS and MERS is from ___________.
   a. Rat b. Bat
   c. Pig d. Owl
4. Which of the following is not a coronavirus?
   a. HKU 1 b. OC 43
   c. 229 E d. OC 33
5. The minimum distance between two sick persons is___________.
   a. 3 feet b. 4 feet
   c. 2 feet d. 9 feet
6. Which is not a nursing inventions ?
   a. Monitor vital signs b. Monitor O_2 saturation
   c. Educate the patients and folks d. None of the above
7. COVID-19 was dangerous for ___________.
   a. Older people b. Older people with disease
   c. The young people d. All of the above
8. Who declared COVID-19 as a global pandemic?
   a. WHO b. IMF
   c. UNICEF d. UN

Answers

1. a	2. c	3. b	4. d	5. a
6. d	7. d	8. a		

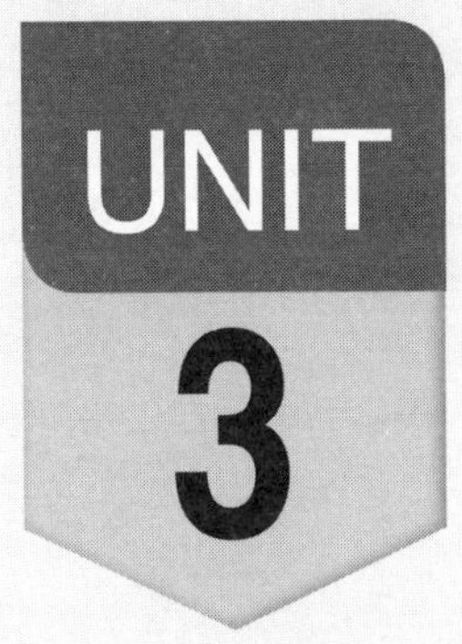

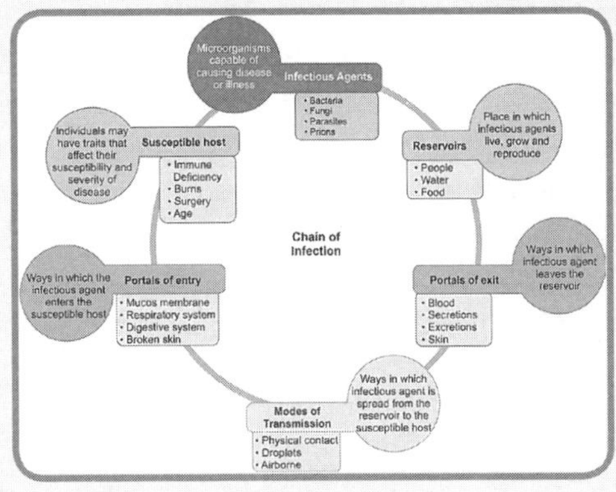

Infection and its Transmission

Learning Objectives

- Sources and types of infection
- Nosocomial infection
- Factors affecting growth of microbes
- Cycle of transmission of infection
- Reaction of body to infection, mechanism of resistance
- Collection of specimen

Infection and Transmission of Pathogenic Microorganisms

INTRODUCTION

An infection is caused by invasion of foreign cells like bacteria in human that causes harm to the host organism. Generally, the host organism is considered "colonized" by cells that don't belong to it. These foreign cells must be harmful to the host organism the colonization be considered as an infection.

WHAT IS INFECTION?

Infection is invasion of a host organism's body tissues by disease-causing organisms, their multiplication, the reaction of host tissues to these organisms and the toxins they produce.

Infectious diseases are also known as transmissible or communicable diseases comprising of clinically evident illness resulted from infection.

SOME IMPORTANT TERMS RELATED TO INFECTION

- **Symptoms:** The subjective sign observed during a disease are called as its symptoms. Here subjective sign mean they can only be felt by the patient. For example, anxiety, back pain and fatigue (tiredness) are all symptoms which can be felt only by the patient.
- **Medical sign:** The objective sign observed during a disease are called as its medical sign. Here objective sign mean they can be observed by the patient, physicians and others. For example, such as blood in the stool, a skin rash, etc. can be seen by all.
- **Syndrome:** This is a group of symptoms which consistently occur together. For example, in Acquired Immunodeficiency Syndrome (AIDS) disease a collection of symptoms is observed in the patient.

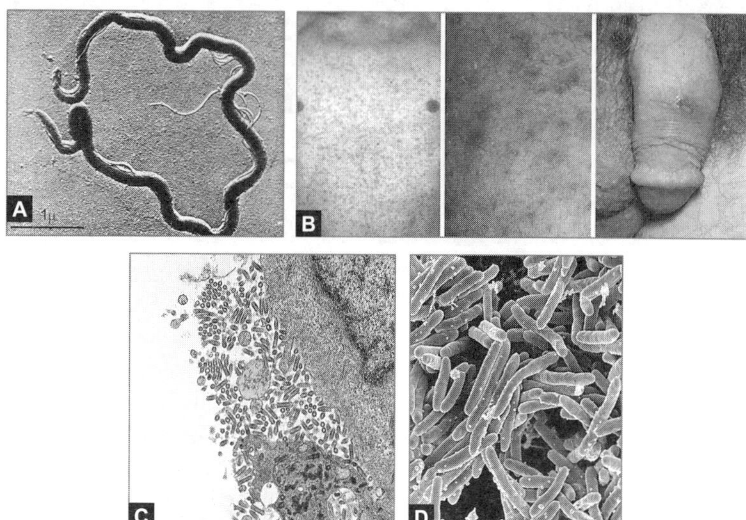

Figures 3.1.1A to D: (A) *Treponema pallidum*, the causal organism of syphilis; (B) Symptoms of syphilis; (C) Rabies virus, the causal organism of rabies; (D) *Mycobacterium tuberculosis*, causal organisms of tuberculosis.

- **Acute illness** are those that will eventually resolve without any medical supervision., e.g. common cold.
- **Chronic illness** are more serious illness that require medical supervision, e.g. Tuberculosis or cancer.

SOURCES OF INFECTION

The sources of infection can be divided into two main groups viz:

a. **Endogenous sources:** A source of infection is endogenous when the infectious agent comes from the patient's own body usually from his own normal flora. Endogenous source of infection becomes important when person's own immunity against his normal flora becomes compromised such as in case of contamination during surgery, malnutrition, impairment of blood supply and debilitating diseases such as AIDS, diabetes or any other accompanying infection. Examples are genera of *Staphylococci* and *Streptococci* which are normally found in the body but can become pathogenic in certain circumstances.

b. **Exogenous sources:** Exogenous sources of infection introduce organisms anywhere from outside to inside of the body. In addition to being exogenous most of the time, infections are transmitted from person-to-person or from animal to man. To be more specific, exogenous source of infections can either be human, animal or environmental in origin.

- *Human origin:* Human can be source of infection in three cases, (1) either when they are clinically infected (symptomatic infection), (2) when they are asymptomatically infected, or (3) when they are carriers. Human can be a source of organisms which cause diseases that are sexually transmitted such as *Treponema pallidum* that causes Syphilis and *N. gonorrhoeae* that causes Gonorrheal infections. Infection may also occur through blood when vectors act as vehicles as in the case of transmission. For example, *Borrelia* that causes relapsing fever.
- *Animal origin:* Animals are another source of infection and an infection derived from this source is called zoonotic infection. Such infections are usually maintained in animals and are acquired accidentally. An example of such infections could be Brucellosis caused by Brucella mainly from cows and their products such as milk; Rabies caused by Rabies Virus from wild animals and Plague which is caused by *Pasteurella pestis*. Moreover, animal products such as meat, milk and eggs can be sources of infection. Example: *Salmonella* species and *Campylobacter*.
- *Environmental origin:* Environmental sources are numerous and few environmental saprophytes are pathogenic for man unless in cases of individuals with severely compromised immune system. But still some parasites may result in complications if introduced into the body from environment. Examples are *Bacillus* and *Clostridium*. Food is another important and very common source of infection due to everyday pattern of dealing with such material. Food can be contaminated and hence a source of infection at several stages. At its origin (infected animal or plant), or at the time of processing when handled with hands or contaminated tools. It is not only a vehicle when transmission is considered but it is also a good environment where bacteria or any other pathogen can multiply and produce toxins.

There is another type of infection called as nosocomial infection or hospital acquired infections. Nosocomial infection is acquired in hospitals and other healthcare facility centers. These infections can be seen in patients acquired during their stay in a healthcare facility or it can manifest after discharge. Such infections are considered more difficult to prevent and treat more unpredictable and more resistant to cure than infections contracted in the community. Patients who undergo surgical procedures have a higher incidence of nosocomial infections than others. The source of microorganisms that cause nosocomial infections can be the patients themselves, healthcare facility or the healthcare personnel.

CHAIN OF INFECTION

1. In order for infection to occur in an individual, a process involving six related components must occur. This process has been referred to as the "Chain of Infection." The six steps or "links" in the chain are:
   a. Infectious agents
   b. Reservoir
   c. Portal of exit
   d. Mode of transmission
   e. Portal of entry
   f. Susceptible host

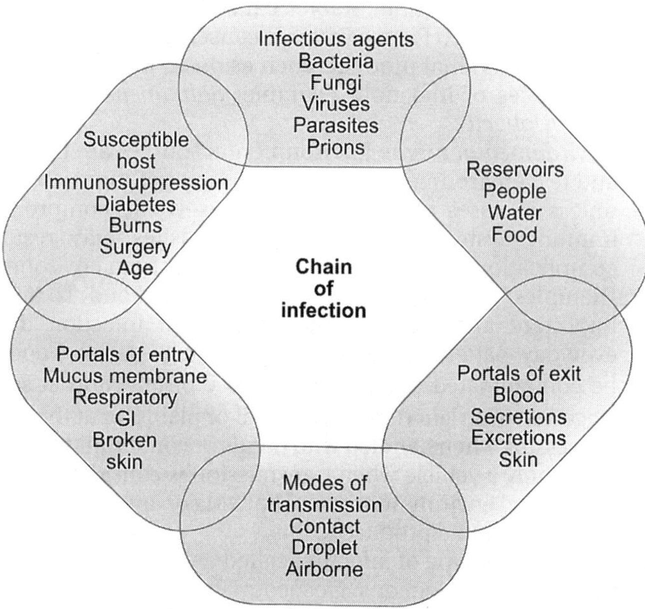

Figure 3.1.2: Chain of infection.

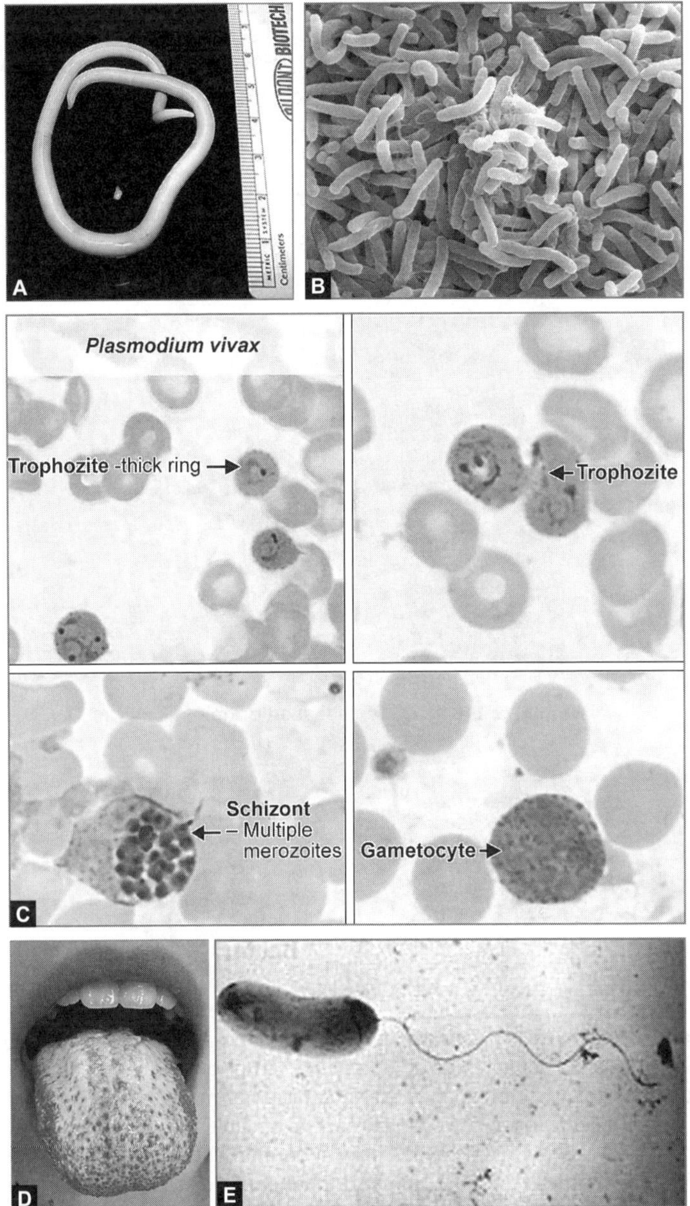

Figures 3.1.3A to E

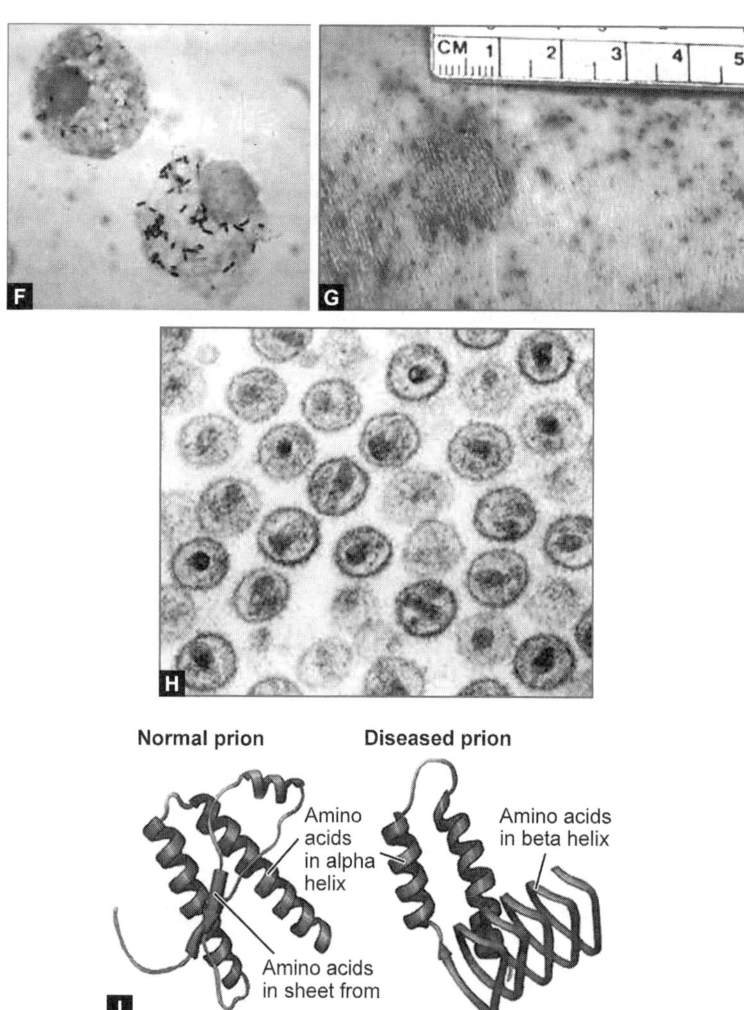

Figures 3.1.3A to I: (A) *Ascaris lumbricoides* (metazoa), causal organisms of Ascariasis; (B) *Vibrio cholerae* (bacteria), causal organism of cholera; (C) *Plasmodium vivax* (protozoa), causal organisms of malaria; (D) Candidiaisis; (E) *Vibrio cholerae* (bacteria), causal organism of cholera; (F) *Rickettsia rickettsii* (Rickettsia), causal organism of Rocky mountain soptted fever; (G) Rocky mountain spotted fever; (H) Human immunodeficiency virus; (HIV), causal organisms of acquired Immunodeficiency syndrome (AIDS); (I) Prions, causal agent of Kuru, BSE and CJD.

INFECTIOUS AGENTS

There are seven categories of biological agents that can cause infectious diseases. Each has its own particular characteristics. The types of agents are as follows:

a. **Metazoa:** These are multicellular animals, most of which are parasites. They cause diseases viz:
   - Trichinellosis, also called trichinosis is caused by an intestinal roundworm transmitted through undercooked meat.
   - Chronic anemia is caused by hookworms which are transmitted through feces-contaminated water and soil. Infection results in retarded mental and physical development of children.
   - Schistosomiasis is caused by a blood fluke and transmitted through contaminated water. Symptoms are related to the number and location of eggs in human body and may involve liver, intestines, spleen, urinary tract, and reproductive system.

b. **Protozoa:** These are single-cell organisms with a well-defined nucleus. Some of these are human parasites. Examples of diseases caused by protozoa include:
   - Malaria which is a mosquito-borne disease (that is one of the top three infectious diseases in the world) along with Tuberculosis and HIV.
   - Giardiasis is an infection of the upper small intestine that causes a diarrheal illness. Outbreaks can be difficult to control especially in child care settings.
   - Toxoplasmosis is transmitted to human from cats and undercooked meat. When this systemic disease infects a pregnant woman, it can cause the death of the fetus.
   - *Pneumocystis carinii* causes Pneumonia or PCP which is often fetal, especially in people with compromised immune systems such as those infected with HIV.

c. **Fungi:** These are nonmotile, filamentous organisms that cause diseases which are very difficult to be treated. Some examples important to public health are as follows:
   - Histoplasmosis is transmitted by inhaling dust from soil that contains bird droppings. The severity varies widely with the lungs, the most common site of infection.
   - Candidiasis is transmitted by contact with human patients and carriers. This fungus causes lesions on the skin or

mucus membranes including "thrush" and vulvovaginitis. Symptoms can be severe in immunocompromised people.

d. **Bacteria:** These are single-celled organisms that lack true nuclei. They are responsible for wide range of human diseases including:
   - Tuberculosis is a chronic lung disease that is a major cause of disability and death in many parts of the world.
   - Staphylococcal disease can affect almost every organ system. Severity ranges from a single pustule of impetigo through pneumonia, arthritis, endocarditis, etc. to sepsis and death.
   - Chlamydia and Gonorrhea are the most widespread sexually transmitted diseases.
   - Tetanus and Diphtheria are two diseases those were once major public health problems but are now well controlled through immunization.

e. **Rickettsia** is a genus of bacteria usually found in the cells of lice, ticks, fleas and mites. They are smaller than most bacteria and share some characteristics of viruses. Diseases cause by rickettsia include:
   - Rocky mountain spotted fever, a tick-borne systemic disease that can be hard to diagnose and that leads to death in 3–5% of US cases.
   - Typhus, a louse-borne rash illness with a high case-fatality rate that has occurred historically in poor living conditions brought on by war and famine.

f. **Viruses** are very small, consisting of RNA or DNA core and an outer coat of protein. They can reproduce and grow only inside living cells. Many viral illness is significant to public health including:
   - Influenza, a respiratory illness that contributes to development of pneumonia and occurs in annual epidemics during the winter months.
   - HIV (Human Immunodeficiency Virus), that causes Acquired Immunodeficiency Syndrome (AIDS). This severe, life-threatening pandemic disease has spreaded worldwide within the past 20–30 years.
   - Rabies is spreaded to human from animal bites or scratches. Rabies is almost always fatal in human but is preventable by a vaccine.
   - Measles, Mumps, Rubella, and Poliomyelitis are other diseases caused by viruses. These diseases are well controlled in the US through immunization.

g. **Prions** are infectious agents that do not have any genes. They seem to consist of a protein with an aberrant structure which somehow replicates in animal or human tissues. Prions cause severe damage to the brain. Diseases associated with prions include:
   - Chronic Wasting Disease (CWD) seen in Mule, Deer and Elk
   - Bovine Spongiform Encephalopathy (BSE) seen in Cows
   - Creutzfeld Jacob Disease (CJD) seen in human

RESERVOIRS

Next essential link in the chain of infection is reservoir, usual habitat in which the agent lives and multiplies. Depending upon the agent, the reservoirs may be:

Human Reservoirs

There are two types of human reservoirs:

1. **Acute clinical cases:** Acute clinical cases are people who are infected with the disease agent and become ill.
2. **Carriers:** They are people who carry infectious agents but are not ill. Depending on the disease, any of the following types of carriers may be of following types:
   - *Incubatory carriers* are people who are going to become ill, but begin transmitting their infection before their symptoms start. For example, measles—a person infected with measles begins to shed the virus in nasal and throat secretions a day or two before any cold symptoms or rash are noticeable.
   - *Inapparent carriers:* People with inapparent infections never develop an illness, but are able to transmit their infection to others. For example, of every 100 individuals infected with the Poliomyelitis virus, only one becomes paralyzed. Four others will have a mild illness with fever, malaise, headache, nausea and vomiting. But 95 out of the 100 will have no symptoms at all although they pass the virus in their feces.
   - *Convalescent carriers* are people who continue to be infectious during and even after their recovery from illness. For example, *Salmonella* patients may excrete the bacteria in feces for several weeks and rarely even for a year or more. This is the most common in infants and young children.
   - *Chronic carriers* are people who continue to harbour infections for a year or longer after their recovery. For

example, the chronic carrier state is not uncommon following Hepatitis B infection, whether or not the person became ill and may be lifelong.

Animal Reservoirs

Animal reservoirs of infectious agents can be described in the same way as human reservoirs. They may be:

- Acute clinical cases or
- Carriers

Depending upon the disease different carrier phases may be important in transmission.

Environmental Reservoirs

Plants, soil and water may serve as reservoir of infection for a variety of diseases.

Examples:

- The organism that causes Histoplasmosis lives in soil with high organic content and undisturbed bird droppings.
- The agents that cause Tetanus, Anthrax and Botulism are widely distributed in soil.
- The agent of Legionnaire's disease lives in water including hot water heaters.

PORTAL OF EXIT

Next link in the chain of disease transmission is portal of exit. Portal of exit is the route by which the disease agent may escape from human or animal reservoir. While many disease agents have only one portal of exit, others may leave by various portals.

The portals most commonly associated with human and animal diseases are given below:

a. **Respiratory:** This is the route of many disease agents that cause respiratory illnesses such as the Common Cold, Influenza, and Tuberculosis. It is also the route used by many childhood Vaccine-preventable diseases, including Measles, Mumps, Rubella, Pertussis, *Haemophilus influenzae* type b (Hib) and Pneumococcal disease. This is the most important portal and the most difficult to control.

b. **Genitourinary:** This portal of exit is the route of sexually transmitted diseases including Syphilis, Gonorrhea, Chlamydia, and HIV. Schistosomiasis—a parasitic disease and

Leptospirosis—a bacterial infection, are both spread through urine released into the environment.

c. **Alimentary:** The alimentary portal of exit may be the mouth, as in rabies and other diseases transmitted by bites. More commonly, disease agents are spread by the other end of intestinal tract. These are referred to as enteric diseases. In general, enteric diseases may be controlled through good hygiene, proper food preparation and sanitary sewage disposal. Examples include:
   - Hepatitis A
   - Typhoid
   - Cholera
   - Giardiasis
d. **Skin:** Skin may serve as a portal of exit through superficial lesions or through percutaneous penetration.
   - Superficial skin lesions that produce infectious discharges are found in Smallpox, Varicella (chickenpox), Syphilis, Chancroid, and Impetigo.
   - Percutaneous exit occurs through mosquito bites (Malaria, West Nile virus) or through the use of needles (Hepatitis B and C, HIV).
e. **Transplacental:** This portal of exit from mother to fetus is important in the transmission of microorganisms such as Rubella, HIV, Syphilis and Cytomegalovirus (the most common infectious cause of developmental disabilities). It is fortunately not a factor for most diseases.

MODE OF TRANSMISSION

A mode of transmission is necessary to bridge the gap between the portal of exit from the reservoir and portal of entry into the host. Two basic modes are direct and indirect.

a. **Direct transmission:** Occurs more or less immediately. Many diseases are transmitted by direct contact with the human, animal or environmental reservoir. Prime examples are sexually transmitted diseases and enteric diseases caused by *Shigella* and *Campylobacter*. Contact with soil may lead to mycotic (fungal) diseases. Droplet spread is also considered direct transmission. Infectious aerosols produced by coughing or sneezing can transmit infection directly to susceptible people up to three feet away. Many respiratory diseases are spread this way.

b. **Indirect transmission:** May occur through animate or inanimate mechanisms.
   - **Animate mechanisms:** Involve vectors. Flies may transmit infectious agents such as *Shigella* in a purely mechanical way by walking on feces and then on food. Mosquitoes, ticks or fleas may serve as reservoirs for the growth and multiplication of agents, for example, in Malaria or Lyme disease.
   - **Inanimate mechanisms:** When disease agents are spread by environmental vehicles or by air, this is referred to as indirect transmission by inanimate mechanisms. Anything may be a vehicle, including objects, food, water, milk, or biological products.
     - Food is a common vehicle for *Salmonella* infections
     - Water is the usual vehicle in Cholera outbreaks
     - Surgical instruments and implanted medical devices may be the vehicles of *Staphylococcal* infections

PORTALS OF ENTRY

The point where infectious agent enters new host is known as the portal of entry such as:

- Non-intact skin, e.g. broken skin such as bed sores or wounds coming in contact with contaminated material
- Respiratory tract, e.g. inhaling air having pathogen
- Gastrointestinal tract, e.g. eating contaminated food
- Mucus membranes, e.g. eyes, nose or mouth exposures with infectious agents

SUSCEPTIBLE HOST

All individuals may be susceptible depending on the exposure and their own general health status. Individuals who have never been exposed to the organism may become ill because they do not have antibodies to protect them (e.g., communicable diseases) either through immunization or previous infection.

Factors that increase the risk of susceptibility are:

- Age (either very young or very old)
- Underlying medical conditions
- Treatments or invasive devices
- Poor nutrition/general health

POSSIBLE QUESTIONS

1. What are the different modes of entry of microorganisms into the body?
2. Define infection and classify it.
3. Write an essay on transmission of infection.
4. What are the different types of sources of infection?
5. Explain about the mode of transmission of infection.
6. What are the principles of infection control?
7. Write short notes:
   a. Susceptible host
   b. Portals of entry
   c. Direct and Indirect modes of disease transmission
   d. Portals of exit
   e. Carriers
   f. Infectious agent
   g. Chain of infection
   h. Endogenous and exogenous sources of infection
   i. Syndrome and symptom
   j. Acute and chronic illness
   k. Reservoir

MULTIPLE CHOICE QUESTIONS

1. *Treponema pallidum* causing syphilis are primarily of:
   a. Animal origin b. Human origin
   c. Environmental origin d. None of the above
2. How many links are there in the chain of infection?
   a. 7 b. 9
   c. 3 d. 6
3. Candidiasis in immunosuppressed patients causing lesions on skin or mucus is caused by:
   a. Virus b. Fungus
   c. Protozoans d. Bacterium
4. If an infectious agent can only multiply inside living cells it would likely to be?
   a. Virus b. Bacteria
   c. Fungi d. Prions
5. The area where the causative agents live is called:
   a. Portal of entry b. Hoard
   c. Reservoir d. Cenote
6. Which are examples of environmental reservoirs for diseases?
   a. Contaminated food b. Soil
   c. Water d. All of the above

7. Which of the following statement about "reservoir" of an infection is not correct?
   a. Reservoir can transmit infection to a susceptible host
   b. Reservoir and source of infection are synonymous
   c. Non-living things can act as reservoirs
   d. Reservoirs can be animals
8. The route by which a causative agent escapes the biological reservoir is:
   a. Portal of entry b. Portal of exit
   c. Susceptible host d. Reservoir
9. Sexually transmitted diseases are an example of:
   a. Direct transmission b. Indirect transmission
   c. Opportunistic transmission d. None of the above
10. Most of the respiratory diseases spread through?
    a. Direct transmission b. Indirect transmission
    c. Nosocomial transmission d. Opportunistic transmission
11. A mosquito bites a person who subsequently develops a fever. What type of transmission would this be?
    a. Mechanical vector transmission b. Biological vector transmission
    c. Direct contact transmission d. Vehicle transmission
12. When a pathogen transmitted through air, soil, food or feces it is called:
    a. Direct transmission b. Indirect transmission
    c. Endogenous transmission d. Exogenous transmission
13. A person infected with measles is considered as a:
    a. Inapparent carrier b. Incubatory carrier
    c. Convalescent carrier d. Chronic carrier
14. Lyme diseases are transmitted to humans to through:
    a. Mosquito b. Flies
    c. Ticks d. None of the above
15. Which of the following acts as a vehicle in indirect transmission?
    a. Food b. Water
    c. Milk d. All of the above
16. A person who gets a disease because of weak defenses is called:
    a. Reservoir b. Bank of pathogen
    c. Causative agent d. Susceptible host

Answers

1. b	2. d	3. b	4. a	5. d
6. b	7. b	8. a	9. a	10. b
11. b	12. b	13. c	14. d	15. d
16. d				

Nosocomial Infection

The **nosocomial infection** is a type of infection which mainly occurs in hospitals or other medical facilities. Nosocomial infection is also known as hospital-acquired infection (HAI). The term nosocomial is derived from the Greek words "nosos", which means "disease," and komeo, means "to take care of."

This type of infection only contracted in a hospital environment. This infection affects all the patients, healthcare-associated infections (HCAIs) can affect nurses, physicians, aides, visitors, salespeople, delivery personnel, custodians, and anyone else who has contact with the hospital.

DEFINITION

Nosocomial infections are produced by the infectious pathogen that developed within a hospital or other type of medical care facility and is acquired by patients while they are in their facility.

EXAMPLE OF NOSOCOMIAL INFECTION

A small group of organisms responsible for this infection, including:

- Methicillin-resistant *Staphylococcus aureus*
- *Candida albicans*
- *Pseudomonas aeruginosa*
- *Acinetobacter baumannii*
- *Stenotrophomonas maltophilia*
- *Clostridium difficile*
- *Escherichia coli*
- *Mycobacterium tuberculosis*
- Vancomycin-resistant *Enterococcus Legionnaires'* disease.

Source of Nosocomial Infection

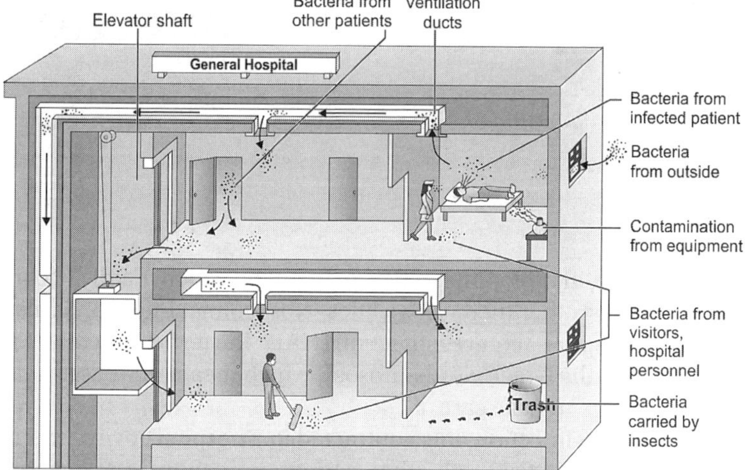

Nosocomial infection divided into two classes based on their source:
1. Exogenous infections
2. Endogenous infections

Exogenous Infections

The source of this type of pathogen is patient, visitors, nurse, or others who enter into the hospital facility.

This type of pathogen can be transmitted by insects, from fomites to patients, equipment used in respiratory or intravenous therapy, catheters, bathroom fixtures and soap, and water systems, also can be a source of exogenous infections.

Endogenous Infections

This type of infections is caused by opportunists among the patient's own normal microflora. In this type the source of pathogen is the patient's own microbiota.

Nosocomial Infections Treatment

The treatment procedure of nosocomial infection is based on the type of infection. The doctor will be recommended antibiotics and bed rest.

Risk for Nosocomial Infection

1. The patients in hospitals are much more susceptible to this infection. Many patients have breaks in the skin (membranes like surgical and accidental wounds, or bed sores) and mucus. The lack of intact skin and mucous membranes will help to easy access for infectious organisms. Sometimes patient's immune system remains weak, the pathogen can take this advantage and can cause infection.
2. The Roommate of a patient can be infected with nosocomial infection.
3. Elderly people, especially those over the age of 70 who are inside the treatment facility, have a higher risk of nosocomial infections.

Transmission of Nosocomial Infection

Hospital-acquired infection can be transmitted by all modes of transmission that occur in the community, such as:

Contact Transmission

The most important and common transmission pathway for nosocomial infection is contact with the infected patient.

There are presently two types of contact transmissions such as:

Direct contact transmission, in this type of transmission the pathogen can be transmitted from an infected person to a normal person when the person came in direct contact with the body surface of the patient.

Indirect contact transmission, in this type the pathogen can be transmitted when a normal person came in contact with a contaminated intermediate object (usually inanimate) from infected patients. For example, contaminated instruments, needles, or dressings, or contaminated gloves that are not changed between patients, saline flush syringes, vials, and bags, etc.

Droplet

Droplets mainly produce during coughing, sneezing, and talking. Nosocomial infection can be transmitted through if the droplets contain infectious pathogens from the infected person.

Airborne Transmission

The nosocomial infection pathogen can be transmitted through droplet nuclei (The remaining particles after the evaporation of the droplet) or dust particle which are remain suspended in the air.

Vehicle Transmission

This type of pathogen can be transmitted from a host to a person through inanimate objects, such as food, water, medications, devices, and equipment.

Vector-borne Transmission

In this type, the pathogens are transmitted through living objects such as mosquitoes, flies, rats, etc.

Prevention and Control of Nosocomial Infection

The transmission of hospital-acquired infection can be prevented by following these precautions:

Precaution for Hospital Staffs

- Wear gloves and gowns in the medical facility or hospital
- Wear masks and protective eyewear during surgery.
- Wash hand before and after contact with a patient and every time change gloves for each patient.
- Always use disposable mouthpiece/airway for cardiopulmonary resuscitation.
- Dispose of contaminated needles and other sharp items immediately after use.

Precaution for Patients

- Proper care should be taken at the patient's wound.
- The patient's cut area must be kept clean.
- Clean spills of blood or contaminated fluids.
- Proper handling of excreta and food
- Safety techniques
- Proper handling of surgical wound care and dressing
- When a new patient arrives at the hospital, he should always be isolated.
- The hospital has to be sanitized every day.
- Every surface of the hospital should be sanitized.

Sites of Nosocomial Infection

Nosocomial infection can be occurring in these following sites of a person, such as urinary tract, surgical wounds, respiratory tract, skin (especially burns), blood (bacteremia), gastrointestinal tract, and central nervous system.

POSSIBLE QUESTIONS

1. Describe nosocomial infection. Give a detail account on its sources, modes of transmission and control measures.

SHORT NOTES

1. Types of nosocomial infection?
2. Contact transmission of HAI?
3. Factors contributing to HAI?
4. Preventive measures for Patients for HAI?

MULTIPLE CHOICE QUESTIONS

1. Hospital acquired infection is otherwise called:
   a. Nosocomial infection
   b. Nostocomial infection
   c. Nosocongenial infection
   d. Nasochomial infection
2. The only infection that can be contaminated in hospital environment is:
   a. Bacterial infection
   b. Fungal infection
   c. Viral infection
   d. Nosocomial infection
3. The most likely agents to cause a nosocomial infection include:
   a. *Staphylococcus* spp.
   b. *Clostridium* spp.
   c. *Mycobacterium tuberculosis*
   d. All of the above
4. Depending upon the sources nosocomial infection can be categorized as:
   a. Outdoor and indoor infection
   b. External and internal infection
   c. Exogenous and endogenous infection
   d. Foreign and domestic Infection

5. Which of the following age groups are most susceptible to Nosocomial infections:
    a. Children 5–10 years old
    b. All hospitalized patients
    c. Adults above 70 years old
    d. Human infants
6. An example of endogenous infection would be:
    a. Infection of a surgical wound from another patient
    b. A surgical site infection
    c. Infection relating to genetic abnormality
    d. Infection in the urinary tract
7. *Pseudomonas aeruginosa* is commonly associated with nosocomial infections of:
    a. Cardiac patients
    b. Burn patients
    c. Patients with stomach infection
    d. HIV patients

Answers

1. a	2. d	3. d	4. c	5. c
6. d	7. b			

Collection of Specimen by Nurses

INTRODUCTION

One means of gathering information about patient's health status is by identifying pathogens and analyzing urine, blood, sputum, and feces. Nurses are responsible for collecting and labeling specimen for analysis and ensuring their delivery to the laboratory.

WHAT IS A SPECIMEN?

A specimen is a sample collected from patient's tissue, fluid or other material for laboratory analysis. This is necessary to carry out medical diagnosis of a disease.

Common examples of specimen include:

- Throat swabs
- Sputum
- Urine
- Blood
- Surgical drain fluids
- Tissue biopsies

PRINCIPLES OF SPECIMEN COLLECTION

A laboratory depends on nurses to collect specimen in an accurate manner. The welfare of patient rests not only on laboratory analysis and physician's interpretation but also on the way in which a specimen is obtained and transmitted to the laboratory by nurses. Factors that must be considered while collecting specimens are as follows;

a. **Moisture:** Moist specimens must always be submitted to a laboratory for analysis. Most bacteria cannot survive in a dry environment, especially the pathogenic ones. Dry swabs are of no value. Hence, when a specimen is taken a nurse must be sure the swab is moist and then delivered to laboratory immediately before it dries out.

b. **Time of collection:** Specimens must be taken possibly before antibiotics are administered. If antibiotics have already been started, then the laboratory sheet must be marked so that everyone is aware of. The timing of blood specimen is very important. Detection of positive blood culture depends on the pathogenic process of the organism.

c. **Labeling and handling of containers:** All containers used for specimen collection must be sterile. The patient should be instructed to handle the container as aseptically as possible, i.e., not to touch the inside of container, laying the lid down in such a way as to contaminate it, leaving the lid off for an excessive length of time, etc. If any of the specimen is spilled on outside, it should immediately be cleaned with a disinfectant. The lid should be secured tightly and the container transported with care to insure against spillage. All containers must be labeled clearly with the patient's name, hospital number, room number and the source of specimen. All specimens are to be sent in ziplock bags to the laboratory. It is absolutely necessary that the specimen be accompanied by a requisition sheet completely filled out which should include information on the specimen container as well as physician, examinations requested, time specimen was collected, clinical diagnosis, current antibiotic therapy. Specimens and sheets improperly identified should be refused by the laboratory.

d. **Effect of temperature:** Most of the microorganisms found in clinical specimens have an optimal temperature of 37°C. Most have a broad range of temperature tolerance; however, some very important pathogens die rapidly when subjected to temperature below their optimal requirement. Therefore, it is better never to refrigerate any specimen especially spinal fluids, vaginal and urethral discharges but deliver them immediately to the laboratory after collection.

e. **Effect of atmosphere:** The atmosphere plays a very important role in isolating and identifying pathogenic bacteria. The two principal gases that affect metabolism of the bacteria are Oxygen and Carbon dioxide. Some bacteria require Oxygen, some require small amounts with varying concentration of Carbon dioxide and some, the anaerobes, must have an atmosphere completely devoid of any trace of Oxygen. Again, it is most important to get the specimen to the laboratory immediately. Anaerobic organisms must be placed in an Oxygen-free environment within 30 minutes after collection.

General Considerations for Specimen Collection

- Collect specimen before antibiotic therapy whenever possible.
- Collect material from where the suspected organism will most likely be found.
- Observe asepsis in collection of all specimens.
- Consider the stage of disease.
- Instruct patients clearly.
- Use proper containers and/or transport media.
- Deliver specimen promptly.
- Provide sufficient information to the laboratory.

THROAT CULTURE

A sample of mucus and secretions from back of the throat is collected on a cotton-tipped applicator and applied to a slide or culture. A determination of which drug is most effective against a particular organism may also be done. A full culture and sensitivity test takes several days because the organisms must have time to grow.

When to Perform?

A throat culture or Strep test is performed by using a throat swab to detect the presence of group of *Streptococcus* bacteria, the most common cause of Strep throat. These bacteria can also cause other infections, including pneumonia, tonsillitis, and meningitis.

Supplies and Equipment

The supplies and equipment required to obtain a sample for throat culture are:

- Sterile cotton-tipped applicator specimen collection kit
- Tongue depressor
- Laboratory request form
- Flashlight.

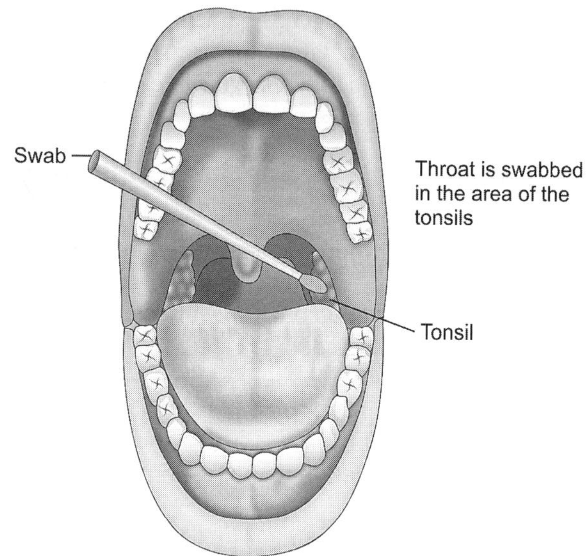

Figure 3.3.1: Taking sample for throat culture.

Procedure for a Throat Culture

Always wash your hands before the procedure. Explain to the patient what you are going to do. Have the patient sit comfortably on a bed or chair and tilt his head back.

- Use flashlight to illuminate the back of the throat. Check for inflamed areas using tongue depressor.
- Ask the patient to say "Ahhh" as you swab the tonsil areas from side to side. Be sure to include any inflamed sites.
- Avoid touching the tongue, cheeks or teeth with the applicator as this will contaminate it with oral bacteria.
- Place the cotton-tipped applicator into the culture tube immediately.
- Label culture tube with the patient's name, SSN, and ward number if applicable.
- Complete the request form.

SPUTUM CULTURE

Sputum is a mixture of saliva and mucus coughed up from the respiratory tract. The sputum specimen should be collected early in the morning before the patient eats, brushes his teeth or uses mouthwash. The specimen is more likely to contain sputum at this time rather than just saliva. Specimens are often taken for three consecutive days because it is difficult for the patient to cough up enough sputum at one time and an organism may be missed if only one culture is done.

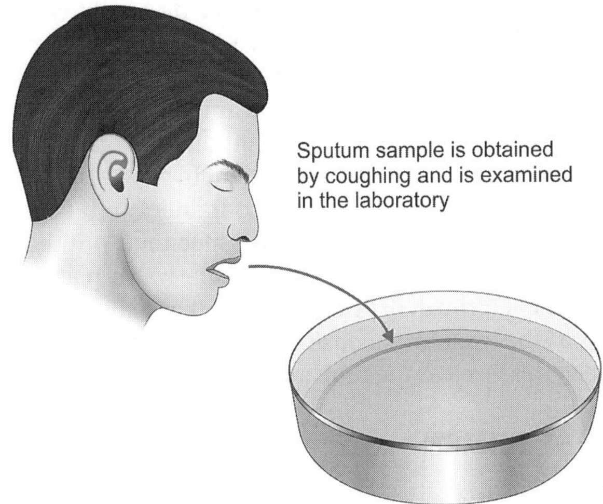

Figure 3.3.2: Taking sample for sputum culture.

When to Perform?

A sputum culture is done to:

- Find and identify bacteria or fungi that are causing an infection (such as Pneumonia or Tuberculosis) of the lungs.
- Identify the best antibiotic to treat the infection (sensitivity testing).
- Monitor treatment of an infection.

Supplies and Equipment

Supplies and equipment required to collect a sputum specimen are

- Sterile container with tight-fitting lid.
- Box of tissues.
- Gloves.
- Laboratory request form.

Procedure for Sputum Specimen

- Wash your hands and gather the equipment.
- Explain the procedure to the patient.

- Place the tissues nearby and have the patient rinse his mouth with clear water to remove any food particles.
- Assist the patient to a sitting position. If necessary ask him to cough deeply and spit into the container. Tell the patient to avoid touching inside of the container because it is sterile.
- A sputum specimen is considered to be highly contaminated and must be treated with caution. To prevent contamination by particles in air, keep the container closed until the patient is ready to spit into it. Close the container immediately after collecting the specimen to prevent the spread of any organisms from the Specimen. Offer tissues for the patient to wipe his mouth.
- Wash your hands, label the container and complete the laboratory request form. Take the specimen to the laboratory immediately allowing it to remain in a warm place which will result in overgrowth of any organisms that may be present.
- Record the amount, consistency and color of the sputum collected, as well as the time and date in the nursing notes.

STOOL SPECIMEN

A stool analysis is a series of tests done on a stool (feces) sample to help diagnose certain conditions affecting the digestive tract. These conditions can include infection (such as from parasites, viruses or bacteria), poor nutrient absorption, or cancer.

When to Perform?

Stool analysis is done to:

- Help identifying diseases of digestive tract, liver, and pancreas.
- Help finding the cause of symptoms affecting digestive tract, including prolonged diarrhea, bloody diarrhea, an increased amount of gas, nausea, vomiting, loss of appetite, bloating, abdominal pain and cramping and fever.
- Screen for colon cancer by checking for hidden (occult) blood.
- Look for parasites such as pinworms or Giardia.
- Look for the cause of an infection such as bacteria, fungus, or virus.
- Check for poor absorption of nutrients by the digestive tract (malabsorption syndrome).

Supplies and Equipment

Supplies and equipment required to collect a stool specimen are:

- Gloves
- Clean bedpan and cover (an extra bedpan or urinal if the patient must void).
- Specimen container and lid.
- Wooden tongue blades.
- Paper bag for used tongue blades.
- Labels.
- Plastic bag for transport of container with specimen to the laboratory.

Procedure for Stool Specimen

- Explain the reason for the test and procedure to patient. Ask the patient to tell you when he feels the urge to have a bowel movement.
- Wear gloves when handling any bodily discharge.
- Give the bedpan when the patient is ready. If the patient wants to urinate first, give a male the urinal or give a female the extra bedpan.
- Remove the bedpan. Use the tongue blade to transfer a portion of the feces to the specimen container. Do not touch the specimen because it is contaminated. It is not necessary to keep this specimen sterile however because the gastrointestinal tract is not sterile.
- Cover the container and label it with the patient's name and social security number.
- Complete the appropriate laboratory request form, noting any special examination ordered.
- Take the specimen to the laboratory immediately; examination for parasites, ova and organisms must be made while the stool is warm.

URINE SPECIMENS

Simple urine tests, such as for sugar and acetone, are often performed by the nurse in the hospital or by the patient at home.

When to Perform?

- Urine tests are very useful for providing information to assist in the diagnosis, monitoring and treatment of a wide range of diseases.

- In addition, a urine test can determine whether or not a woman is ovulating or pregnant.
- Urine can also be tested for a variety of substances relating to drug abuse, both as part of rehabilitation program and in the world of professional sport.
- The urine can be tested very quickly using a strip of special paper which is dipped in the urine just after urination.
- This will show if there are any abnormal products in the urine such as sugar, protein, or blood.
- If more tests are needed to get more details, the urine will be analyzed in a laboratory.

Physical Appearance Test

Urine is assessed first for its physical appearance:

a. **Color:** Freshly voided urine is transparent and light amber in color. The amount and kinds of waste in the urine make it lighter or darker. Blood in the urine colors it. If the amount of blood in the urine is great, the urine will be red.

b. **Odor:** Freshly voided urine has a characteristic odor. When urine stands, decomposition from bacterial activity gives it an ammonia-like odor. Refrigerate the urine sample if it is not to be examined at once.

Midstream Urine Specimen

Midstream urine collection is the most common method of obtaining urine specimens from adults, particularly men. This method allows a specimen which is not contaminated from external sources to be obtained without catheterization.

Supplies and Equipment

- Sterile specimen cup
- Zephiran, a soap solution
- Three cotton balls (to use with zephiran or soap solution)
- Laboratory request form

Procedure

- Instruct the patient to clean urethral area thoroughly. This will prevent external bacteria from entering the specimen. The female should wipe from front to back to avoid contaminating the vaginal and urethral area from anal area. She should clean

each side with a separate cotton ball then use the last one for the urethral area itself. The male should cleanse the penis using the first cotton ball for the urethral, the next cotton ball to clean the end of the penis and the last to cleanse the urethral opening.
- Instruct the patient to void a small amount of urine into the toilet to rinse out the urethra, void the midstream urine into the specimen cup and the last of the stream into the toilet. The midstream urine is considered to be bladder and kidney washings; the portion that the physician wants to be tested.
- Complete the laboratory request form, label the specimen container with patient identifying information and send to the laboratory immediately. A delay in examining the specimen may cause a false result when bacterial determinations are to be made.
- Wash your hands and instruct the patient to do likewise.
- Record that the specimen was collected. Note any difficulties the patient had or if the urine had an abnormal appearance.

24-hour Urine Specimen

A 24-hour urine collection always begins with an empty bladder so that the urine collected is not "left over" from previous hours. This specimen shows the total amounts of wastes the kidneys are eliminating and the amount of each.

Supplies and Equipment

- Large, clean bottle with cap or stopper
- Measuring graduate
- Bedpan or urinal
- Refrigerated storage area
- Gloves

Procedure

- Label the bottle with patient identifying information, the date and note the time of collection at beginning and end.
- Instruct the patient to void all urine into a bedpan or urinal. Measure each specimen of urine voided and pour into the refrigerated bottle. Wash your hands before and after each collection. Record each amount on the intake and output (I and O) sheet.

- Exactly 24-hour after beginning the collection, ask the patient to void. This will complete the specimen collection.
- Send the bottle and laboratory request form to the laboratory.

BLOOD CULTURES

Blood cultures are done to identify a disease-causing organism, especially in patients who have an elevated temperature for an unknown reason. Drawing blood from HIV positive patients is done in accordance with the hospital or clinic's local policy.

When to Perform?

Blood test is performed for:
- Knowing general state of health
- Confirming the presence of a bacterial or viral infection
- Seeing how well certain organs, such as the liver and kidneys, are functioning.
- Screening for certain genetic conditions such as cystic fibrosis or spinal muscular atrophy.

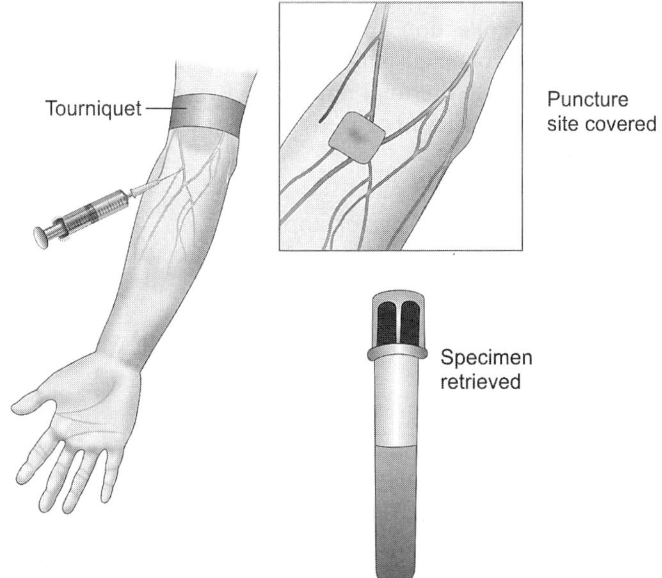

Figure 3.3.3: Collection of blood sample for testing.

Supplies and Equipment

Supplies and equipment required for a blood culture are:

- Sterile syringe (20 cc) and three needles (usually 20 gauge)
- Two blood culture bottles (one for anaerobic and one for aerobic specimens)
- Betadine solution
- Sterile cotton balls or gauze pads
- Gloves
- Tourniquet
- Band-aid
- Chux (to protect the bed)
- Laboratory request form.

Procedure for Blood Cultures

- Explain the procedure and the reason for doing such to the patient.
- Gather all supplies and equipment and bring to the patient's bedside.
- Assist the patient to a comfortable position. If the patient is noncooperative or disoriented, get someone to help you.
- Carefully wash your hands
- Clean the top of both culture bottles with betadine solution.
- Put the needle on the syringe.
- Apply the tourniquet.
- Put on gloves and clean the drawing site with betadine solution.
- Draw at least 10 cc of blood from the patient (5 cc is needed for each bottle).
- Loosen the tourniquet.
- Remove the syringe and needle while applying pressure to the venipuncture site with cotton ball or gauze pad. Have the patient apply pressure to the site.
- Replace needle on the syringe with another sterile needle.
- Inject 5 cc of blood into anaerobic bottle; do not allow air to enter the bottle.
- Replace needle on the syringe with another sterile needle.
- Inject 5 cc of blood into the aerobic bottle and while the needle is still in the bottle, disconnect it from the syringe so that air enters the aerobic bottle.
- Gently mix the blood with the solution in both bottles.
- Label both bottles with patient identifying information and the type of culture that is, aerobic or anaerobic.

- Complete laboratory request forms and send the specimens to the laboratory immediately.
- Place a band-aid over the patient's venipuncture site.

POSSIBLE QUESTIONS

1. What are Specimens? Give a detail account of the principles for collection of Specimens.
2. Give a detail account of the process of urine specimen collection.
3. What is Sputum? When we take sputum specimen for laboratory testing? Discuss its steps.
4. Write an essay on the procedure and precautions involved in the collection of blood sample.
5. Write Short Notes:
   a. Specimen collection
   b. Throat culture
   c. Fecal culture
   d. Urine test
   e. Blood test
   f. Sputum culture

MULTIPLE CHOICE QUESTIONS

1. Which of the following information must be put on the specimen label?
   a. Patients name
   b. Source of specimen
   c. Hospital number
   d. All of the above
2. The best time for collecting a sputum specimen is:
   a. At night
   b. Early morning when the patient awakens
   c. After eating
   d. Before eating
3. A sputum specimen is collected in order to determine infection in the:
   a. Alimentary canal
   b. Urinary tract
   c. Respiratory system
   d. Liver
4. In clinical specimens the optimal temperatures of microorganisms is found as:
   a. 31 degrees
   b. 27 degrees
   c. 37 degrees
   d. None of the above
5. Which of the following commonly causes Strep throat?
   a. *Aspergillus* spp.
   b. *Streptococcus* spp.
   c. *Pseudomonas* spp.
   d. *Escherichia coli*
6. A throat culture or Strep test is also performed for the diagnosis of:
   a. Acute pharyngitis
   b. Bacterial pneumonia
   c. Meningitis
   d. Ascariasis

7. Which of the following are the most common culture specimens used in microbiology?
   a. Sputum
   b. Stool
   c. Urine
   d. All of the above
8. Which of the following diseases can be diagnosed through blood cultures?
   a. Polio
   b. Covid
   c. AIDS
   d. Elephantiasis
9. Freshly voided urine shows which of the following character?
   a. Transparent and light amber colored
   b. Transparent with tints of red
   c. Dark yellow colored
   d. Deep amber colored
10. Midstream urine collection method is commonly used in cases of:
    a. Adults
    b. Infants

Answers

1. d	2. b	3. c	4. c	5. b
6. c	7. d	8. c	9. a	10. a

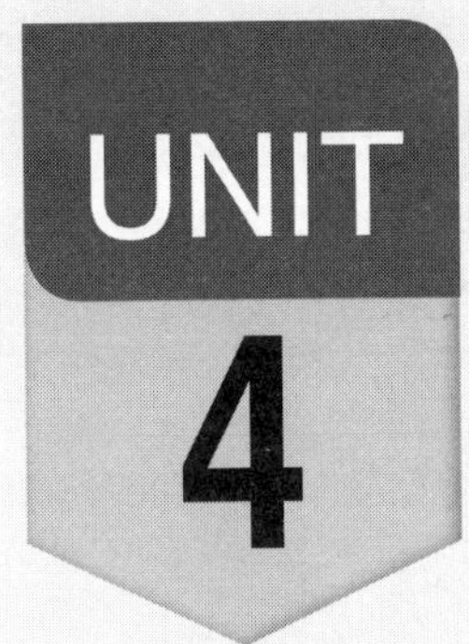

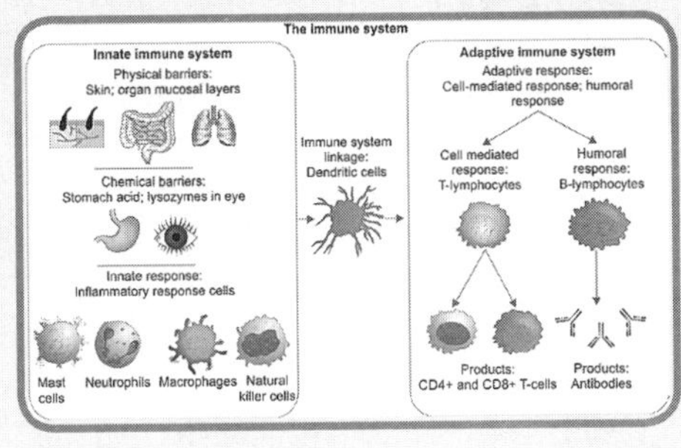

Immunity

Learning Objectives

- Types of immunity—innate and acquired
- Hypersensitivity and autoimmunity
- Immunoprophylaxis (vaccines, sera, etc.)
- Immunization schedule
- Principles and uses of serological tests

Fundamentals of Immunity

INTRODUCTION

Our body is constantly under attack by bacteria, fungi, viruses and other dangerous pathogenic organisms. But we remain healthy most of the time only because we have a good defence system within our body which is referred as the Immune system. Immunity (derived from Latin term Immunis, meaning exempt) is the ability of an organism to resist infection by pathogens or state of protection against foreign organisms or substances called as antigens. Various cells, tissues and organs that carry out this activity constitute the immune system.

TYPES OF IMMUNITY (FLOWCHART 4.1.1)

Humans have two types of Immunity: Innate (Non-specific) and Adaptive (Specific). There are three lines of defences systems that the organisms has to cross to invade the host (humans).

- First line of defences (physical and chemical barriers)
- Second line of defense (Blood and lymph systems, cellular defenses and molecular defenses)
- Third line of defense (T-lymphocytic cells and B-Lymphocytic cells).

INNATE IMMUNITY

The type of immunity inherited by the organism from parents and protects it from birth throughout life is known as Innate or Inborn Immunity. Everyone is born with innate (or natural) immunity, a type of general protection. Innate immunity acts as the first line of defense which prevents pathogens or infectious agents from entering the body.

Innate immunity includes:

- First line of defense
  a. Physical barriers
  b. Chemical barriers
- Second line of defense
  a. Blood and lymph systems
  b. Cellular defenses
  c. Molecular defenses

Note: Innate immunity is also called as nonspecific or natural immunity.

Flowchart 4.1.1: Types of immunity.

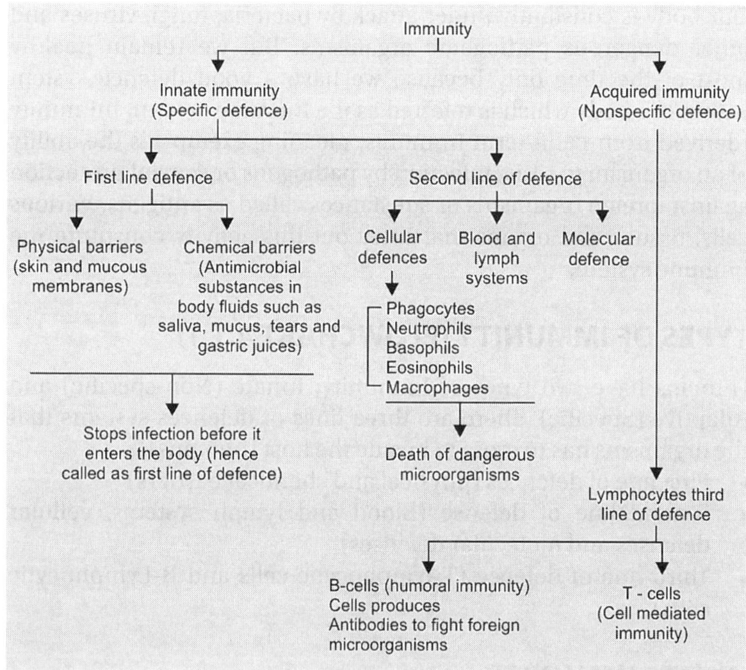

PHYSICAL BARRIERS

Skin

- The outermost layer of the skin is composed of epithelial cells that have been keratinized meaning that they have become compacted, cemented together and filled with an insoluble protein called keratin. Keratin doesn't normally allow the penetration of bacteria and viruses through it.

- Continuous shedding (desquamation) of the outer squamous epithelial cells within the skin removes organisms that try to enter the skin
- Relative dryness on the skin also slows microbial growth
- Secretions from sebaceous and sweat glands keep the skin acidic in a pH range of 3 to 5. This acidic pH kills most microbes
- Normal flora present on skin exert their inhibitory effects on harmful pathogens.

Mucous Membranes

- Mucous membranes are like digestive, respiratory, and genito-urinary tracts
- Prevents entry of harmful microbes
- Mucus (a viscous fluid) traps microbes and particles
- In the trachea, ciliated epithelial cells sweep out mucus, trap microbes and prevents these from entering the lungs
- Exposes them to the acidic environment of the stomach that kills most microbes.

CHEMICAL BARRIERS

- Microbial colonization is also inhibited by saliva, tears, and mucus secretions that continually released on exposed epithelium. All of these secretions contain antimicrobial proteins. For example: lysozyme, an enzyme found in tears, digests the cell walls of many bacteria.
- Sweat has high acid and electrolyte concentrations and this acidic pH is inhibitory to many microbes.
- The HCL in the stomach renders protection against pathogens that are swallowed. The intestine's digestive juices and bile are potentially destructive to microbes too.
- Even semen contains an antimicrobial chemical (spermine) that inhibits bacteria and the vagina has a protective acidic pH maintained by the normal flora.
- Urine has a low pH and the presence of urea and other metabolic end products (Uric acid, Fatty acids, Enzymes)

BLOOD AND LYMPH SYSTEMS

Two interrelated fluid systems support the body's immune response- the blood system and the lymphatic system. These two systems provide a transportation network for the cellular defences against infection.

Blood System

- The blood system produces body's leukocytes (White Blood Cells) and transports these immune cells to the sites of infection (Figure 12.1, Tables 12.1 and 12.2)
- These cells circulate in the blood and are moved between arteries, capillaries and veins by the pumping of heart
- Leukocytes are defensive cells that are important to both specific and nonspecific host defences. These cells are divided into two groups: polymorphonuclear leukocytes or granulocytes and mononuclear leukocytes or agranulocytes:
  - Granulocytes- Basophils, Neutrophils and Eosinophils
  - Agranulocytes - Lymphocytes (B-Cells and T-cells). These are the third line of defence system.

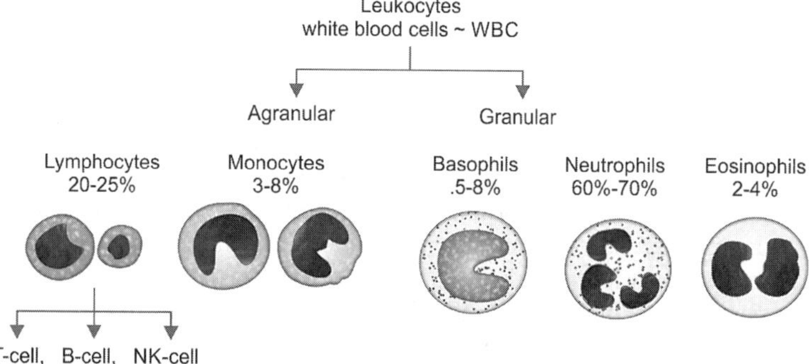

Figure 4.1.1: Types of leukocytes.

Lymphatic System

- The lymph system is a secondary transport system that serves to protect and maintain the internal fluid environment by producing and filtering lymph
- Lymph is a clear fluid that contains White Blood Cells and arises from the drainage of fluid from the bloodstream and surrounding tissue

Table 4.1.1: Cells of leukocytes and their functions.

Leukocytes	% in WBC count	Function	Carry out phagocytosis (engulfment of foreign proteins)
Leukocytes	% in WBC count	Function	Carry out Phagocytosis (engulfment of foreign proteins)
Granulocytes (have prominent cytoplasmic granules)			
Neutrophils	Makes up to 55–90%	These cells carry digestive enzymes and chemicals for phagocytosis	Yes
Eosinophils	1-3%	High level of these cells is seen in parasitic and fungal infections. Contain digestive enzymes to kill foreign particles	Yes, weakly phagocytic.
Basophils	Comprise of < 0.5%	Associated with allergy and inflammation reactions	No
Mast Cells		Not found in circulation and are located in tissues near blood vessels and nerves. They release chemicals such as Histamine and Serotonin	No
Agranulocytes (Consists of Lymphocytes and Natural Killer cells- The Third line of Defence, that comes under Adaptive or Specific Immunity)			

Contd...

Contd...

Leukocytes	% in WBC count	Function	Carry out phagocytosis (engulfment of foreign proteins)
B-cells	Lymphocytes Comprises of 20-30% of WBCs	Producers of antibodies	No. It provides specific Immunity
T-cells		Recognize foreign particles (antigens)	No. It provides specific Immunity
Natural Killer cells	5-10% of lymphoid cells	Recognize and kill infected cells	Yes
Monocytes (when mature and capable of phagocytosis, these cells are called as macrophages)	Largest of all WBC and the third most common in circulation (3-7%)	Cleaning up messes caused by infections and inflammation-even self tissues that are injured. Contains various enzymes and reactive oxygen species to kill engulfed microorganisms	Yes. Very effectively performs phagocytosis

Table 4.1.2: Primary functions of important immune cells.

	Basophils and mast cells	Neutrophils	Eosinophils	Monocytes and macrophages	Lymphocytes and plasma cells	Dendritic cells
	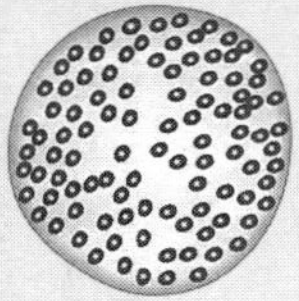 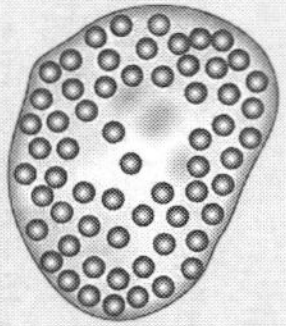	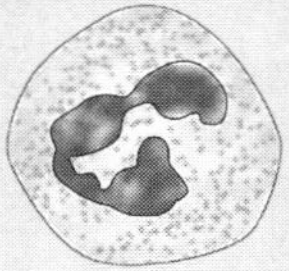	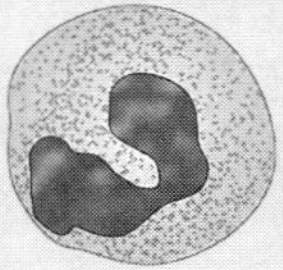	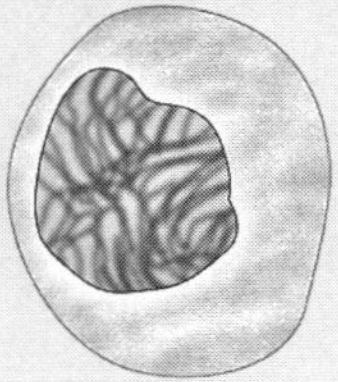 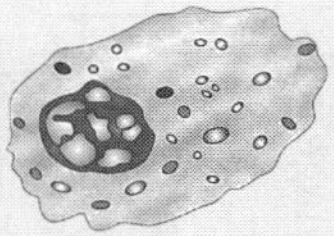	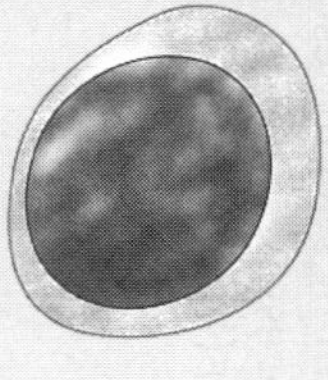 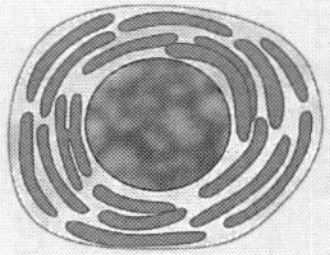	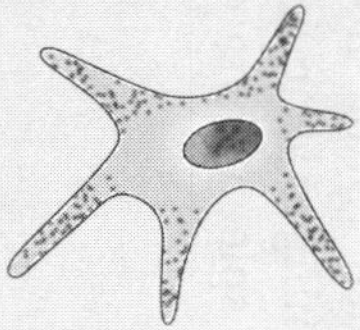
Primary function(s)	Release chemicals that mediate inflammation	Ingest and destroy invaders	Destroy invaders, particularly antibody-coated parasites	Ingest and destroy invaders antigen presentation	Specific responses to invaders, including antibody production	Recognize pathogens and activate other immune cells by antigen presentation

- The fluid is filtered at points called lymph nodes - where pathogens are removed before returning to venous circulation
- Major lymphatic organs include the spleen, thymus, tonsils and adenoids.

CELLULAR DEFENCES

The cellular defences of the innate immune system describe the types of cells employed along with the processes initiated by these cells. These defences include inflammation (by mast cells), phagocytosis, fever and clotting (by platelets).

Inflammation (Figure 4.1.2)

- The inflammatory response is the way in which the body reacts when pathogens damage cells.

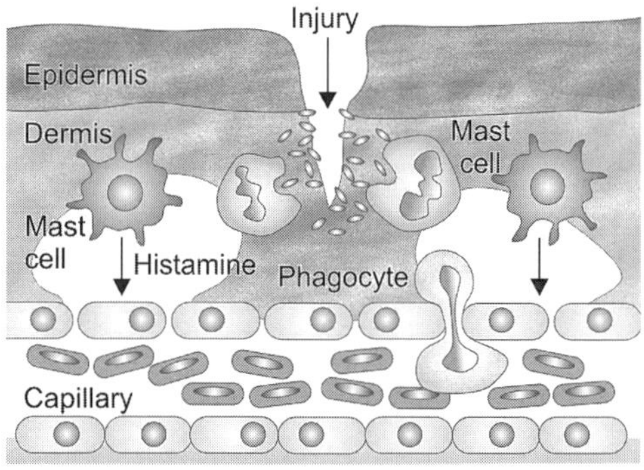

Figure 4.1.2: Overview of the inflammatory response. Histamine release by mast cells leading to inflammation.

- When tissue damage occurs, mast cells release a chemical called histamine, which causes local vasodilation and increased capillary permeability.
- It also releases chemotactic factors which recruit wandering macrophages (phagocytes) to the site of damage to fight the infection.
- While inflammation is necessary to allow immune cells to access infected tissue, side effects include redness, swelling, heat and pain.
- Inflammation can either be short-term (acute) or long-term (chronic).

Phagocytosis (Figure 4.1.3)

- Phagocytic leucocytes circulate in the blood but may move into body tissue in response to infection.
- They concentrate at sites of infection due to the release of chemicals (such as histamine) from damaged body cells.
- Pathogens are engulfed when cellular extensions (pseudopodia) surround the pathogen and then fuse, sequestering it in an internal vesicle.
- The vesicle may then fuse with the lysosome to digest the pathogen
- Some of the pathogens antigenic fragments may be presented on the surface of the macrophage, in order to help stimulate antibody production.
- This mechanism of endocytosis is called phagocytosis ('cell-eating').

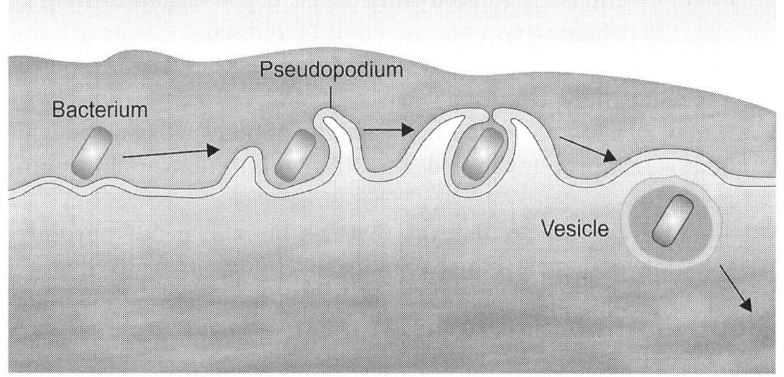

Figure 4.1.3: Overview of phagocytosis by a leucocyte.

Phagocytic Cells

Macrophages

- Large, long-lived phagocytes
- Cells extend long pseudopodia, engulf the microbe into a vacuole which fuses with a lysosome.
- Lysosomes kill in two ways
  - by generating Toxins such as Nitric oxide
  - by digetsing microbes with lysozyme
- Some microbes have outer capsules to which macrophages cannot attach. Others, like *Mycobacterium tuberculosis,* are resistant to lysosomal destruction.

Eosinophils

- Help fight large parasitic invaders, e.g. *Schistosoma mansoni* (blood fluke)
- They position themselves alongside the parasite and discharge destructive enzymes from cytoplasmic granules

Neutrophils

- Usually the first to arrive
- Attracted to chemical signals released by infected tissue
- Self-destruct while destroying invaders

Fever

- A fever is an abnormally high body temperature associated with infection and is triggered by the release of prostaglandins.
- Fever may help to combat infection by reducing the growth rate of pathogens (via the inactivation of enzymes and toxins required by the invader).
- It may also increase metabolic activity of body cells and activate heat shock proteins in order to strengthen the overall immune response.
- Up to a certain point fever may be beneficial but beyond a tolerable limit it can cause damage to a body's own enzymes.

Blood Clotting (Figure 4.1.4)

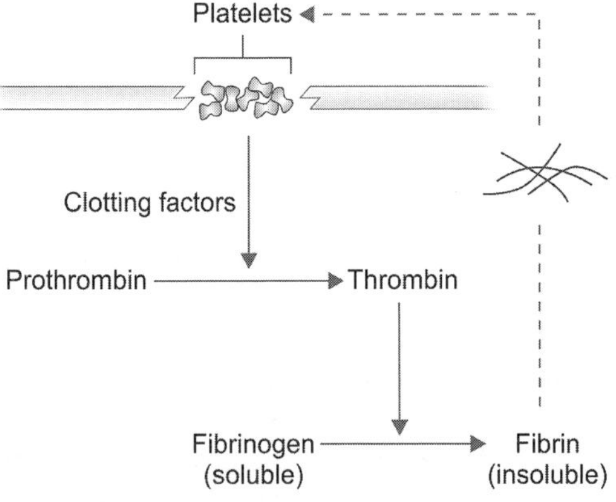

Figure 4.1.4: Mechanism of blood clotting.

- Clotting (hemostasis) is a mechanism that prevents the loss of blood from broken vessels.
- Damaged cells and platelets release chemical signals called clotting factors which trigger a coagulation cascade.
- Clotting factors convert the inactive zymogen prothrombin into the activated enzyme thrombin.
- Thrombin catalyses the conversion of the soluble plasma protein fibrinogen into an insoluble form (fibrin).
- Fibrin forms an insoluble mesh of fibres that trap blood cells at the site of damage.
- Clotting factors also cause platelets to become sticky, which then adhere to the damaged region to form a solid plug called a clot
- The clot prevents further blood loss and blocks entry to foreign pathogens.

MOLECULAR DEFENCES

Molecular defences involves a number of proteins that either attack invading microbes directly or hinder their ability to reproduce.

These defences include complement proteins, cytokinetics and interferons

Complement Proteins

- Complement proteins are produced by macrophages, monocytes and other body cells (particularly liver cells).
- These proteins are normally inactive in the blood but in response to immune activation initiate a cascade of reactions that help protect the body.
- Activation of the complement system may provide protection in the following ways:
  - Assist in the destruction of pathogenic organisms by destroying cell membranes.
  - Recruiting phagocytes to the site of infection (chemotaxis).
  - Aid in identification of pathogens (opsonization).
  - Intensifying the inflammatory response.

Cytokines

- Cytokines are proteins produced in response to antigens and function as chemical messengers in the immune response
- They may facilitate immunity in three main ways:
  - They may regulate the innate immune response (via chemotaxis and activation of the inflammatory response)

- They may regulate the adaptive immune response (via activation of lymphocytes)
- They may activate hematopoiesis (production and differentiation of new white blood cells)

Interferons

- Interferons are a specific type of cytokine that provide protection against viruses and tumor cells.
- Infected cells release interferons which alert surrounding cells to reduce their susceptibility to infection (e.g., by activating antiviral agents).
- Interferons will also recruit natural killer cells (NK cells) which target and destroy infected cells.

ADAPTIVE IMMUNE SYSTEM: THIRD LINE OF DEFENCE (FLOWCHARTS 4.1.2 AND 4.1.3)

The secondkind of protection is adaptive (or specific) immunity, which develops throughout our lives. This is also called as acquired immunity. Adaptive immunity involves the lymphocytes and develops as people are exposed to diseases or immunized against diseases through vaccination

Flowchart 4.1.2: Types of adaptive immunity.

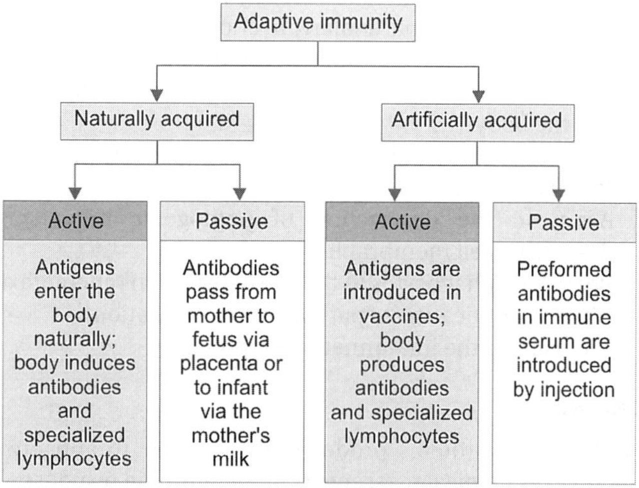

Adaptive immunity

Naturally acquired		Artificially acquired	
Active	Passive	Active	Passive
Antigens enter the body naturally; body induces antibodies and specialized lymphocytes	Antibodies pass from mother to fetus via placenta or to infant via the mother's milk	Antigens are introduced in vaccines; body produces antibodies and specialized lymphocytes	Preformed antibodies in immune serum are introduced by injection

(few years – life long) (weeks - months) (few years – life long) (~ 3 weeks)

Natural= Normal Environmental exposure

Artificial= Medically provided

Active: Immune response, antibody production and T-cell activation

Passive: Delivery of Preformed antibodies, not long term immunity, no development of an everlasting immune response

Adaptive immune system is responsible for the destruction of foreign particles (antigens) once they have entered the body. The cells of the acquired immune system are mainly the B-cells and T-cells.

Flowchart 4.1.3: Classification of adaptive immunity.

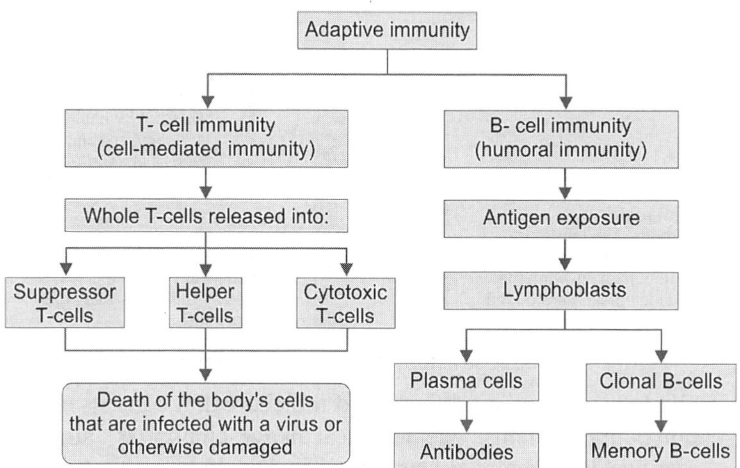

Humoral and Cellular Immunity

Adaptive immunity has two components: B-cells producing antibodies and T-cells both of which protect against infection. Antibodies are proteins that are produced by B-cells, circulate in the blood and bind to antigens on infectious agents. This interaction can result in direct inactivation of the microorganisms. Antibodies are primarily responsible for protection against many bacteria and viruses. This part of the immune response is termed as Humoral Immunity. B-cells produce specialized subpopulations of memory cells and plasma cells. Memory cells are capable of remembering the specific antigen and respond more rapidly and efficiently against future infections. Memory cells are long lived where as plasma cells are short lived. Plasma cells produce antibodies in the blood.

ANTIBODIES (FIGURE 4.1.5)

Antibodies are antigen-reactive glyco-proteins, designated as immunoglobulins, present in the plasma and in extracellular fluids. They bind to specific antigens and potentially neutralize their harmful effects.

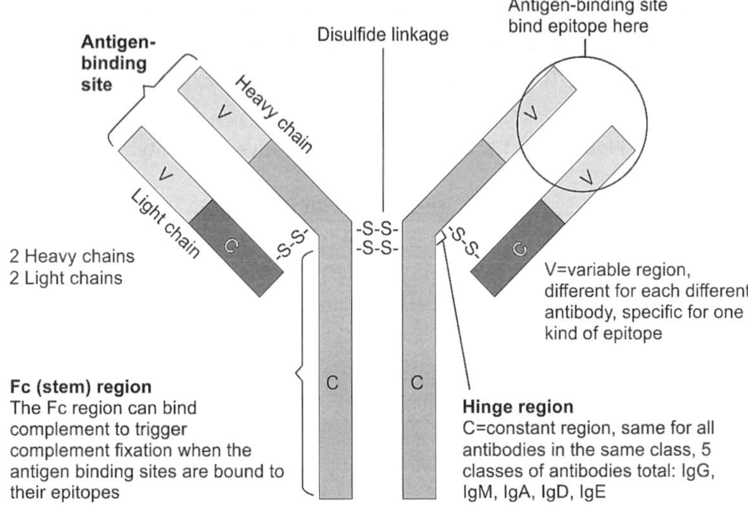

Figure 4.1.5: Basic structure of an antibody (immunoglobulin).

- The Ig monomer is a "Y"-shaped molecule that consists of four polypeptide chains; two identical heavy chains (H) and two identical light chains (L) connected by Disulfide bonds.
- Each heavy and light chain is made-up of a number of domains (i.e Ig folding or Ig domain).
- Each domain is about 110 Amino acids in length and contains an interchain Disulfide bond.
- Each chain in antibody consists of two regions- Constant (C) and Variable (V) region. Amino acid sequence in the C-terminal regions of the H and L chains is the same whereas the amino acid sequence in the variable region of H and L chains is different.
- The regions of variable domains actually contact the antigen and hence make up the antigen-binding site.
- Some parts of an antibody have unique functions. The arms of the Y for example, contain the sites that can bind two antigens (in general identical) and therefore recognize specific foreign objects. This region of the antibody is called the Fab (Fragment, antigen binding) region. It is composed of one constant and one variable domain from each heavy and light chain of the antibody.

- The variable domain is referred to as the FV region and is the most important region for binding to antigens.
- Fc region of the antibody is the region that triggers complement fixation reaction.

Classes of Antibodies/Immunoglobulins (Figure 4.1.6)

IgG Antibodies

- Monomer
- 80% of serum antibodies
- Produced on second+exposure
- In blood, lymph
- Can enter tissue, cross placenta
- Fix complement, enhance phagocytosis, neutralize toxin and viruses, protects fetus and newborn, antiserum

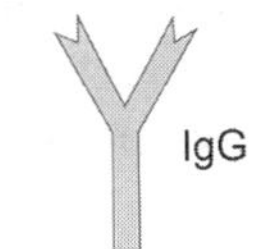

IgM antibodies

- Pentamer
- 5–10% of serum antibodies
- Produced only on first exposure
- In blood, lymph, on B cells
- Fix complement, agglutinates antigen

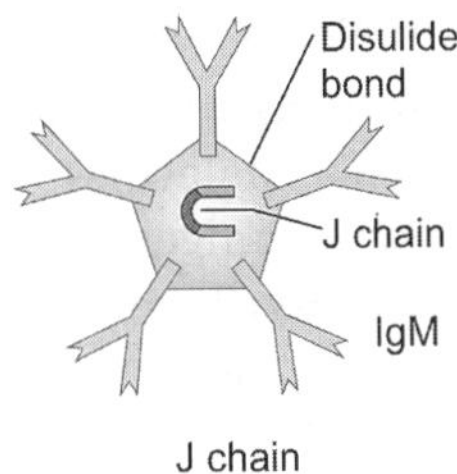

IgA Antibodies

- Dimer
- 10–15% of serum antibodies
- In secretions
- Mucosal protection

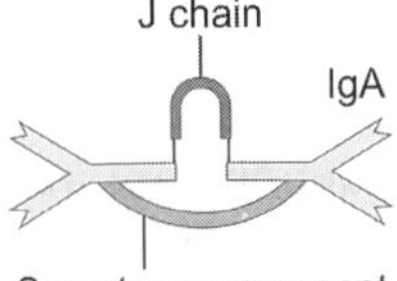

IgD Antibodies

- Monomer
- 0.2% of serum antibodies
- Surface receptor on B cells
- Initiate humoral immune response by B cells

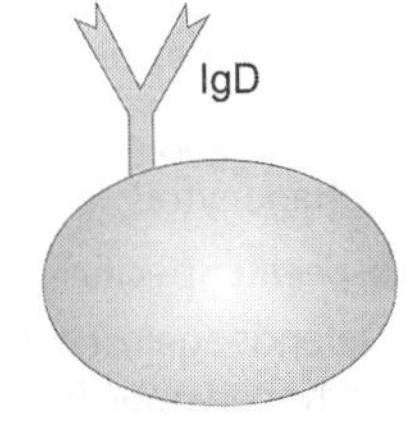

IgE Antibodies

- Monomer
- 0.002% of serum antibodies
- Surface receptor on mast cells and basophils
- Inflammation allergic reaction; lysis of parasitic worms

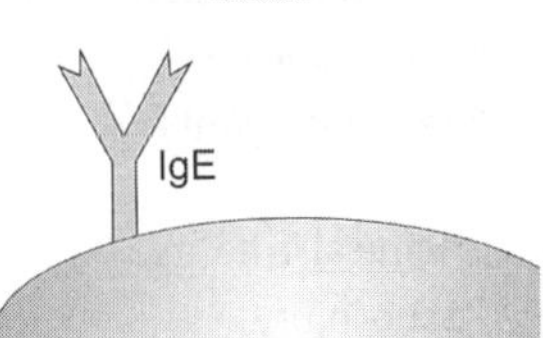

Figure 4.1.6: Classes of immunoglobulins.

T-cells are the constituent of lymphocytes that undergo differentiation during immune response and develop into several sub-populations of effector T-cells that have an effect on many other cells. Some develop into T–Cytotoxic cells that attack and kill targets directly. Targets for Tc-cells include cells infected by viruses and cancerous cells. Other T-cells may develop into T-Helper cells and T-Suppressor cells that stimulate the activities of other leukocytes through cell to cell contact or through secretion of cytokines. This part of immune response is called as Cellular or Cell-mediated immunity.

The collaboration between B-cells and T-cells (Specially T-Helper cells) is important for almost all antibody responses to antigens.

Features of Adaptive Immunity (Figure 4.1.7)

- **Specificity:** Lymphocytes (B- and T-cells) bind and respond to foreign molecules (antigens) via antigen receptors: each to a specific antigen
- **Diversity:** The body possesses millions of lymphocytes that can recognize and respond to millions of antigens (one each)
- **Memory:** 1" exposure to an antigen generates lymphocytes and long-lived memory cells — next exposure to the same antigen, memory cells react more quickly and stronger response (acquired immunity')
- **Self-Tolerance**: Lymphocytes can distinguish self (our normal antigens) from non- sell (antigens from foreign material).

Table: 4.1.3: Difference between innate and adaptive immunity.

Innate vs adaptive immunity	
Innate (phagocytois, inflammation)	Adaptive (lymphocytes)
• Nonspecific specific	• Specific
▪ Defends against *any* pathogen upon first exposure	▪ Responds to specific pathogens on 2nd or later exposure
▪ Responds to:	
• Infectious agents	▪ Comes into play after nonspecific responses have begun
• Chemical irritants	
• Tissue injury	
• Burns	

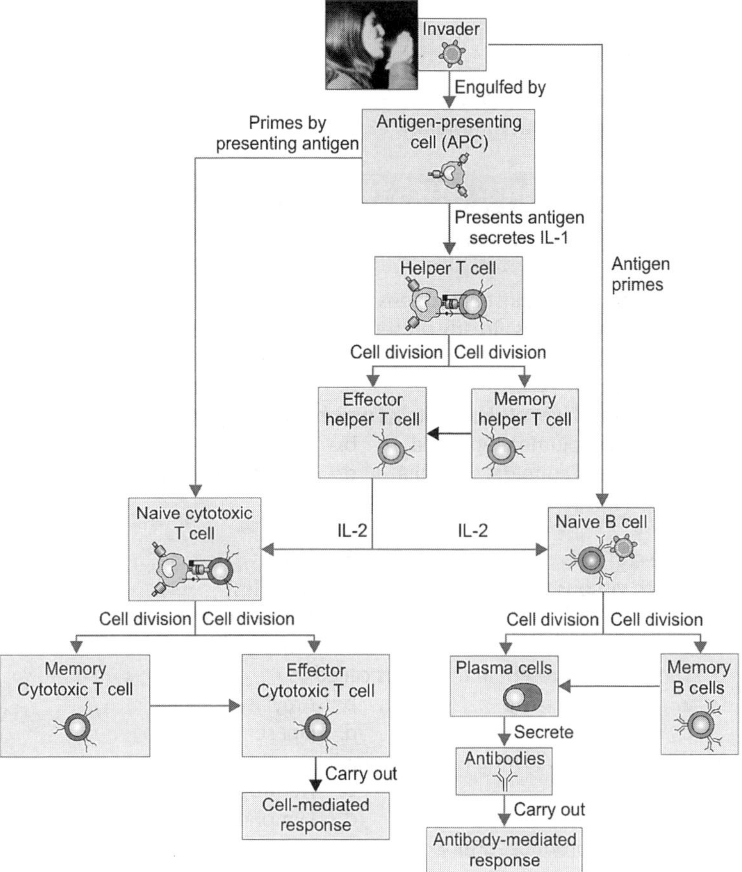

Figure 4.1.7: Summarizes an example of adaptive immune response when exposed to a microbial antigen.

POSSIBLE QUESTIONS

1. Describe innate immunity
2. What is immunity? Describe adaptive immunity with its features.

SHORT NOTES

1. Mucous membrane
2. Lymphatic system
3. Phagocytosis

4. Types of phagocytic cells
5. Cytokinesis
6. Interferons
7. Classes of immunoglobulins
8. Features of adaptive immunity.

MULTIPLE CHOICE QUESTIONS

1. The word immunis refers to ____________.
   a. Exempt
   b. Having high degree to resist
   c. Protecting against pathogens
   d. All of the above
2. Which immunity is already present in the body since birth?
   a. Adaptive
   b. Innate
   c. Acquired
   d. All of the above
3. Outer most layer of skin contains which type of epithelial cell?
   a. Simple columnar epithelia
   b. Stratified squamous epithelia
   c. Stratified cuboidal epithelia
   d. Simple cuboidal epithelia
4. The pH range of skin is in between ______.
   a. 3-4
   b. 3-5
   c. 2-4
   d. 5-6
5. Which viscous fluid traps microbes and particles?
   a. Cell membrane
   b. Mucous membrane
   c. Plasma membrane
   d. None of the above
6. The enzyme present in the tear is called as _____________.
   a. Lysozyme
   b. Amylase
   c. Protease
   d. Lipase
7. Which of the following is not a granulocytes?
   a. Basophils
   b. Neutrophils
   c. Eosinophils
   d. Lymphocytes
8. Which cell produces antibodies?
   a. B-cells
   b. T-cells
   c. Mast cells
   d. None of the above
9. The word Homeostasis refers to __________.
   a. Blood clotting
   b. Blood realising
   c. Both a and b
   d. None of the above
10. IgG antibodies are present in:
    a. Blood
    b. Lymph
    c. Both a and b
    d. B cells

Answers

1. d	2. b	3. b	4. b	5. b
6. a	7. d	8. a	9. a	10. c

CHAPTER 4.2

Hypersensitivity and Autoimmunity

Hypersensitivity is increased reactivity or increased sensitivity by the animal body to an antigen to which it has been previously exposed. The term is often used as a synonym for allergy, which describes a state of altered reactivity to an antigen.

Hypersensitivity has been divided into categories based upon whether it can be passively transferred by antibodies or by specifically immune lymphoid cells. The most widely adopted current classification is that of Coombs and Gell which designates immunoglobulin-mediated (immediate) hypersensitivity reactions as types I, II, and III, and lymphoid cell-mediated (delayed-type) hypersensitivity/cell-mediated immunity as a type IV reaction.

"Hypersensitivity" generally represents the "dark side," signifying the undesirable aspects of an immune reaction, whereas the term "immunity" implies a desirable effect. A hypersensitive response (HR) is an anti-pathogen response in plants produced by avr-R system activation that leads to alterations in Ca+ flux, MAPK activation, and NO and ROI formation. There is rapid necrosis of plant cells in contact with the pathogen. This process prevents spread of the pathogen and releases hydrolytic enzymes that facilitate injury to the pathogen's structural integrity.

CAUSES OF HYPERSENSITIVITY

Immune responses that are the cause of hypersensitivity diseases may be specific for antigens from different sources:

- Autoimmunity: reactions against self-antigens.
- Reactions against microbes.
- Reactions against non-microbial environmental antigens.

MECHANISM OF HYPERSENSITIVITY

Hypersensitivity diseases are commonly classified according to the type of immune response and the effector mechanism responsible for cell and tissue injury. These mechanisms include some that are predominantly dependent on antibodies and others predominantly dependent on T cells, although a role for both humoral and cell-mediated immunity is often found in many hypersensitivity diseases.

Immediate (Type I) Hypersensitivity

It is caused by IgE antibodies specific for environmental antigens and is the most prevalent type of hypersensitivity disease. Immediate hypersensitivity diseases, commonly grouped under allergy or atopy, are often caused by activation of interleukin-4 (IL-4), IL-5, and IL-13 producing Th2 cells and the production of IgE antibodies, which activate mast cells and eosinophils and induce inflammation.

Antibody-mediated (Type II) Hypersensitivity

IgG and IgM antibodies specific for cell surface or extracellular matrix antigens can cause tissue injury by activating the complement system, by recruiting inflammatory cells, and by interfering with normal cellular functions.

Immune Complex-mediated (Type III) Hypersensitivity

IgM and IgG antibodies specific for soluble antigens in the blood form complexes with the antigens, and the immune complexes may deposit in blood vessel walls in various tissues, causing inflammation, thrombosis, and tissue injury.

T Cell-mediated (Type IV) Hypersensitivity

In these disorders, tissue injury may be due to T lymphocytes that induce inflammation or directly kill target cells. In most of these diseases, the major mechanism involves the activation of CD4+ helper T cells, which secrete cytokines that promote inflammation and activate leukocytes, mainly neutrophils and macrophages. CTLs contribute to tissue injury in some diseases.

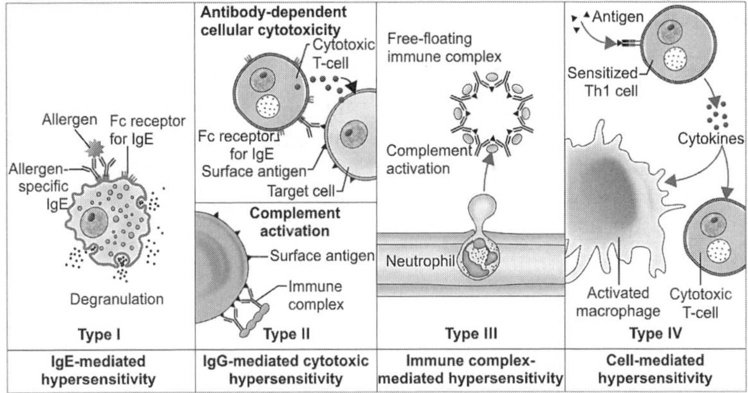

Figure. 4.2.1: Types of hypersensitivity reactions.

TYPES OF HYPERSENSITIVITY REACTIONS

The Gell's and Coombs' classification of hypersensitivity reactions considers four types of reactions. Type I, II, and III reactions are basically mediated by antibodies with or without participation of the complement system; type IV reactions are cell-mediated. While in many pathological processes mechanisms classified in more than one of these types of hypersensitivity reactions may be operative, the subdivision of hypersensitivity states into four broad types aids considerably in the understanding of their pathogenesis.

HYPERSENSITIVITY TYPE I, II, III AND IV- SUMMARY IN TABLE FORM

Alternative Name

Type I	Type II	Type III	Type IV
Allergic hypersensitivity	Cytotoxic hypersensitivity	Immune complex hypersensitivity	Cell-mediated hypersensitivity/ Delayed type of hypersensitivity

Principle

Type I	Type II	Type III	Type IV
Antibody-mediated degranulation of granulocytes leads to the destruction of cells.	Antibody-mediated destruction of healthy cells.	Antigen-antibody complex-mediated destruction of cells.	T lymphocytes mediated the destruction of cells.

Primary Mediator

Type I	Type II	Type III	Type IV
IgE	IgG/IgM	IgG/IgM	Specific subsets of CD4+ helper T cells or CD8+ cytotoxic T cells

Other Components as Mediators

Type I	Type II	Type III	Type IV
Mast cell, basophils, histamine and other pharmacological agents	Complement, neutrophils	Complement, phagocytes, and K cells	Dendritic cells, macrophages, and cytokines

Reaction Time

Type I	Type II	Type III	Type IV
Immediate or within a few hours	5–8 hours	2–8 hours	After 24 hours only, mostly 48–72 hours after contact

Antigen

Type I	Type II	Type III	Type IV
Free in circulation (Soluble)	Fixed on cells	Free in circulation (Soluble)	Soluble or cell-bound

Antigen Origin

Type I	Type II	Type III	Type IV
Exogenous	Endogenous or exogenous	Exogenous or endogenous	Exogenous or endogenous

Antibody

Type I	Type II	Type III	Type IV
Fixed on mast cells and basophils	Free in circulation	Free in circulation	Not applicable

Mechanism

Type I	Type II	Type III	Type IV
Allergen-specific IgE antibodies bind to mast cells via their Fc receptor. When the specific allergen binds to the IgE, cross-linking of IgE induces degranulation of mast cells.	IgG or IgM antibody binds to a cellular antigen, leading to complement activation and cell lysis. IgG can also mediate ADCC with cytotoxic T cells, natural killer cells, macrophages, and neutrophils.	Antigen-antibody complexes are deposited in tissues. Complement activation provides inflammatory mediators and recruits neutrophils. Enzymes released from neutrophils damage tissue.	Th2 cells secrete cytokines, which activate macrophages and cytotoxic T cells.

Complement Activation

Type I	Type II	Type III	Type IV
No	Yes	Yes	No

Appearance

Type I	Type II	Type III	Type IV
Weal and flare	Lysis and necrosis	Erythema and edema	Erythema and induration

Transfer with Serum

Type I	Type II	Type III	Type IV
Passive transfer possible with serum	Passive transfer	Passive transfer	Cannot be transferred with serum; but possible with T cells transfer

Desensitization

Type I	Type II	Type III	Type IV
Easy but short-lived	Easy but short-lived	Easy but short-lived	Difficult but long-lived

Examples

Type I	Type II	Type III	Type IV
Asthma, Rhinitis, Atopic eczema, Bee sting reaction	Rhesus incompatibility (Rh hemolytic disease), Transfusion reactions, cell destruction due to autoantigens, drug-induced hemolytic anemia	Glomerulonephritis, systemic lupus erythematosus, Farmer's lung arthritis, vasculitis	The tuberculin reaction, granuloma formation, allergic contact dermatitis, Type-1 diabetes

HYPERSENSITIVITY TYPE I: IMMEDIATE REACTION

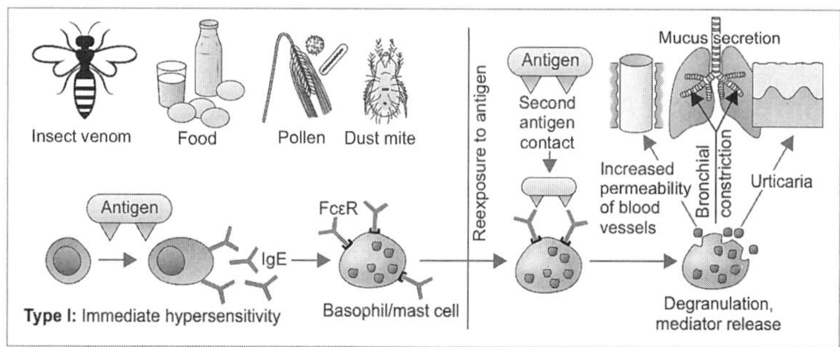

Some antigens (allergens), such as insect venom, foods, pollen, and dust mite, can induce the formation of IgE antibodies in individuals with a corresponding predisposition. The IgE antibodies bind via Fc receptors to mast cells (sensitization). If the individual is re-exposed to the allergen, cross-linkage of the membrane-bound IgE occurs. This results in the immediate release of mediators (e.g., histamine, kininogen), which induce vasodilation, smooth muscle contraction, mucus secretion, edema, and/or skin blisters. Most allergens are small proteins that can easily diffuse through the skin or mucosa. They are frequently proteases and are active at very low doses. IL-4 favors the differentiation of TH2 cells. The exact mechanism that leads B cells to produce IgE is not known.

The allergen stimulates the induction of CD4+T cells. These T cells secrete cytokines that cause IgE production by plasma cells.

The IgE molecule will bind to the Fc receptor on mast cells and basophils which in turn causes vasodilation increased vascular permeability and vascular spasm. This type may occur as a systemic or local reaction:

- **Systemic reactions:** Skin erythema, followed by respiratory difficulty due to bronchial constriction.
- **Local reactions:** Generally on the skin or mucosal surface at the site of Ag exposure. Allergy to penicillin, *Aspergillus* spores, rupture of *Echinococcus* cyst.

HYPERSENSITIVITY TYPE II: ANTIBODY-MEDIATED CYTOTOXIC REACTION

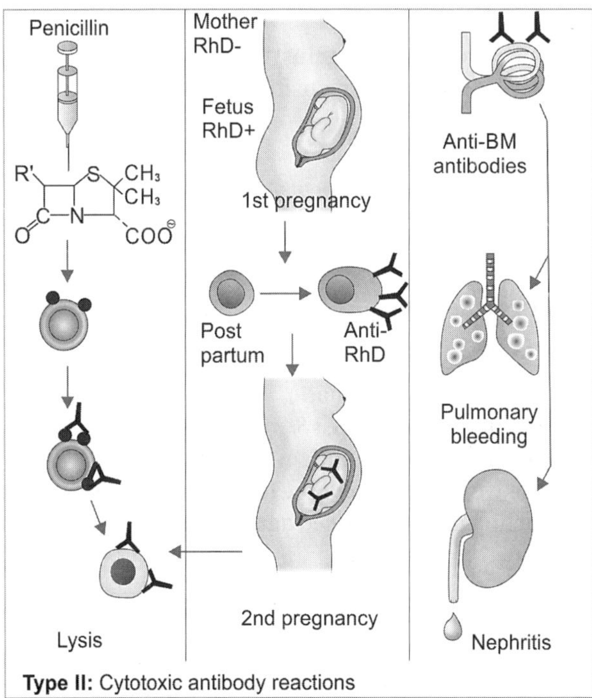

Type II: Cytotoxic antibody reactions

The immunization of individuals to erythrocyte antigens during pregnancy is a typical example of a type II reaction. Children who inherit the RhD erythrocyte antigen from their father can induce immunization against the RhD+ antigen in their RhD-mother. Sensitization usually occurs at birth when fetal blood cells come into contact with the maternal immune system. In any subsequent pregnancies, maternal anti-RhD antibodies of the IgG type can pass into the placenta and cause severe hemolysis of fetal RhD+ erythrocytes.

Other examples: Drugs (e.g., penicillin) can passively bind to erythrocytes. Antibodies directed against penicillin then lead to lysis of the erythrocytes. The formation of antibodies directed against the basement membrane (BM) of the glomerulus can develop during the course of kidney inflammation. Lung damage accompanied by pulmonary hemorrhage and renal inflammation (glomerulonephritis) may occur due to cross-reaction of these antibodies with the basement membrane of the lung (Goodpasture's syndrome).

In this type Ab are formed against target Ag that are cell membrane components. Not really hypersensitivity, but cytotoxic reactions:

Complement-mediated

- Ab reacts with cell surface Ag leading to fixation of the complement system and then cell lysis, e.g., red cells are the most common cells damaged by this mechanism.

Many Cell Types (Macrophages, Neutrophils, NK Cells) Cause Lysis of Target Cell Coated by IgG

- Poststreptococcal rheumatic fever: Molecular mimicry: Antibodies produced against *S. pyogenes* cross-react with various tissue, e.g., heart, joints - inflammation.
- Oncocerca worm infection may lead to blindness because of the cross-reaction of Ab produced against pathogens and proteins of the retina.

Antibody-mediated Cellular Dysfunction

- In some cases Ab is directed against cell surface receptor impairing the function but not cause cell injury.

HYPERSENSITIVITY TYPE III: IMMUNE COMPLEX-MEDIATED REACTION

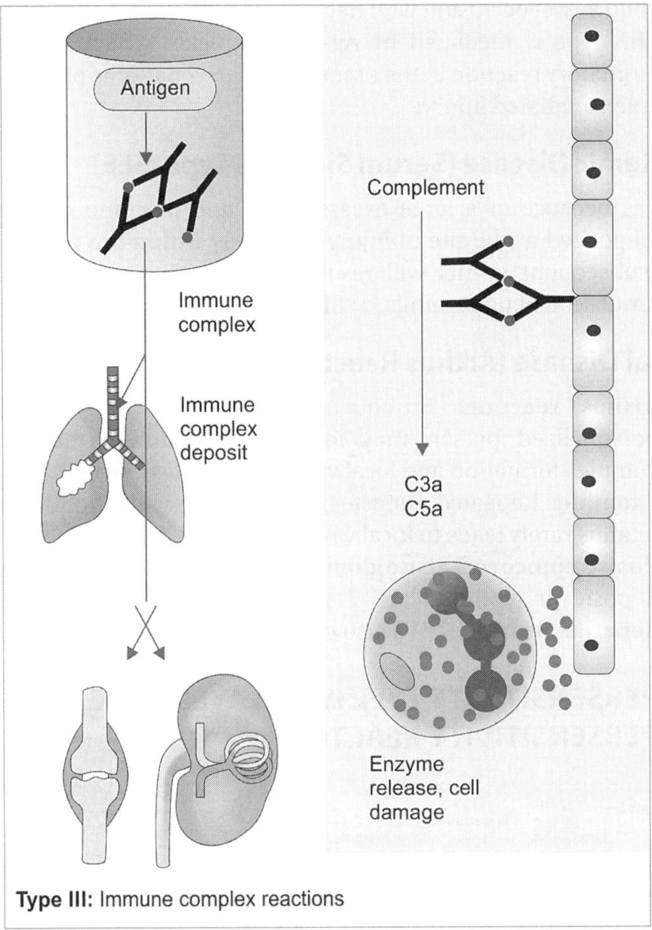

Type III: Immune complex reactions

Antibody-antigen complexes (immune complexes) can form during an immune response. Immune complexes can settle in vessel walls, the basement membrane of the lungs and/or kidneys, and in the joints (synovia). They can induce inflammatory processes in these structures by binding complement factors C3a and C5a (anaphylatoxins). A particular type III reaction is the Arthus reaction: when an antigen has penetrated the skin of an individual who has preformed IgG antibodies, the immune complexes can bind to Fc receptors of most cells inducing degranulation inflammatory cells are recruited and complement is activated, leading to the release of C5a and local inflammation, platelet accumulation, and eventually to blood vessel occlusion with necrosis.

This type is mediated by Ag-Ab complexes which initiate an inflammatory reaction in the tissue. There are 2 patterns of immune-complex mediated injury:

Systemic Disease (Serum Sickness Type, SLE)

This is because of a large excess of Ab and immune complexes are deposited at the site of injury especially within the vessel wall, the subsequent events will result in necrotizing vasculititis and accumulation of neutrophils>>>SLE

Local Disease (Arthus Reaction)

- **Arthus reaction:** Intraductal injection of antigens to a personalized person may lead to local intradermal Ab-Ag complex formation and local vasculitis, redness, swelling.
- **Example:** Repeated (booster) vaccination with diphtheria or tetanus rarely leads to local vasculitis.
- **Poststreptococcal acute glomerulonephritis:** Ab-ag complexes deposit in glomeruli HBV infection: HBsAg-Ab complexes **hepatitis B virus (HBV)** also cause acute glomerulonephritis.

HYPERSENSITIVITY TYPE IV: DELAYED-TYPE HYPERSENSITIVITY REACTION

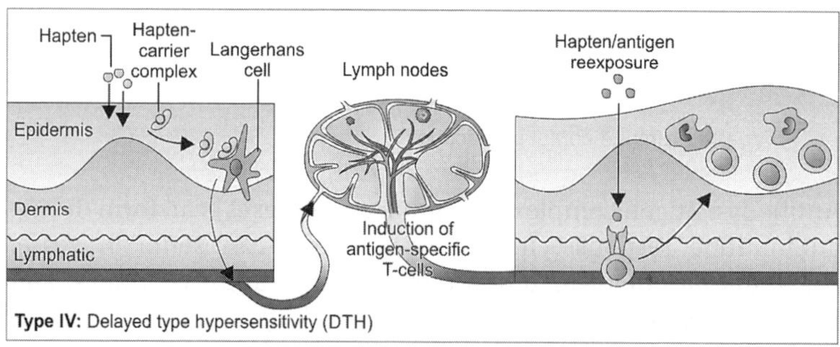

Type IV: Delayed type hypersensitivity (DTH)

Haptens are molecules of very small molecular weight (often < 1 kDa. They are too small to function as antigens, but they can penetrate the epidermis and bind to certain proteins in the skin (carrier proteins).

Hapten-carrier complexes are bound by antigen-presenting cells of the skin (Langerhans cells), which then migrate to regional lymph nodes. T-cell stimulation then occurs at the lymph node. The so-called sensitization phase lasts approximately for 10–14 days. If the individual is reexposed to the hapten, antigen-specific T cells migrate to the skin, where they accumulate and proliferate. They also cause edema formation and local inflammation with the help of cytokines. Compounds containing nickel or chrome and chemicals such as those found in rubber are typical triggers of type IV hypersensitivity reactions.

This is mediated by T-cells. There are 2 types that involve CD4/8+T Cells.

Acute (within 2-3 days)

- Tuberculin test, contact dermatitis: Mediated by CD4+ T helper cells cd4+ cells recognize ag (tuberculin), this leads to the formation of sensitized cd4+ cells.
- Upon cutaneous injection into previously sensitized individual sensitized cd4+cells become activated and secrete cytokines.
- Tuberculin/Manntoux test: Intradermal injection of tuberculin = purified tuberculoprotein leads to swelling after 48–72 h if the patient has been exposed to *Mycobacterium tuberculosis* previously.

Chronic (> 1 week)

- Granuloma formation, graft rejection: Mediated by cd8+ cytotoxic T cell.
- Lymphocytes surrounding epitheloid cells lead to the formation of granuloma.

Autoimmune Diseases

- Autoimmune is a disorder of the body's defense mechanism in which an immune response is generated against component or products of its own tissues treating them as foreign material and attacking them.
- The disorder caused by inflammation and destruction of tissues by the body's immune response as a result of autoimmunity is known as autoimmune disease.

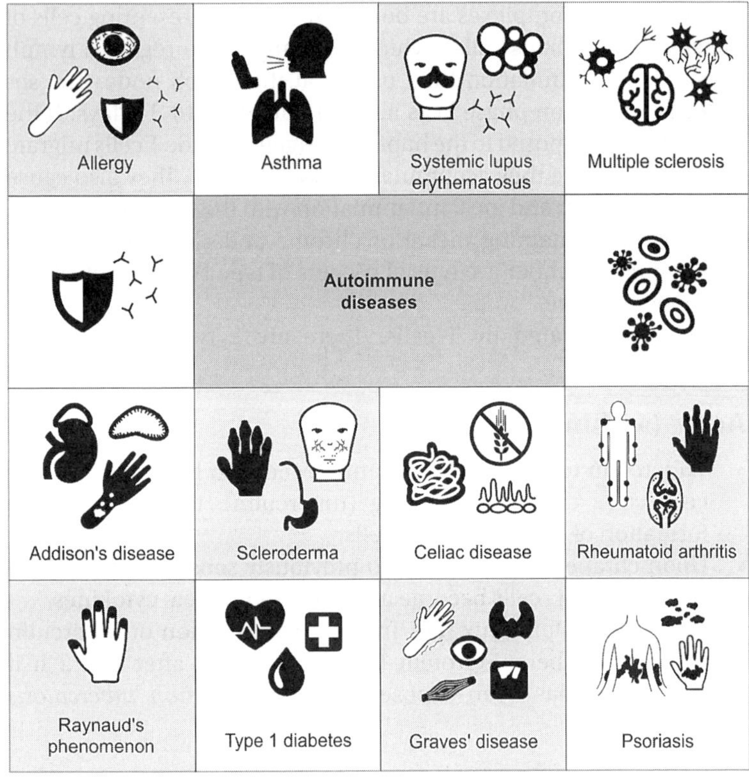

Proposed Mechanism for Induction of Autoimmunity

A variety of mechanisms have been proposed to account for the T-cell mediated generation of autoimmune disease. And it is likely that autoimmune disease does not develop from a single event rather from a number of different events.

Some of the Proposed Mechanisms:

- Forbidden clone
- Altered antigen
- Sequestered antigen
- Immunological deficiency theory
- Genetic influence

Forbidden Clone

Mutation in the lymphocytes may result in the formation of changed or altered clone. These altered clone may recognize host as foreign and lead to development of autoimmunity.

Altered Antigen

Some of the antigens on the host cell get altered by chemical, biological or physical means. Thus formed new antigenic determinants which may be recognized as foreign by the host.

Sequestered Antigen

- Some of the antigens in the body are hidden from cells of immune system.
- If the organs containing such antigens are damaged, it causes exposure of sequestered antigen thus an immune reaction to these antigens may occur.

Immunological Deficiency Theory

- According to this theory, mutation or loss of immune regulatory power, i.e., deficiency in immune system results in a condition in which self-antigen behaves as foreign.

Genetic Influence

- This was determined by family studies. It is well recognized that certain immune disorder predominate in females and families.
- This has strongly supported the role of genetic influence in autoimmunity.
- Genetic links have occurred between disease and HLA antigens.

Types of Autoimmune Disease

On the basis of pathogenic mechanism, autoimmune disease are classified into two types:

Organ Specific Autoimmune Disease

- This autoimmune disease is directed against a component of one particular type of organ.
- The organ specific autoimmune disease can further be divided into two groups:

- **Autoimmune disease mediated by direct cellular damage:**
  - This type of damage occur when lymphocytes or antibodies bind to cell membrane antigens, causing cellular lysis or inflammatory response in affected organ.
  - The damaged cellular structure is then replaced by connective tissue (fibrous) and it losses its function.
  - **Examples**: Hashimoto's thyroiditis, autoimmune anemia, Goodpasture's syndrome, Insulin dependent diabetes mellitus.
- **Autoimmune disease mediated by stimulating or blocking auto antibodies:**
  - In some cases, antibodies act as antagonist and bind to hormone receptor stimulating inappropriate activity. This usually leads to overproduction of mediators or increase cell growth.
  - They also bind to hormone receptor function and thereby block receptor function. This causes impaired secretion of mediators and gradual atrophy of the affected organ.
  - **Examples**: Grave's disease, Myasthenia gravis.

Systematic Autoimmune Disease

- It is the type of autoimmune disease which is directed against an antigen that is present in many different sites and can include involvement of several organs and tissues.
- These disease reflect a general defect in immune regulation that result in hyperactive T-cells and B-cells.
- **Examples**: Rheumatoid arthritis, Systematic lupus erythematosus (SLE), multiple sclerosis.

Some Examples of Autoimmune Diseases

Graves Disease

- The production of thyroid hormones is carefully regulated by thyroid stimulating hormone (TSH) produced by pituitary gland. The binding of TSH to receptor on thyroid cell activates adenylate cyclase enzyme stimulating synthesis of thyroxine and tri-iodo thyroxine.
- A patient with Graves' disease produces autoantibody (LATS) that bind to receptor of TSH and mimic the normal action of TSH, activating adenylate cyclase and resulting in production

of thyroid hormones. Unlike TSH, however autoantibody are not regulated and consequently they overstimulate the thyroid gland.

Myasthenia Gravis

- It is an autoimmune disease mediated by blocking antibodies.
- A patient with this disease produces autoantibodies that bind the acetylcholine receptor on motor end plates of muscles, blocking the normal binding of acetylcholine. The result is progressive weakening the skeletal muscles.
- It also inducing complement mediated lysis of cells and the antibodies cause the destruction of the cells bearing receptors.

Hashimoto's Thyroiditis

- In Hashimoto thyroiditis, an individual produces antibodies and sensitized TH1 cell specific for thyroid antigens.
- An attending delayed type hypersensitivity (DTH) response is characterized by an intense infiltration of the thyroid gland by lymphocytes, macrophages and plasma cells which form lymphocytic follicles and germinal centers.
- The ensuring inflammatory response cause goiter or visible enlargement of the thyroid gland, a physiological response to hypothyroidism.
- Hypothyroidism is caused when antibodies are formed to a number of thyroid proteins including thyroglobulin and thyroid peroxidase, both of which are involved in the uptake of iodine.
- Binding of autoantibodies to these protein interfere with thyroid gland functioning.

Goodpasture's Syndrome

- In Goodpasture's syndrome, autoautobodies specific for certain basement membrane antigen bind to basement membrane of kidney glomeruli and alveoli of lungs.
- Subsequent complement activation leads to direct cellular damage and an ensuring inflammatory response meditated by a buildup of complement split products.
- Damage to the glomerulus and alveolar basement membrane leads to progressive kidney damage and pulmonary hemorrhage.
- Death may ensure within several months of the onset of symptoms.

Autoimmune Anemias

- Autoimmune anemias include pernicious anemia, autoimmune hemolytic anemia (AIHA) and drug-induced hemolytic anemia.
  - **Pernicious anemia** is caused by autoantibodies to intrinsic factor, a membrane bound intestinal protein on gastric parietal cells which facilitate uptake of vitamin B_{12} from small intestine. Binding of autoantibody to intrinsic factor block absorption of vitamin B_{12}. In absence of sufficient vitamin B_{12}, which is necessary for proper hematopoiesis, the number of functional mature RBCs decrease below normal.
  - **Autoimmune hemolytic anemia:** An individual with autoimmune hemolytic anemia makes autoantibody to red-blood cell antigen, triggering complement mediated lysis or antibody-mediated opsonization and phagocytosis of RBC.
  - **In drug-induced hemolytic anemia,** certain drugs such as penicillin or anti-hypertensive agents like methyldopa interact with RBC, the cells become antigenic.

Insulin Dependent Diabetes Mellitus (IDDM)

- IDDM is caused by an autoimmune attack on pancreas.
- The attack is directed against specialized insulin producing beta-cell that are location in spherical cluster islets of Langerhans, scattered throughout the pancreas.
- The autoimmune attack destroys beta cell resulting in decreased production of insulin and consequently increased level of blood glucose.
- Several factors are important in destruction of beta cells, first activated CTLs migrate into an islet and begin to attack the insulin producing cells.
- The CTL infiltration and activation of macrophages, frequently referred to as insulitis which is followed by cytokine release and presence of autoantibodies which lead to a cell- mediated DTH.
- The autoantibodies to beta cells may contribute to cell distribution by facilitating either antibody-mediated complement lysis or antibody-dependent cell-mediated cytotoxicity (ADCC).

Systemic Lupus Erythematosus

- One of the best example of a systemic autoimmune disease is systemic lupus erythematosus (SLE).

- The individual affected by SLE may produce autoantibodies to a vast array of tissues, antigens, such as DNA, histones, RBCs, platelets, leukocytes, and clotting factors.
- Interaction of these autoantibodies with their specific antigens produces various symptoms.
- Autoantibody specific for RBC and platelets for examples, can lead to complement mediated lysis resulting in hemolytic anemia and thrombocytopenia, respectively.
- When immune complex of autoantibodies with various nuclear antigens are deposited along the walls of small blood vessels, a type III hypersensitivity reaction develops.
- The complexes activates the complement system and generate membrane-attack complexes and complement split produces that damage the wall of the blood vessel, resulting in vasculitis and glomerulonephritis.

Multiple Sclerosis

- Multiple sclerosis (MS) is the most common cause of neurologic disability associated with autoimmune disease in western country.
- With this disease production of auto-reactive T-cell that participate in the formation of inflammatory lesions along the myelin sheath of nerve fibers.
- The cerebrospinal fluid of patient with active MS contains activated T lymphocytes, which infiltrate the brain tissue and cause characteristic inflammatory lesions, destroying the myelin.
- Since myelin function to insulate the nerve fibers, a breakdown in the myelin sheath leads to numerous neurologic dysfunctions.

Rheumatoid Arthritis

- Rheumatoid arthritis is common autoimmune disorder.
- Many individuals with rheumatoid arthritis produce a group of autoantibodies called rheumatoid factors that are reactive with determinants of Fc region of IgG antibody.
- The classic rheumatoid factor is an IgM antibody with that reactivity. Such autoantibodies bind to normal circulating IgG, forming IgM–IgG complexes that are deposited in the joints.
- The immune complexes can activate the complement cascade, resulting in type III hypersensitive reaction which leads to chronic inflammation of the joints.

POSSIBLE QUESTIONS

1. What is Hypersensitivity ? Discuss its mechanism and causes.
2. Discuss immediate and antibody-mediated cytotoxic reaction.
3. What is autoimmunity? Discuss the proposed mechanisms and give 2 examples of autoimmune disease.

SHORT NOTES

1. Rheumatoid arthritis.
2. Graves disease.
3. Causes of hypersensitivity.

MULTIPLE CHOICE QUESTIONS

1. Hypersensitivity refers to ______________.
   a. Increased sensitivity to an antigen
   b. Excessively sensitivity to an antigen
   c. Inappropriate immunologic response to antigen
   d. All of the above
2. Immediate hypersensitivity is caused by ____________.
   a. IgE b. IgG
   c. IgB d. All of the above
3. Which secrete cytokines?
   a. Th cells b. Macrophages
   c. Both a and b d. None of the above
4. IDDM is caused by autoimmune attack on ______________.
   a. Liver b. Pancreas
   c. Heart d. Stomach
5. Which of the following is not a systematic autoimmune disease?
   a. Multiple sclerosis b. Rheumatoid arthritis
   c. SLE d. Asthma
6. Which of the following is an organ specific autoimmune disease?
   a. Thyroiditis b. IDSM
   c. Autoimmune anemia d. All of the above
7. Which molecule can bind to protein in skin?
   a. Haptens b. Actin
   c. Ferritin d. None of the above
8. Which disease occurs due to bronchial constriction?
   a. Skin erythema b. Asthma
   c. Emphysema d. All of the above
9. Which of the following immunoglobin is specific for soluble antigens ?
   a. IgM b. IgG
   c. IgE d. Both a and b

10. Which of the following types of hypersensitivity has lowest time of reaction?
    a. Type I
    b. Type II
    c. Type III
    d. Type IV

Answers

1. d	2. a	3. c	4. b	5. d
6. d	7. a	8. d	9. d	10. a

Immunoprophylaxis of Infectious Diseases and Immunization Schedule

Prophylaxis of infectious diseases represents the actions taken before or shortly upon exposure of an individual to an infectious agent or its product (e.g. toxin), aimed to prevent infection and disease development. The most important prophylactic method is **immunoprophylaxis** in which a process of **immunization** is used for preventing infections. The goal of immunization is to induce immunity (i.e. state of resistance to an infection) in an immunized person for a certain period of time (that may vary from several weeks to several decades).

- Immunization can be achieved spontaneously without any intentional human activity (called **natural immunization**) or by a deliberate action of men (so-called **artificial immunization**), and both of them can be actively induced in an individual by exposure to a pathogen or its components or products (**active immunization**) or passively adopted through immunoglobulin transfer (**passive immunization).**
- Natural immunity is actively induced after each infection, whereas the neonatal protection by maternal antibodies transported across the placenta to the fetus (IgG) and via immunoglobulins in milk (breastfeeding - predominantly IgA) is an example of natural passive immunization.
- On the other hand, **artificial active immunization** is most commonly done by exposure of an individual to nonpathogenic forms or microbes or their components and/or products, a process called **vaccination**, while **artificial passive immunization** represents the induction of immunity through administration of human immunoglobulins or animal sera specific for the pathogen or its toxins. In the text that follows, these two forms of immunization performed by medical workers will be described in more details.

PASSIVE IMMUNIZATION

- Artificial passive immunization is mediated by the administration of antibodies of human or animal origin to an individual.
- These products have **immediate action**, but induce **short-lived immunity** that lasts weeks to several months, which is determined by the half-life of immunoglobulins (around three weeks for IgG and only few days for the other isotypes).
- In general, passive immunization is used for **prophylactic purposes**, to protect immunodeficient patients (prematurely born children or patients with defects in humoral immunity) against various infections or to prevent disease development after exposure of an individual to a particular pathogen (for example, after accidental injury by the HBV- contaminated needle or bite by the animals infected by rabies virus).
- However, in some cases, passive immunization (owing to its immediate action) can also be used for **therapy** with the aim to reduce the clinical symptoms of the disease and often represents the life-saving therapeutic method.
- For example, it is used for toxin-mediated diseases such as diphtheria and botulism, or when the person is exposed to some toxins from animals, such as snake venoms.
- Passive immunity is most commonly induced by the administration of human immunoglobulins, but animal sera and monoclonal antibodies are also sometimes used for the passive immunization of individuals.

The immunoglobulins of human origin contain primarily IgG antibodies extracted from the plasma of great number of blood donors and usually are given via intravenous or intramuscular routes of administration. Depending on the method of production and the purpose of their application, two groups of products are available:

- **Human serum globulin** (**gammaglobulin** or **intravenous immunoglobulins**, **IVIG**) contains antibodies that are specific for various pathogens that are commonly encountered by the majority of people and are present in the blood of most adults (the normal repertoire of antibodies in human population). They are extracted from the plasma of thousands of randomly selected blood donors. These products are used for the prophylaxis of infectious diseases in patients with a deficit in antibody production (hypo- or agammaglobulinemia). Also, they are sometimes used for prevention of specific infectious diseases (e.g. measles, hepatitis A, rubella in the first trimester of pregnancy, etc.) in cases when the products with high titer of specific immunoglobulins (see below) are not available. In addition to prevention of infectious disease, intravenous immunoglobulins (IVIG) are also being increasingly used for hematological diseases (for example, idiopathic thrombocytopenia, ITP) and various autoimmune diseases.

- **Specific immunoglobulins** or **high-titer immunoglobulins** (also called **hyperimmune globulins**) contain high titer of antibodies specific for particular pathogen and they are used in the prophylaxis or therapy for specific infectious disease. They are extracted from the plasma of seropositive people with high-titer antibodies for a certain pathogen, i.e., those who were vaccinated or recently suffered from the disease caused by that pathogen. These products have been developed for hepatitis B, tetanus, rabies, respiratory syncytial virus (RSV), varicella (chickenpox) and other pathogens/diseases.

Apart from human immunoglobulins, animal sera are also sometimes used for passive immunization. **Animal sera** are obtained from animals (usually horses) immunized with specific antigen (mostly toxin of interest) and contain animal immunoglobulins specific for that antigen (such sera are called **antisera** or **antitoxins**). Animal proteins, including horse immunoglobulins, usually induce strong humoral response in humans, which may lead to a formation of circulating immune complexes and their deposition in kidney and other organs and cause serum disease (type III hypersensitivity). Therefore, human immunoglobulins are used always when it is possible. However, in cases when production of human preparations is not convenient and human products are not available (e.g. against snake venoms or botulinum toxin), horse antisera are still used to block the toxicity of animal venoms or in therapy of some diseases, such as botulism.

Finally, **monoclonal antibodies** that are being increasingly used for the treatment of autoimmune and chronic inflammatory diseases can also be used for the prophylaxis or therapy of specific infectious diseases. For example, monoclonal antibodies are occasionally used for prevention of RSV infection in prematurely born children.

ACTIVE IMMUNIZATION (VACCINATION)

- **Vaccination** is the most commonly used form of artificial immunization aimed to **actively induce** protective immune response against a certain pathogen in an individual and, in the event of subsequent exposure to that pathogen, prevent disease development in an immunized person.
- The term **vaccine** is derived from the Latin word *vacca* (cow), given that the first recorded successful vaccination of a child against smallpox (Edward Jenner, 1796) was carried out using vaccinia virus that causes cowpox.
- Since then, the development of many efficient vaccines against various pathogens has led to the striking decrease in the incidence of many common infectious diseases in the last 50 years.
- Moreover, the only human disease that has been eradicated by human intervention was smallpox, and this was achieved by a worldwide program of vaccination.
- Therefore, vaccination is considered to be one of the greatest successes of immunology and medicine in general.
- Unfortunately, occasional interruptions of vaccination programs in developing countries and in regions of social conflicts, as well as the increasing anti-vaccination movement have led to a local reemergence of some infectious diseases and represent constant threat to public health today.
- As previously noted, vaccination is based on the principle of an exposure of an individual to a pathogen or its components and/or products, that are modified in a way that they can induce an immune response in vaccinated persons, but not the disease.
- The aim of vaccination is to **induce pathogen-specific adaptive immune response** that results in **immunological memory** through the generation of **memory T and B cells** and **long-lived plasma cells**.
- Since days or even weeks are needed for the development of memory cells, the vaccines are **not efficient right after their administration** (contrary to immunoglobulins that have immediate action), but they induce **long-lasting immunity** (usually for years and sometimes life-long protection).
- The majority of vaccines induce **T-cell dependent humoral immune response** and a production of **high-affinity antibodies**.
- These antibodies can neutralize or block pathogen binding to host cells or activate some of the effector mechanisms, such as the complement system. On the other hand, most vaccines are

unable to induce strong cellular response mediated by $CD8^+$ cytotoxic T lymphocytes (CTLs), probably because exogenous proteins that enter the cell through endocytosis are not efficiently presented by class I MHC molecules.

- Still, some vaccines (mainly live, attenuated viral vaccines) induce good **cytotoxic response** in addition to T-dependent humoral response, while some other vaccines, such as polysaccharide vaccines against pneumococci and meningococci, induce **T-cell independent humoral immune response** to bacterial capsular polysaccharides.

Although vaccines are usually administered before exposure to pathogen (for **prophylactic purposes**), in some cases, when the incubation of disease is long enough, post-exposure vaccine administration is possible, too (rabies vaccine can be given soon after the infected animal bite and still be effective).

Also, post-exposure administration can be efficient when given in combination with specific immunoglobulins (e.g. after accidental injury by the HBV-contaminated needle or protection against tetanus in non-vaccinated persons). As for the vaccine administration, the most common route of administration is **parenteral** (using subcutaneous or intramuscular injections), although mucosal (**oral** and **nasal**) vaccines that induce local production of protective IgA antibodies have been developed (e.g. Sabin oral polio vaccine and nasal flu vaccine). Each vaccine must meet certain criteria in order to be suitable for the widespread use **(Table 4.3.1)**:

Table 4.3.1: Characteristics of high-quality vaccines.

Characteristic	Explanation
Safety	Vaccine must not cause disease or serious side effects
Efficacy of protection	Vaccine has to provide protection against disease after exposure to pathogen in majority of people
Sustained protection	Protection against disease must last for several years
Induction of neutralizing antibodies	Provides neutralization of toxins and their harmful effects
Induction of cytotoxic T cell response	Intracellular pathogens are more effectively eliminated by CTL
Practical considerations	Low cost, stability, ease of application (e.g. oral vaccine), etc.

- First of all, it has to be efficient (i.e. able to induce a protective immune response in the vast majority of vaccinated subjects) and safe (it should not cause disease or serious adverse effects).
- Next, good vaccines should induce both humoral and cell-mediated immunity (i.e. to activate CTLs), which is particularly important for the intracellular pathogens residing in cytosol.
- Also, it is important that the vaccine should induce a long-lasting immunity, thereby avoiding or reducing to a minimum the need for its re-application (booster doses).
- Finally, the vaccine has to fulfill certain practical requirements, such as stability (so that it can be easily transported and last for longer periods), ease of application (advantage of oral and nasal administration in comparison to injection), low price (vaccines should be available in developing countries), etc.

Note: In general, vaccines that contain one or few antigens of a pathogen, such as subunit vaccines (see below), are associated with less adverse effects compared with whole-cell vaccines, but are less immunogenic (i.e. induce weaker immune response). There are two ways for overcoming this disadvantage, either by adding **adjuvants** that increase the immunogenicity of the vaccines or by **revaccination** (administration of several additional doses, so called **booster doses**, over a longer period of time). Adjuvants are believed to stimulate innate immunity by acting on dendritic cells and other antigen-presenting cells, through their accumulation, increased expression of costimulators and production of cytokines, which all results in activation of adaptive immunity to antigens present in vaccines. Adjuvants may also cause side effects, such as inflammation at the site of inoculation, but are rarely associated with more serious adverse events.

Finally, vaccines provide protection not only for the vaccinated people, but also for unvaccinated ones, if the majority of people in the population have been vaccinated, a phenomenon called **herd immunity** (also called herd effect, community immunity, or population immunity). It is a form of indirect protection from infectious disease that occurs when a large percentage of a population has become immune to an infection, thereby providing protection for individuals who are not immune. In other words, widespread vaccination reduces the number of susceptible people in the population, disrupts the transmission of infection and diminishes the probability for susceptible individuals to be exposed to a pathogen and develop disease.

Types of Vaccines, their Properties and Mechanisms of Action

All vaccines can be divided, based on their properties, into several groups or **types**: live, inactivated, subunit, conjugated and combined vaccines (Features of different vaccine types are presented in **Table 4.3.2**).

Live Vaccines

- **Live vaccines** are composed of viable microorganisms with limited capacity to induce disease in humans.
- These strains of pathogens usually infect other animal species (e.g. cow in case of smallpox vaccine) or their virulence has been reduced through a process called attenuation (so called attenuated strains), so these vaccines are also called **attenuated vaccines**.
- **Attenuation** is usually performed by repeated pathogen passage in cell cultures in the absence of host immune mechanisms under conditions that are different from those present in human body (e.g. on lower temperature or in animal cells which normally cannot be infected by that pathogen).
- During that process, the accumulation of mutations and the adaptation of a pathogen to such new conditions results in a loss of its capacity to induce disease in humans.
- In general, live vaccines are safe and provide **complete immune response** since they induce not only production of neutralizing and other antibodies but also T cell-mediated response (both CTLs and helper T cells).
- They also provide **long-lasting immunity**, so they are usually administered in one or two doses.
- Most of these vaccines are given to children in the second year of life (with the exception of BCG that is given at birth), because of the immunological immaturity of the infants and the presence of the maternal antibodies that can reduce immunogenicity of the vaccine and inhibit immune response of the host and consequently reduce efficacy of live vaccines. Live vaccines have certain limitations: they are **relatively unstable**, especially on the higher temperatures (that is why the transport and storage of these vaccines are complicated, especially in rural regions) and there is the **risk of causing disease** if given to **people with immunodeficiencies**.

Table 4.3.2: Features of different vaccine types.

Type of vaccine	Examples	Immunization principle	Form of protection	Advantages	Limitations
Live (Attenuated)	Measles Mumps Rubella Varicella Polio (Sabin) Tuberculosis (BCG)	Weakened (attenuated) pathogen	Antibody production Cell-mediated immune response	Complete immune response Long-lasting immunity	Instability risk in immunocompromised persons
Inactivated (Killed)	Influenza Polio (Salk) Pertussis	Killed (inactivated) pathogen			
Subunit (Antigenic)	Diphtheria Tetanus HBV Influenza	Modified toxin (toxoid) Recombinant antigen Purified antigens (H and N)	Antibody production	Stability Safety	Low immunogenicity (adjuvants) Shorter immunity (booster administration)
Conjugated	Pneumococci Meningococci *Haemophilus influenzae* type B	Capsular polysaccharide linked to a protein (toxoid)	Antibody production (T-dependent humoral response)		
Combined (Polyvalent)	Pneumococci	Different serotypes of the same pathogen	As in single vaccines	As in single vaccines Very practical	As in single vaccines
	DTP, MMR	Different pathogens			

(BCG, Bacillus Calmette-Guerin, attenuated strain of *Mycobacterium bovis*; HBV, Hepatitis B virus; HBsAg, surface antigen of HBV; H, Hemagglutinin; N, Neuraminidase; DTP, Diphtheria, Tetanus, Pertussis; MMR, Measles, Mumps, Rubella)

- Therefore, live vaccines are not generally given to immunocompromised patients and pregnant women (for them, inactivated and subunit vaccines, although less effective, are safer choice).

Inactivated Vaccines

- **Inactivated vaccines** (also called **killed vaccines**) contain whole microorganisms that were killed using various chemicals (e.g. formaldehyde) or high temperatures, but their antigenic properties and immunogenicity were preserved. These vaccines are usually used for preventing disease where pathogen cannot be successfully attenuated. Inactivated vaccines are **stable** and **safe** (except for the people allergic to vaccine components, e.g., egg) and they act mainly through **induction of antibodies** and are less potent in activation of CTLs.
- On the other hand, inactivated vaccines are less immunogenic than attenuated ones, so they are usually **administered with adjuvants** in more than one dose (frequent revaccination). Vaccines for whooping cough (pertussis), typhoid fever, polio (Salk vaccine) and influenza are examples of inactivated vaccines. Although inactivated vaccines are good and efficient, there is a tendency for these vaccines to be replaced by subunit vaccines (when they are available).

Subunit Vaccines

- **Subunit vaccines** represent a special form of inactivated vaccines. They are composed of structural components of microorganisms or their products (e.g. toxins) that can induce protective immune response in recipients, which is mediated primarily by **antibodies, mainly neutralizing**.
- Since they are composed of individual antigens, these vaccines are also called **antigenic vaccines**.
- Those antigens are obtained by **isolation and purification** of pathogen products, or, more often, by using **recombinant DNA techniques** (as recombinant proteins produced by yeast cells). They are typically **surface antigens**, mainly proteins, which are important for the adherence of virus or bacteria to host cells, or polysaccharide antigens in the capsules of encapsulated bacteria. Examples of such subunit vaccine are the vaccines against influenza (containing hemagglutinin and neuraminidase) and polysaccharide vaccines against pneumococci and meningococci.

- Subunit vaccines also include vaccines against diseases mediated by toxins, such as diphtheria and tetanus. These vaccines do not contain bacteria that cause disease, but inactivated forms of their toxins, called **toxoids**. *Conjugated vaccines*

Conjugated Vaccines

- This is a special type of subunit vaccines, have been recently developed as result of our better understanding of the process of T cell-B cell cooperation in which CD4$^+$ helper T cells stimulate B cells to produce high-affinity antibodies in T-dependent humoral immune response.
- Typically, conjugated vaccines are those against encapsulated bacteria, such as pneumococci, meningococci and *Haemophilus influenzae* type B (HiB).

Combined Vaccines

- **Combined** (or **combination**) **vaccines** are also called **polyvalent vaccines** (vaccines that contain only one antigen sometimes are called monovalent), since they contain several **antigens of different serotypes** of the same pathogen or a number of antigens from **different pathogens**.
- Examples for the first are above mentioned vaccines against pneumococci, i.e., polysaccharide vaccine that contain antigens of 23 the most common serotypes in population, or conjugated vaccine containing antigens of 10 or 13 serotypes that cause severe invasive infections in children.

IMMUNIZATION SCHEDULE

This schedule of recommended immunizations may vary depending upon where you live, your child's health, the type of vaccine, and the vaccines available.

Some of the vaccines may be given as part of a combination vaccine so that a child gets fewer shots **(Table 4.3.3).** Talk with your doctor about which vaccines your kids need.

Birth

HepB: Hepatitis B vaccine. Ideally, the first dose is given within 12–24 hours of birth, but kids not previously immunized can get it at any age. Some low birth weight infants will get it at 1 month or when they are discharged from the hospital.

Table 4.3.3: National immunization schedule (NIS) for infants, children and pregnant women (vaccine-wise).

Vaccine	When to give	Dose	Route	Site
For pregnant women				
TT-1	Early in pregnancy	0.5 mL	Intra-muscular	Upper arm
TT-2	4 weeks after TT-1*	0.5 mL	Intra-muscular	Upper arm
TT- Booster	If received 2 TT doses in a pregnancy within the last 3 yrs*	0.5 mL	Intra-muscular	Upper arm
For infants				
BCG	At birth or as early as possible till one year of age	0.1 mL (0.05 mL until 1 month age)	Intra-dermal	Left upper arm
Hepatitis B - Birth dose	At birth or as early as possible within 24 hours	0.5 mL	Intra-muscular	Anterolateral side of mid-thigh
OPV-0	At birth or as early as possible within the first 15 days	2 drops	Oral	Oral
OPV 1, 2 and 3	At 6 weeks, 10 weeks and 14 weeks (OPV can be given till 5 years of age)	2 drops	Oral	Oral
Pentavalent 1, 2 and 3	At 6 weeks, 10 weeks and 14 weeks (can be given till one year of age)	0.5 mL	Intra-muscular	Anterolateral side of mid-thigh
Rotavirus#	At 6 weeks, 10 weeks and 14 weeks (can be given till one year of age)	5 drops	Oral	Oral
IPV	Two fractional dose at 6 and 14 weeks of age	0.1 mL	Intra-dermal two fractional dose	Intradermal: Right upper arm
Measles/MR 1st Dose$	9 completed months–12 months (can be given till 5 years of age)	0.5 mL	Sub-cutaneous	Right upper arm

Contd...

Contd...

Vaccine	When to give	Dose	Route	Site
JE - 1**	9 completed months–12 months	0.5 mL	Sub-cutaneous	Left upper arm
Vitamin A (1st dose)	At 9 completed months with Measles-Rubella	1 mL (1 lakh IU)	Oral	Oral
For Children				
DPT booster-1	16–24 months	0.5 mL	Intra-muscular	Anterolateral side of mid-thigh
Measles/ MR 2nd dose $	16–24 months	0.5 mL	Sub-cutaneous	Right upper arm
OPV Booster	6–24 months	2 drops	Oral	Oral
JE-2	16–24 months	0.5 mL	Sub-cutaneous	Left upper arm
Vitamin A*** (2nd to 9th dose)	16–18 months. Then one dose every 6 months up to the age of 5 years	2 mL (2 lakh IU)	Oral	Oral
DPT Booster-2	5–6 years	0.5 mL	Intra-muscular	Upper arm
TT	10 years and 16 years	0.5 mL	Intra-muscular	Upper arm

- *Give TT-2 or Booster doses before 36 weeks of pregnancy. However, give these even if more than 36 weeks have passed. Give TT to a woman in labor, if she has not previously received TT.
- **JE Vaccine is introduced in select endemic districts after the campaign.
- *** The 2nd to 9th doses of Vitamin A can be administered to children 1–5 years old during biannual rounds, in collaboration with ICDS.
- #Phased introduction, at present in Andhra Pradesh, Haryana, Himachal Pradesh and Orissa from 2016 and expanded in Madhya Pradesh, Assam, Rajasthan, and Tripura in February 2017 and planned in Tamil Nadu and Uttar Pradesh in 2017.
- $ Phased introduction, at present in five states namely Karnataka, Tamil Nadu, Goa, Lakshadweep and Puducherry (As of Feb' 2017).

1–2 months

HepB: Second dose should be given 1 to 2 months after the first dose.

2 months

- **DTaP:** Diphtheria, tetanus, and acellular pertussis vaccine
- **Hib:** *Haemophilus influenzae* type b vaccine
- **IPV:** Inactivated poliovirus vaccine
- **PCV:** Pneumococcal conjugate vaccine
- **RV:** Rotavirus vaccine

4 months

- **DTaP**
- **Hib**
- **IPV**
- **PCV**
- **RV**

6 months

- **DTaP**
- **Hib:** This third dose may be needed, depending on the brand of vaccine used in previous Hib immunizations.
- **PCV**
- **RV:** This third dose may be needed, depending on the brand of vaccine used in previous RV immunizations.

6 months and annually

- **Influenza (Flu):** The flu vaccine is recommended every year for children 6 months and older:
  - Kids younger than 9 who get the flu vaccine for the first time (or who have only had one dose before July 2021) will get it in 2 separate doses at least a month apart.
  - Those younger than 9 who have had at least 2 doses of flu vaccine previously (before July 2021) will only need 1 dose.
  - Kids older than 9 need only 1 dose.
- The vaccine is given by injection with a needle (the flu shot) or by nasal spray. Both types of vaccine can be used this flu season (2021–2022) because they seem to work equally well. Your doctor will recommend which to use based on your child's age and general health. The nasal spray is only for healthy people

ages 2–49. People with weak immune systems or some health conditions (such as asthma) and pregnant women should **not** get the nasal spray vaccine.

6–18 months

- **HepB**
- **IPV**

12–15 months

- **Hib**
- **MMR:** Measles, mumps, and rubella (German measles) vaccine. Sometimes given together with the varicella vaccine and called MMRV.
- **PCV**
- **Varicella (chickenpox)**

12–23 months

- **HepA:** Hepatitis A vaccine; given as 2 shots at least 6 months apart

15–18 months

- **DTaP**

4–6 years

- **DTaP**
- **MMR**
- **IPV**
- **Varicella**

9–16 years

- **Dengue vaccine:** This vaccine is given in 3 doses to children who have already had dengue fever and who live in areas where it is common (such as Puerto Rico, American Samoa, and the U.S. Virgin Islands).

11–12 years

- **HPV:** Human papillomavirus vaccine, given in 2 shots over a 6- to 12-month period. It can be given as early as age 9. For teens and young adults (age 15–26), it is given in 3 shots over 6 months. It is recommended for both girls and boys to prevent genital warts and some types of cancer.

- **Tdap:** Tetanus, diphtheria, and pertussis booster. Also recommended during each pregnancy a woman has.
- **MenACWY:** Meningococcal vaccine. Protects against meningococcal bacteria types A, C, W, and Y. A booster dose is recommended at age 16.

16–18 years

- **MenB:** Meningococcal vaccine. Protects against meningococcal bacterium type B. The MenB vaccine may be given to kids and teens in 2 or 3 doses, depending on the brand. Unlike the meningococcal conjugate vaccine, which is recommended for all, the decision to get the MenB vaccine is made by the teens, their parents, and the doctor. It is only recommended as routine for kids 10 years and older who have specific conditions that weaken their immune system, or during an outbreak.

Other Things to Know

- The **HepA vaccine** can be given as early as 6 months of age to babies who will travel to a place where hepatitis A is common (they will still need routine vaccination after their first birthday). It is also recommended for older kids who did not get it in the past.
- **The MMR vaccine** can be given to babies as young as 6 months old if they will be traveling internationally. These children should still get the recommended routine doses at 12–15 months and 4–6 years of age, but can get the second dose as early as 4 weeks after the first if they will still be traveling and at risk.
- **The flu vaccine** is especially important for kids who are at risk for health problems from the flu. High-risk groups include, but are not limited to, kids younger than 5 years old and those with chronic medical conditions, such as asthma, heart problems, sickle cell disease, diabetes, or HIV.
- **Pneumococcal vaccines** can be given to older kids (age 2 and up) who have conditions that affect their immune systems, such as asplenia or HIV infection, or other conditions, like a cochlear implant, chronic heart disease, or chronic lung disease.
- **The meningococcal vaccines** can be given to kids as young as 8 weeks old (depending on the vaccine brand) who are at risk

for a meningococcal infection, such as meningitis. This includes children with some immune disorders. Kids who live in (or will travel to) countries where meningitis is common, or where there is an outbreak, also should get the vaccine.

- Safe and effective COVID-19 vaccines are available for adults and all children ages 5 and older. Booster shots are recommended for adults and kids 12 and older. Everyone who is eligible should get the COVID-19 vaccine and booster shot as soon as possible.

POSSIBLE QUESTIONS

1. What is immunization? Discuss on active immunization.
2. Discuss briefly about passive immunization .
3. Give an account details of live vaccines and inactivated vaccines.

SHORT NOTES

1. Conjugated vaccines.
2. Combined vaccines.
3. Immunization schedule for both birth and 2 months kid.

MULTIPLE CHOICE QUESTIONS

1. The process of immunization which is used for preventing infection is called as__________
   a. Immunoprophylaxis b. Prophylactic
   c. Natural immunization d. Passive immunization
2. The process by which an individual is exposed to a nonpathogenic forms of microbes is called as ____________
   a. Vaccination b. Immunization
   c. Monoclonal antibodies d. None of the above
3. Animal sera which contains animal immunoglobulin for a specific antigen is called as ______
   a. Antisera b. Antitoxins
   c. Both a and b d. Monoclonal antibodies
4. Full form of HPV is __________
   a. Human protective vaccination
   b. Human papillomavirus
   c. Human public vaccination
   d. All of the above

5. Tdap stands for
   a. Tetanus, diphtheria and polio
   b. Tetanus, dengue, pertussis booster
   c. TB, diphtheria, pertussis booster
   d. Tetanus, diphtheria, pertussis booster
6. Vaccine protest against meningococcal is ______
   a. HPV
   b. Tdap
   c. MenACWY
   d. MMR
7. What is Attenuation?
   a. Weakened bacteria use for vaccination
   b. Long lasting immunity
   c. Relatively unstable
   d. None of the above
8. Polyvalent vaccine is otherwise called as ________
   a. Combined vaccine
   b. Subunit vaccine
   c. Conjugated vaccine
   d. Both a and b
9. HBV is a __________ type of vaccine.
   a. Combined vaccine
   b. Subunit vaccine
   c. Conjugated vaccine
   d. Live vaccines
10. MenB is used for which type of meningococcal?
   a. A
   b. B
   c. W
   d. Y

Answers

1. a	2. a	3. c	4. b	5. d
6. c	7. a	8. a	9. b	10. b

Principles and Uses of Serological Tests

Serology is the scientific study of serum and other body fluids. In practice, the term usually refers to the diagnostic identification of antibodies in the serum. Such antibodies are typically formed in response to an infection (against a given microorganism), against other foreign proteins (in response, for example, to a mismatched blood transfusion), or to one's own proteins (in instances of autoimmune disease). In either case, the procedure is simple.

PRINCIPLE OF ANTIGEN–ANTIBODY INTERACTIONS

In the field of immunology, many serologic techniques are used to detect the interaction of antigens with antibodies. These methods are suitable for the detection and quantitation of antibodies to infectious agents, as well as microbial and non-microbial antigens. In antigen antibody interaction determination of either antigen or antibody is possible, this determination follows a general principle: know antigen suspension or antiserum is used to detect and measure unknown antibody or microbial antigen.

IN VITRO ANTIGEN–ANTIBODY REACTIONS AND THEIR ROLE IN THE DIAGNOSIS OF DISEASE

There are different types of antigen antibody interaction these include:

- Precipitation reaction
- Agglutination reaction
- Complement fixation reaction
- Enzyme immuno assay (EIA)
- Radio immuno assay (RIA)

Precipitation Reaction

Precipitins can be produced against most proteins and some carbohydrates and carbohydrates- lipid complexes. Various system are available in which precipitation tests are performed in semisolid media such as agar or agarose, or nongel support medium such as cellulose acetate. Agar has been found to interfere with the migration of charged particles and has been largely replaced as an immunodiffusion medium by agarose. Agarose is a transparent, colorless, neutral gel. In the clinical laboratory several applications of the precipitation reaction are used. These methods include:

- Immunodiffusion
- Electroimmunodiffusion

Immunodiffusion

These are of two types: single and double immuodiffusion.

Double Diffusion

This technique also referred to as the Ouchterlony method, may be used to determine the relationship between antigen and antibodies.

Principle: Antibody dilutions and specific soluble antigens are placed in adjacent wells. If the well size and shape, distance between wells, temperature, and incubation time are optimal, these solutions diffuse out, bind to each other, cross-link, and form a visible precipitate at the point of equivalence perpendicular to the axis line between the wells the precipitation bands will be compared with a standard antigen.

The precise location of the band depends on the concentration and rate of diffusion of antigen and antibody. In a condition of antibody excess, the band will be located nearer the antigen well. If two antigens are present in the solution that can be recognized by the antibody, two precipitin bands form independently.

Antibodies associated with autoimmune disorders such as rheumatoid arthritis and systemic lupus erythematosus can be identified by double diffusion.

Identity

An identity reaction is indicated when the precipitin band forms a single smooth area. This precipitin is formed between the antibody and the two test antigens fuses, indicating that the antibody is precipitating identical antigen specificities in each preparation. This does not mean that the antigens are necessarily identical*; they are only identical insofar as the antibody can distinguish the difference.*

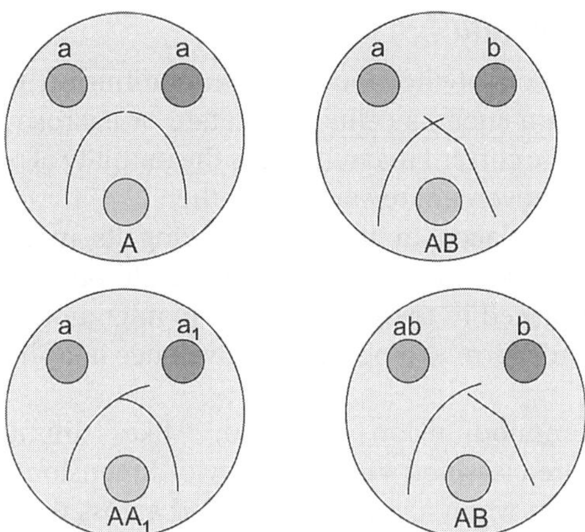

Figure 4.4.1: Precipitation pattern of ouchterlony type of immunodiffusion. (From Mary LT: Immunology and serology in laboratory medicine, 2nd ed,st Louis, 1996,Mosby)

Nonidentity

A non-identity pattern is expressed when the precipitation line cross each other. They intersect or cross because the sample contain no antigenic determinants in common.

Partial identity

In a partial identity pattern, the precipitation lines merge with spur formation. This merger indicated that the antigen are non-identical but possess common determinants.

Single Radial Immunodiffusion

This is a simple and specific method for identification and quantitation of a number of proteins found in human serum and other body fluids.

Principle: Radial immunodiffusion is based on a technique using a precipitin reaction in which specific antibody is added to a buffered agarose medium, serum containing the test antigen is placed in a well centered in the agarose. The diameter of the resulting precipitin zone is related to the concentration of antigen placed in a well.

The unknown antigen is in the wells and the specific antibody in the agar, the greater the antigen concentration the larger the circle of precipitation.

Electroimmunodiffusion (EID)

EID is a variation of the double immunodiffusion reaction in a support medium such as cellulose acetate or agarose through the use of an electric current that enhances the mobility of reactants and increase their movement toward each other.

Antibody is placed in the well favoring its migration in the direction of the cathode; antigens that tend to be more negatively charged and placed in the well that favors migration of the anode. Precipitin bands form at a point of equivalence in a shorter periods of time.

Electroimmunodiffusion method, like immunodiffusion procedures, are classified into one-or-two-dimensional, singles, or double diffusion when a voltage is applied across the gels to move the antigens and antibodies together, immuno-double diffusion becomes counter current immuno electrophoresis (CIE) radial immunodiffusion (RID) becomes electro immunoassay (EIA).

Counter current immunoelectrophoresis (CIE) is a variation of the classic precipitin procedure; it merely adds an electrical current to help antigens and antibodies move toward each other more quickly than in simple diffusion. The procedure takes advantage of the net electric charge of the antigens and antibodies being tested in a particular test buffer. Variables such as types of gel, amount of current, a concentration of antigen and antibody must be carefully controlled for maximum reactivity. The sensitivity of CIE is 10 to 20 times greater than in immuno-double diffusion, however, it is more expensive than other techniques such as immunodiffusion.

Electroimmunoassay

Antigens may be quantitiated by electrophoresis than in an antibody-containing gel electroimmunoassay. This technique combines the speed of electrophoresis with the accuracy and sensitivity of radioimmunoassay.

Agglutination Reaction

Precipitation and agglutination are the visible expression of the aggregation of antigens and antibodies through the formation of a framework in which antigen particles or molecules alternate with antibody molecules.

Agglutination of particles to which soluble antigen has been absorbed produces a serum method of demonstrating precipitins.

Example of artificial carriers includes latex particles and colloidal charcoal. Cells unrelated to the antigen, such as erythrocytes coated with antigen in a constant amount can be used as a biologic carriers. Whole bacterial cells can contain an antigen that will bind with antibodies produced in response to that antigen when it was introduced into the host.

Agglutination tests are easy to perform and in some cases are the most sensitive tests currently available. These tests have a wide range of applications in the clinical diagnosis of non-infectious immune disorders and infectious diseases.

Latex Agglutination

In latex agglutination procedures, antibody molecules can be bound to the surface of latex beads. Many antibody molecules can be bound to each latex particle, increasing the potential number of exposed antigen-binding sites. If an antigen is present in a test specimen, the antigen will bind to the combining sites of the antibody exposed on the surface of the latex heads, forming visible cross-linked aggregates of latex beads and antigen. In some test systems, latex particles can be coated with antigen. In the presence of serum antibodies, these particles agglutinate into large visible clumps.

Examples of tests based on latex agglutination reaction include C-reactive protein, IgG rheumatoid factors, and IgM rheumatoid factors.

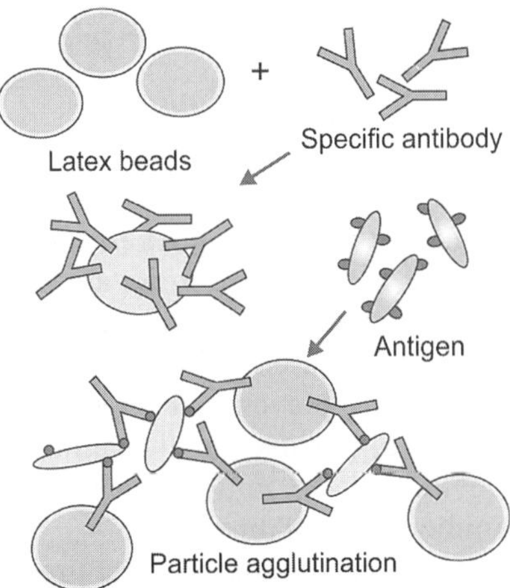

Figure 4.4.2: Latex agglutination reaction.

Direct Bacterial Agglutination

Direct whole pathogens can be used to detect antibodies directed against pathogens. The most basic tests are those that measure the antibody produced by the host to determinants on the surface of a bacterial agent in response to infection with that bacterium. In a thick suspension of the bacteria, the binding of specific antibodies to surface antigens of the bacteria causes the bacteria to clump together in visible aggregates. This type agglutination is called bacterial agglutination. Because tube testing allows more time for antigen-antibody reaction, it is considered to be more sensitive than slide testing.

Indirect or Passive Hemagglutination

Hemagglutination is agglutination of red blood cells, and tests for antibody detection. In the indirect or passive hemagglutination technique, erythrocytes are coated with substances such as extracts of bacterial cells, protozoa or purified polysaccharides or proteins.

Erythrocyte of animals such as sheep or rabbits, or from group "O" humans, function as carrier for detecting and titrating the corresponding antibodies by agglutination. This technique is called indirect or passive hemagglutination testing because it is not the antigen of the erythrocytes themselves but the passively attached antigens that are bound by antibody. For example, in rubella antibody test, erythrocytes are coated with rubella antigen. In the presence of antibody, agglutination occurs.

Hemagglutination Inhibition Technique

Hemagglutination inhibition test is used to detect some viral antibodies, for example, rubella. A known quantity of rubella viral antigen is mixed with dilutions of the patient's serum, to which red blood cells are added. If the serum lucks antibody, the virus will spontaneously attach to the red cells, link together, and agglutinate. If antibody to the virus is present, all of the virus particles will be bound by antibody, which prevents or inhibits hemagglutination. The serum is, therefore, positive for the antibodies. The highest dilution of serum that totally inhibits agglutination of red cells determines the antibody titer of the serum.

Disadvantage of this technique include: time consuming, and subjective bias in the interpretation for results. Negative results do not always indicate the absence of antibody. In some case, false negative results can occur from a low titer of antibody. Non-specific inhibitors can cause false positive results.

Complement Fixation Reaction

Complement fixation is a classic method for demonstrating the presence of antibody in serum. This method consists of two components: The first component is an indicator system consisting of a combination of sheep red cells; complement-fixing antibody produced against the sheep red cells in another animal, and an exogenous source of complement, usually guinea pig serum. When these three components are combined in an optimal concentration, the antisheep cell antibody, hemolysin, can bind to the surface of the red cells. Complement can subsequently bind to this antigen antibody complex and cause cell lysis. The second component consists of a known antigen and patient serum, which are added to a suspension of sheep erythrocytes, hemolysin, and a complement.

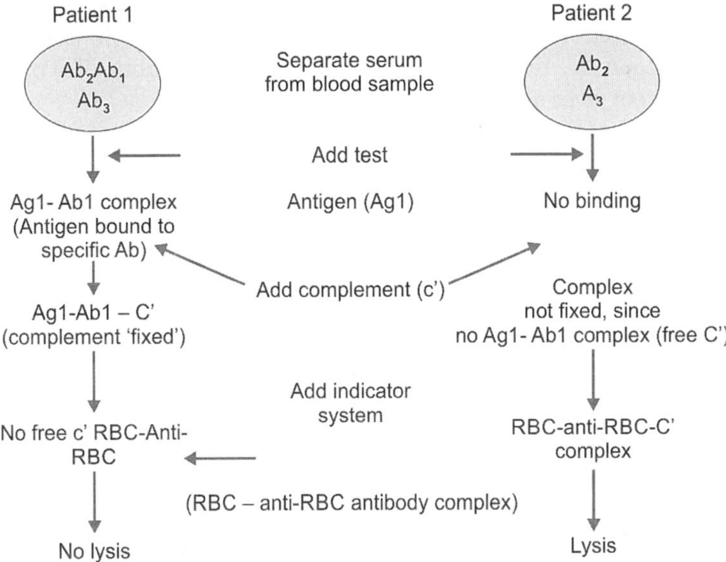

Figure 4.4.3: Complement fixation test.

The two components of the complement fixation procedure are tested in sequence. Patient serum is first added to the known antigen, and complement is added to the solution. If the serum contains antibody to the antigen, the resulting antigen–antibody complexes will bind all of the complement. Sheep red cells and hemolysin are then added. If complement has not been bound by an antigen-antibody complex formed from the patient serum and known antigen, it is available to bind to the indicator system of indicates both a lack of antibody and a negative complement fixation test. If the patient's serum does contain a complement-fixing antibody appositive result will be demonstrated by the lack of hemolysis.

Immunofluorescent Test (IFT)

The fluorescent techniques are extremely specific and sensitive. This technique consists of labeling antibody with fluorescein isothiocyanate, a fluorescent compound with an affinity for proteins to form a complex, conjugate. The fluorescent assay includes: direct immunofluorescent assay and indirect immunofluorescent assay.

Direct Immunofluorescent Assay

In this technique, fluorescein-conjugated antibody is used to detect antigen–antibody reactions. This method can be applied to the detection of hepatitis B virus and chlamydia. A fluorescent microscope is required to observe the production of color; fluorescein gives a yellow-green light.

Indirect Immunofluorescent Assay (IFA)

This method is based on the fact that antibodies not only react with homologous antigens but can act as antigens and react with antibody.

In the indirect immunofluorescent assay, the antigen source to the specific antibody being tested is fixed to the surface of a microscopic slide. The patent's serum is diluted and placed on the slide to cover the antigen source. If antibody is present in the serum, it will bind to its specific antigen unbound antibody is then removed by washing the slide, finally antihuman globulin conjugated to a fluorescent substance that will fluoresce when exposed to a fluorescent substance that will fluoresce when exposed to ultraviolet light is placed on the slide. This conjugated marker of human antibody will bind to the antibody already bound to the antigen on the slide and will serve as a marker for the antibody when viewed under a fluorescent microscope.

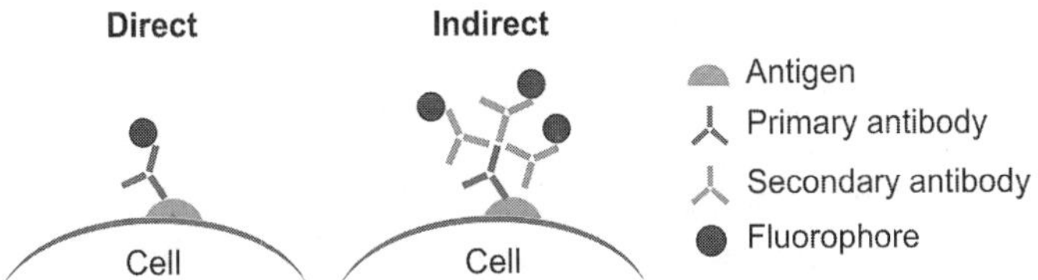

Figure 4.4.4: Direct and indirect immunofluorescent test.

Enzyme Immunoassay (EIA)

An enzyme labeled antibody or enzyme labeled antigen conjugate is used in immunologic assays for detection of antigens or antibodies, in a patient's serum, e.g. HIV antibody, HIV antigen, hepatitis A antibody.

Various enzymes are employed in enzyme immunoassay. The most commonly used enzymes are peroxidase and alkaline phosphatase. In EIA, a plastic bead or plastic plate is coated with antigen. The antigen reacts with antibody in the patient serum. The bead or plate is then incubated with an enzyme-labeled antibody conjugate, if antibody is present on the bead or plate. The enzyme activity is measured spectrophotometrically after the addition of the specific chromogenic substrate. Test result is calculated by comparing the spectrophotometer reading of patient serum to that of a control serum.

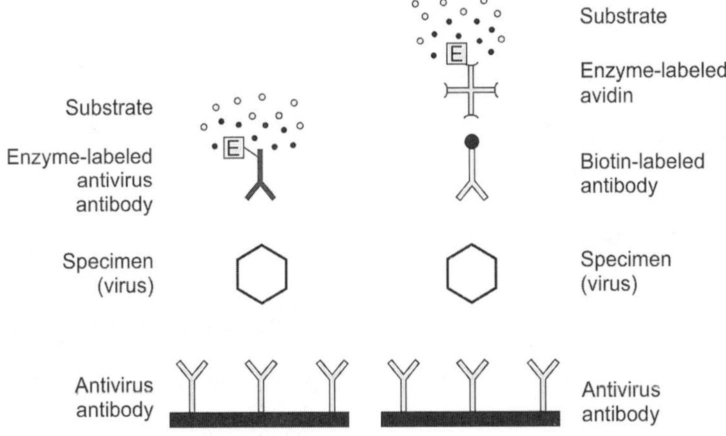

Figure 4.4.5: Enzyme immunoassay.

Radioimmunoassay (RIA)

In radioimmunoassay, radioisotopes can be used to measure the concentration of antigen or antibody in serum sample. If antibody concentration is being measured, radioactive labeled antibody competes with patient unlabeled antibody for binding sites on a known amount of antigen.

The main advantage of the radioimmunoassay method is the extreme sensitivity and ability to detect trace amounts of antigen or antibody. In addition, a large number of tests can be performed in a relatively short time period. The disadvantage is the hazards and instability of isotopes.

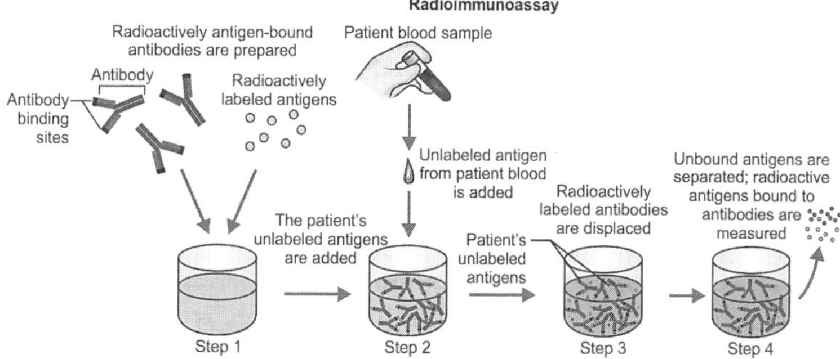

Figure 4.4.6: Radio immunoassay.

POSSIBLE QUESTIONS

1. Briefly discuss about different types of antigen–antibody interaction.

SHORT NOTES

1. Latex agglutination
2. Enzyme Immunoassay
3. Hemagglutination inhibition technique
4. Electroimmunodiffusion

MULTIPLE CHOICE QUESTIONS

1. The study of serum and other body fluids are called as ______________.
   a. Fluid mechanism
   b. Serology
   c. Agglutination
   d. Immunology

2. In vitro condition refers to ________________.
   a. Within living organism
   b. Outside living organism
   c. Growing in an artificial environment
   d. Both b and c
3. Which of the following can be identified by double diffusion?
   a. Rheumatoid arthritis
   b. Systemic lupus erythematosus
   c. Both a and b
   d. All of the above
4. Agarose is ____________
   a. Transparent
   b. Colorless
   c. Neutral
   d. All of the above
5. Which of the following is used to measure the concentration of antigen or antibody in serum?
   a. Isotopes
   b. Radioisotope
   c. Isobars
   d. None of the above
6. In Enzyme Immunoassay, which of the following enzymes is not used?
   a. Alkaline phosphate
   b. Peroxidase
   c. Amylase
   d. All of the above

Answers

1. b
2. d
3. d
4. d
5. b
6. c

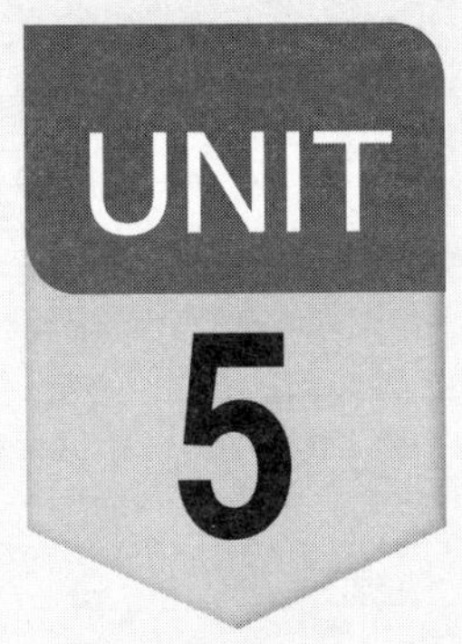

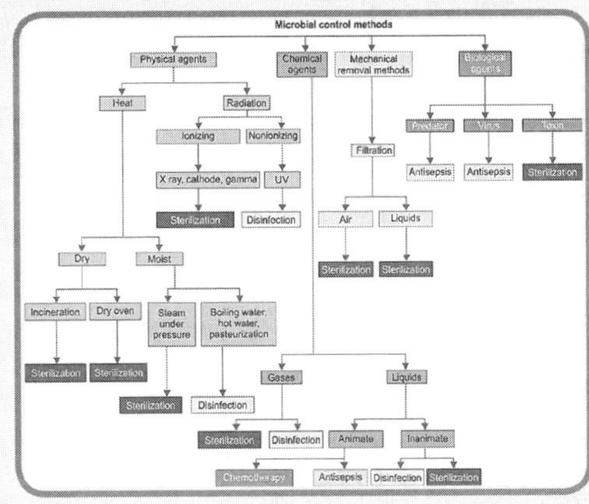

Control and Destruction of Microbes

Learning Objectives

- Principles and methods of microbial control
  - Sterilization
  - Disinfection
  - Chemotherapy and antibiotics
  - Pasteurization
- Medical and surgical asepsis
- Bio-safety and waste management

Fundamentals of Control and Destruction of Microorganisms

INTRODUCTION

The main reasons to control and destroy microorganisms are:
i. to prevent transmission of disease and infection
ii. to prevent decomposition and spoilage
iii. to prevent contamination
This can be achieved by various ways.

IMPORTANT TERMS USED IN THE CONTROL OF MICROORGANISMS

Terms related to destruction of microorganisms are:

Sterilization: Destruction of all microorganisms, including endospores on an object or in a material.

Disinfection: The destruction of pathogens but not endospores on an object or in a material. The number of pathogens is reduced or growth is inhibited to a level that does not produce disease.

Antisepsis: Chemical disinfection of the skin, mucosal membranes or other living tissues.

Germicide ("cide" = kill): A chemical agent that rapidly kills microorganisms. Specific germicides include:
- Sporicide—kills spores
- Bactericide—kills bacteria
- Viricide—kills viruses
- Fungicide—kills fungi

Chemotherapy: Chemicals used internally to kill or inhibit growth of microorganisms within host tissue.

Terms Related to Suppression of Microorganisms

i. **Asepsis:** It means "without infection". It is the absence of pathogens from an object or area. Aseptic techniques prevent the entry of pathogens into the body.
   There are two types of asepsis:
   Surgical asepsis: Techniques designed to remove all micro-organisms. It prevents infectious agents from reaching a wound.
   Medical asepsis: Techniques designed to exclude micro-organisms associated with communicable diseases. It includes dust control, handwashing, use of individualized equipment and instruments, waste disposal, care of instruments, syringes, needles, thermometers and dressings.
ii. **Sanitization:** The reduction or removal of pathogens on inanimate (non-living) objects by chemical or mechanical cleansing.
iii. **Bacteriostasis ("static" = halt):** Bacterial growth and multiplication are inhibited, but the bacteria are not killed.

Terms for Destruction or Suppression of Microorganisms

- **Antimicrobial agents**—any substances that destroy or suppress microorganisms
- **Antibiotic**—a product formed by microorganisms that destroy or suppress microorganism

PRINCIPLES OF MICROBIAL CONTROL

Methods used to control and destroy the growth of microorganisms and their transmission of infectious disease aim at:

- Stopping the growth of microorganism for a period of time
- Reducing the number of microorganisms to a safe level
- Destroying the microorganisms

The degree of effectiveness of this process depends on following factors:

- Number of microorganisms
- Type of microorganism
- Their physiological state, such as the stage of growth or formation of endospores
- Environment in which they are growing (glassware, instruments, tissue, food):

The microorganisms can be controlled either by one or more of the following ways:

- Destroying the cell wall, or stopping the cell wall synthesi
- Destroy the cell membrane
- Denaturing (destroying the structure) protein and DNA
- Stopping the protein synthesis
- Stopping the DNA replication and transcription process

METHODS OF MICROBIAL CONTROL

The methods of microbial control fall in one of the following categories:

- Disinfection
- Sterilization
- Antisepsis
- Chemotherapy

Microbial control could be achieved by following ways:

- Physical agents
- Chemical agents
- Mechanical removal methods

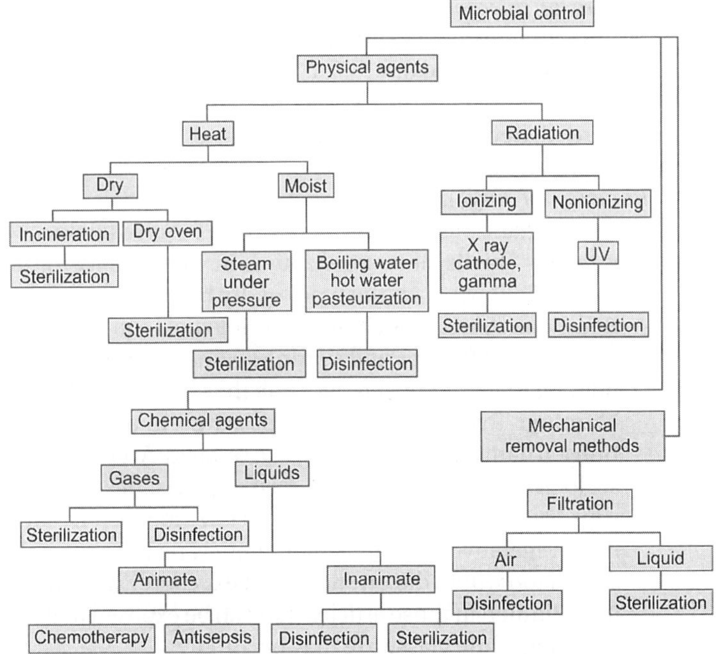

Figure 5.1.1: Microbiology control methods.

Physical Agents

Heat

Heat is the most common, inexpensive, simplest, reliable and effective method used to destroy microorganisms. When heat is used for sterilization process in the presence of moisture then it is called as moist heat whereas in the absence of moisture, it is called as dry heat.

i. Basic Principle: Heat denatures (destroys the structure) Nucleic acids (DNA and RNA), proteins and enzymes of the microorganism. In absence of these molecules microorganisms can't survive.
ii. Factors influencing sterilization by heat:
   - *Nature of heat:* Moist heat is more effective than dry heat.
   - Temperature and time: Temperature and time are inversely proportional. As temperature increases, the time taken is decreased.
   - *Number of microorganisms:* More the number of micro-organisms, higher the temperature or longer the duration required.
   - *Nature of microorganism:* Depends on species and strain of microorganism, sensitivity to heat may vary. Spores are highly resistant to heat.
   - *Type of material:* Articles that are heavily contaminated require higher temperature or prolonged exposure. Certain heat sensitive articles must be sterilized at lower temperature.
   - *Presence of Organic material:* Organic materials such as protein, sugars, oils and fats increase the required time.
   - **Dry heat** - This is heat sterilization in the absence of any moisture. Following are the types of dry heat sterilization:
     - **Red heat:** Articles such as bacteriological loops, straight wires, tips of forceps and searing spatulas are sterilized by holding them in Bunsen flame till they become red hot.
     - **Flaming:** This is a method of passing the article over a Bunsen flame, but not heating it to redness. Articles such as scalpels, mouth of test tubes, flasks, glass slides and cover slips are passed through the flame a few times. Even though most vegetative cells are killed, there is no guarantee that spores too would die on such short exposure. This method too is limited to those articles that can be exposed to flame. Cracking of the glassware may occur.

- **Incineration:** This is a method of destroying contaminated material by burning them in incinerator. Articles such as soiled dressings; animal carcasses, pathological material and bedding, etc. should be subjected to incineration. This technique results in the loss of the article, hence is suitable only for those articles that have to be disposed. Burning of polystyrene materials emits dense smoke and hence they should not be incinerated.
- **Hot air oven:** This method was introduced by Louis Pasteur. Articles to be sterilized are exposed to high temperature (160°C) for duration of one hour in an electrically heated oven. Since air is poor conductor of heat, even distribution of heat throughout the chamber is achieved by a fan. The heat is transferred to the article by radiation, conduction and convection. The oven should be fitted with a thermostat control, temperature indicator, meshed shelves and must have adequate insulation.

Articles Sterilized

Metallic instruments (like forceps, scalpels, scissors), glasswares (such as petri-dishes, pipettes, flasks, all-glass syringes), swabs, oils, grease, petroleum jelly and some pharmaceutical products.

Sterilization Process

Articles to be sterilized must be perfectly dry before placing them inside to avoid breakage. Articles must be placed at sufficient distance so as to allow free circulation of air in between. Mouths of flasks, test tubes and both ends of pipettes must be plugged with cotton wool. Articles such as petri dishes and pipettes may be arranged inside metal canisters and then placed. Individual glass articles must be wrapped in kraft paper or aluminum foils.

Advantages: It is an effective method of sterilization of heat stable articles. The articles remain dry after sterilization. This is the only method of sterilizing oils and powders.

Disadvantages:

- Since air is poor conductor of heat, hot air has poor penetration.
- Cotton wool and paper may get slightly charred.
- Glasses may become smoky.
- Takes longer time compared to autoclave.
- **Infrared Rays:** Infrared rays bring about sterilization by generation of heat. Articles to be sterilized are placed in a

moving conveyer belt and passed through a tunnel that is heated by infrared radiators to a temperature of 180ºC. The articles are exposed to that temperature for a period of 7.5 minutes. Articles sterilized included metallic instruments and glassware. It is mainly used in central sterile supply department. It requires special equipment, hence is not applicable in diagnostic laboratory.

- **Moist Heat:** This is heat sterilization in the presence of any moisture. Following are the types of moist heat sterilization:

At Temperature Below 100ºC

- **Pasteurization:** This process was originally employed by Louis Pasteur. Currently, this procedure is employed in food and dairy industry. There are two methods of pasteurization:
  - *Holder method:* Heated at 63ºC for 30 minutes
  - *Flash method:* Heated at 72ºC for 15 seconds followed by quickly cooling to 13ºC

  Ultra-high Temperature (UHT) Heated for 140ºC for 15 sec and 149ºC for 0.5 sec.
  - This method is suitable to destroy most milk borne pathogens like *Salmonella, Mycobacteria, Streptococci, Staphylococci* and *Brucella,* however *Coxiella* may survive pasteurization.
- **Vaccine bath:** The contaminating bacteria in a vaccine preparation can be inactivated by heating in a water bath at 60ºC for one hour. Only vegetative bacteria are killed and spores survive.
- **Serum bath:** The contaminating bacteria in a serum preparation can be inactivated by heating in a water bath at 56ºC for one hour on several successive days. Proteins in the serum will coagulate at higher temperature. Only vegetative bacteria are killed and spores survive.

At Temperature 100°C

- **Boiling:** Boiling water (100ºC) kills most vegetative bacteria and viruses immediately. Certain bacterial toxins such as Staphylococcal enterotoxin are also heat resistant. Some bacterial spores are resistant to boiling and survive; hence this is not a substitute for sterilization.

Steam at 100°C: Instead of keeping the articles in boiling water, they are subjected to free steam at 100ºC. A steamer is a metal cabinet with perforated trays to hold the articles and a conical lid. The bottom of steamer is filled with water and is heated. The steam that is generated sterilizes the articles when exposed for a period of 90 minutes. Media such as TCBS, DCA and selenite broth are sterilized by steaming.

At Temperature Above 100°C

- **Autoclave:** Sterilization can effectively be achieved at a temperature above 100°C using an autoclave. Water boils at 100°C at atmospheric pressure, but if pressure is raised, the temperature at which the water boils also increases. In an autoclave, the water is boiled in a closed chamber. As the pressure rises, the boiling point of water also raises. At a pressure of 15 lbs inside the autoclave, the temperature is said to be 121°C. Exposure of articles to this temperature for 15 minutes sterilizes them.
- **Advantages of steam:** It has more penetrative power than dry air, it moistens the spores (moisture is essential for coagulation of proteins), condensation of steam on cooler surface releases latent heat, draws in fresh steam.

Construction and Operation of Autoclave

- A simple autoclave has vertical or horizontal cylindrical body with a heating element, a perforated tray to keep the articles, a lid that can be fastened by screw clamps, a pressure gauge, a safety valve and a discharge tap.
- The articles to be sterilized must not be tightly packed.
- The screw caps and cotton plugs must be loosely fitted.
- The lid is closed but the discharge tap is kept open and the water is heated. As the water starts boiling, the steam drives air out of the discharge tap.
- When all the air is displaced and steam start appearing through the discharge tap, the tap is closed.
- The pressure inside is allowed to rise up to 15 lbs per square inch. At this pressure, the articles are held for 15 minutes, after which the heating is stopped and the autoclave is allowed to cool.
- Once the pressure gauge shows the pressure equal to atmospheric pressure, the discharge tap is opened to let the air in.
- The lid is then opened and articles removed. Articles sterilized: Culture media, dressings, certain equipment, linen, etc.

Precautions

- Articles should not be tightly packed
- The autoclave must not be overloaded
- Air discharge must be complete and there should not be any residual air trapped inside
- Caps of bottles and flasks should not be tight
- Autoclave must not be opened until the pressure has fallen or else the contents will boil over
- Articles must be wrapped in paper to prevent drenching, bottles must not be overfilled.

Advantage: Very effective way of sterilization, quicker than hot air oven.

Disadvantages: Drenching and wetting or articles may occur, trapped air may reduce the efficacy, takes long time to cool.

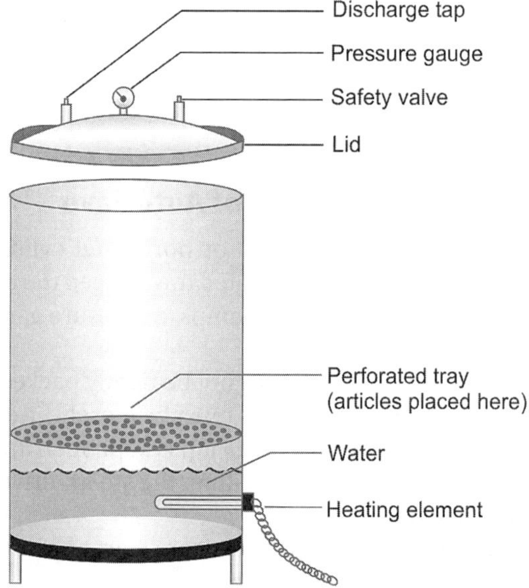

Figure 5.1.2: Autoclave.

Radiation Sterilization

Two types of radiations are used, ionizing and non-ionizing. Non-ionizing rays are low energy rays with poor penetrative power while ionizing rays are high-energy rays with good penetrative power. Since radiation does not generate heat, it is termed "cold sterilization". In some parts of Europe, fruits and vegetables are irradiated to increase their shelf life up to 500 percent.

a. **Non-ionizing rays:** Rays of wavelength longer than the visible light are non-ionizing. Microbicidal wavelength of ultra violet-rays lie in the range of 200–280 nm with 260 nm being most effective. UV-rays are generated using a high-pressure mercury vapour lamp. Ultra violet-rays induce formation of Thymine-Thymine dimers, which ultimately inhibits DNA replication. Ultra violet radiation readily induce mutations in cells irradiated with a non-lethal dose. Microorganisms such as bacteria, viruses, yeasts, etc., that are exposed to an effective UV-radiation are inactivated within seconds.

   Disadvantages
   - Low penetrative power of non-ionizing rays
   - Limited life of the UV-bulb
   - Some bacteria have DNA repair enzymes that can overcome damage caused by UV-rays
   - Rays are harmful to skin and eyes
   - It doesn't penetrate glass, paper or plastic

b. **Ionizing rays:** Ionizing rays are of two types, particulate and electromagnetic rays.
   - **Particulate rays:** High speed electrons are produced by a linear accelerator from a heated cathode. Electron beams are employed to sterilize articles like syringes, gloves, dressing packs, foods and pharmaceuticals. Sterilization is accomplished in few seconds. Unlike electromagnetic rays, the instruments can be switched off. Disadvantage includes poor penetrative power and requirement of sophisticated equipment.
   - **Electromagnetic rays:** These include Gamma rays which are produced from nuclear disintegration of certain radioactive isotopes (Co60, Cs137). They have more penetrative power than electron beam but require longer time of exposure. These high-energy radiations damage the nucleic acid of the microorganism. A dosage of 2.5 megarads kills all bacteria, fungi, viruses and spores. It is used commercially to sterilize disposable petri-dishes, plastic syringes, antibiotics, vitamins, hormones, glasswares and fabrics. Disadvantages include; unlike electron beams, they can't be switched off, glasswares tend to become brownish, loss of tensile strength in fabric.

Chemical Methods

Disinfectants are those chemicals that destroy pathogenic bacteria from inanimate surfaces. Some chemical have very narrow spectrum of activity and some have very wide. Those chemicals that can sterilize are called chemosterilants. Those chemicals that can safely be applied over skin and mucus membranes are called antiseptics.

An ideal antiseptic or disinfectant should have following properties:
- Should have wide spectrum of activity
- Should be able to destroy microbes within practical period of time
- Should be active in the presence of organic matter
- Should make effective contact and be wettable
- Should be active in any pH
- Should be stable
- Should have long shelf life
- Should be speedy
- Should have high penetrating power
- Should be non-toxic, non-allergenic, non-irritative or non-corrosive
- Should not have bad odour
- Should not leave non-volatile residue or stain
- Efficacy should not be lost on reasonable dilution
- Should not be expensive and must easily be available

Such an ideal disinfectant is not yet available.

Classification of Disinfectants

Based on consistency

a. Liquid (e.g. Alcohols, Phenols)
b. Gaseous (Formaldehyde vapour, Ethylene oxide)

Based on spectrum of activity

a. High level
b. Intermediate level
c. Low level

Based on mechanism of action

a. Action on membrane, (e.g. Alcohol, detergent)
b. Denaturation of cellular proteins, (e.g. Alcohol, Phenol)

ALCOHOLS

- **Mode of action:** Alcohols dehydrate cells, disrupt membranes and cause coagulation of protein.

- **Examples:** Ethyl alcohol, Isopropyl alcohol and Methyl alcohol
- **Application:** A 70% aqueous solution is more effective at killing microbes than absolute alcohols. 70% Ethyl alcohol (spirit) is used as antiseptic on skin. Isopropyl alcohol is preferred to Ethanol. It can also be used to disinfect surfaces. It is used to disinfect clinical thermometers. Methyl alcohol kills fungal spores, hence is useful in disinfecting inoculation hoods.
- **Disadvantages:** Skin irritant, volatile (evaporates rapidly), inflammable.

ALDEHYDES

- **Mode of action:** Acts through alkylation of amino-, carboxyl- or hydroxyl group, and probably damages nucleic acids. It kills all microorganisms, including spores.
- **Example:** Formaldehyde, Glutaraldehyde
- **Application:** 40% Formaldehyde (formalin) is used for surface disinfection and fumigation of rooms, chambers, operation theatres, biological safety cabinets, wards, sick rooms, etc.
- **Disadvantages:** Vapours are irritating (must be neutralized by ammonia), has poor penetration, leaves non-volatile residue, activity is reduced in the presence of protein. Glutaraldehyde requires alkaline pH and only those articles that are wettable can be sterilized.

PHENOL

- **Mode of action:** Act by disruption of membranes, precipitation of proteins and inactivation of enzymes.
- **Examples:** 5% Phenol, 1-5% Cresol, 5% Lysol (a saponified cresol), Hexachlorophene, Chlorhexidine, Chloroxylenol (Dettol)
- **Applications:** Act as disinfectants at high concentration and as antiseptics at low concentrations. They are bactericidal, fungicidal, mycobactericidal but are inactive against spores and most viruses. They are not readily inactivated by organic matter. The corrosive phenolics are used for disinfection of ward floors, in discarding jars in laboratories and disinfection of bedpans.
- **Disadvantages:** It is toxic, corrosive and skin irritant. Chlorhexidine is inactivated by anionic soaps. Chloroxylenol is inactivated by hard water.

HALOGENS

- **Mode of action:** They are oxidizing agents and cause damage by oxidation of essential sulfydryl groups of enzymes. Chlorine reacts with water to form Hypochlorous acid which is microbicidal.
- **Examples:** Chlorine compounds (chlorine bleach, hypochlorite) and iodine compounds (tincture iodine, iodophores)
- **Applications:** Chlorine gas is used to bleach water. Household bleach can be used to disinfect floors. 0.5% sodium hypochlorite is used in serology and virology.
- **Disadvantages:** They are rapidly inactivated in the presence of organic matter. Iodine is corrosive and staining. Bleach solution is corrosive and will corrode stainless steel surfaces.

HEAVY METALS

- **Mode of action:** Act by precipitation of proteins and oxidation of sulfhydryl groups. They are bacteriostatic.
- **Examples:** Mercuric chloride, Silver nitrate, Copper sulfate, Organic mercury salts (e.g., Mercurochrome, Merthiolate)
- **Applications:** 1% silver nitrate solution can be applied on eyes as treatment for ophthalmia neonatorum (Crede's method). Silver sulphadiazine is used topically to help to prevent colonization and infection of burn tissues.
- **Disadvantages:** Mercuric chloride is highly toxic are readily inactivated by organic matter.

SURFACE ACTIVE AGENTS

- **Mode of actions:** They have the property of concentrating at interfaces between lipid containing membrane of bacterial cell and surrounding aqueous medium. These compounds have long chain hydrocarbons that are fat soluble and charged ions that are water-soluble. Since they contain both of these, they concentrate on the surface of membranes. They disrupt membrane resulting in leakage of cell constituents.
- **Examples:** These are soaps or detergents.
- **Application:** They are active against vegetative cells, mycobacteria and enveloped viruses. They are widely used as disinfectants at dilution of 1-2% for domestic use and in hospitals.
- **Disadvantages:** Their activity is reduced by hard water, anionic detergents and organic matter. *Pseudomonas* can metabolise cetrimide, using them as a carbon, nitrogen and energy source.

DYES

- **Mode of action:** Acridine dyes are bactericidal because of their interaction with bacterial nucleic acids.
- **Examples:** Aniline dyes such as crystal violet, malachite green and brilliant green.
- **Applications:** They may be used topically as antiseptics to treat mild burns. They are used as paint on the skin to treat bacterial skin infections. The dyes are used as selective agents in certain selective media.

HYDROGEN PEROXIDE

- **Mode of action:** It acts on microorganisms through its release of nascent oxygen. Hydrogen peroxide produces hydroxyl-free radical that damages proteins and DNA.
- **Application:** It is used at 6% concentration to decontaminate the instruments, equipment such as ventilators. 3% hydrogen peroxide solution is used for skin disinfection and deodorizing wounds and ulcers. Strong solutions are sporicidal.
- **Disadvantages:** Decomposes in light, broken down by catalase, proteinaceous organic matter drastically reduces its activity.

ETHYLENE OXIDE (EO)

- **Mode of action:** It is an alkylating agent. It acts by alkylating sulfydryl-, amino-, carboxyl- and hydroxyl- groups.
- **Properties:** It is a cyclic molecule, which is a colorless liquid at room temperature. It has a sweet ethereal odour, readily polymerizes and is flammable.
- **Application:** It is a highly effective chemosterilant, capable of killing spores rapidly. Since it is highly flammable, it is usually combined with CO_2 (10% CO_2+ 90% EO) or Dichlorodifluoromethane. It requires presence of humidity.
- **Disadvantages:** It is highly toxic, irritating to eyes, skin, highly flammable, mutagenic and carcinogenic.

BETA-PROPIOLACTONE (BPL)

- **Mode of action:** It is an alkylating agent and acts through alkylation of carboxyl- and hydroxyl- groups.
- **Properties:** It is a colorless liquid with pungent to slightly sweetish smell. It is a condensation product of ketone with formaldehyde.
- **Application:** It is an effective sporicidal agent and has broad-spectrum activity. 0.2% is used to sterilize biological products.

It is more efficient in fumigation than formaldehyde. It is used to sterilize vaccines, tissue grafts, surgical instruments and enzymes.

- **Disadvantages:** It has poor penetrating power and is a carcinogen.

Table 5.1.1: Common antiseptics and disinfectants.

Chemical	Action	Uses
Ethanol (50–70%)	Denatures proteins and solubilizes lipids	Antiseptic used on skin
Isopropanol (50–70%)	Denatures proteins and solubilizes lipids	Antiseptic used on skin
Formaldehyde (8%)	Reacts with NH_2, SH and COOH groups	Disinfectant, kills endospores
Tincture of Iodine (2% I_2 in 70% alcohol)	Inactivates proteins	Antiseptic used on skin Disinfection of drinking water
Chlorine (Cl_2) gas	Forms hypochlorous acid (HClO), a strong oxidizing agent	Disinfect drinking water; general disinfectant
Silver nitrate ($AgNO_3$)	Precipitates proteins	General antiseptic and used in the eyes of newborns
Mercuric chloride	Inactivates proteins by reacting with sulfide groups	Disinfectant, although occasionally used as an antiseptic on skin
Detergents (e.g., quaternary ammonium compounds)	Disrupts cell membranes	Skin antiseptics and disinfectants
Phenolic compounds (e.g., Carbolic acid, lysol, Hexylresorcinol, Hexachlorophene)	Denature proteins and disrupt cell membranes	Antiseptics at low concentrations; disinfectants at high concentrations
Ethylene oxide gas	Alkylating agent	Disinfectant used to sterilize heat-sensitive objects such as rubber and plastics
Ozone	Generates lethal oxygen radicals	Purification of water, sewage

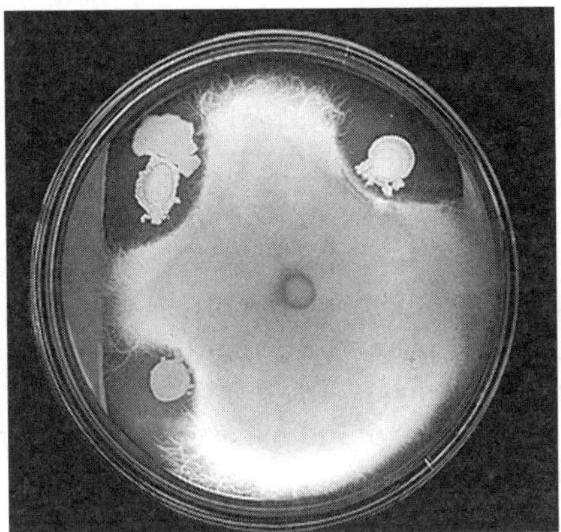

Figure 5.1.3: Three bacterial colonies growing on this plate secrete antibiotics that diffuse into the medium and inhibit the growth of a mold.

CHEMOTHERAPY AND ANTIBIOTICS

Chemotherapeutic agents (synthetic antibiotics): Antimicrobial agents of artificial origin are useful in the treatment of microbial or viral disease.

Examples are Sulfanilamides, Isoniazid, Ethambutol, AZT, Nalidixic Acid and Chloramphenicol.

Antibiotics: Antimicrobial agents produced by microorganisms that kill or inhibit other microorganisms. Most clinically-useful antibiotics are produced by microorganisms and are used to kill or inhibit infectious bacteria.

Properties of Antibiotics

- Antibiotics are low molecular-weight (non-protein) molecules produced as secondary metabolites, mainly by microorganisms that live in the soil.
- Most of these microorganisms form some type of a spore or other dormant cell and there is thought to be some relationship (besides temporal) between antibiotic production and the processes of sporulation.
- Among the molds, the notable antibiotic producers are *Penicillium* and *Cephalosporium* which are the main source of the beta-lactam antibiotics (Penicillin and its relatives).
- In the bacteria, the Actinomycetes, notably *Streptomyces* species, produce a variety of types of antibiotics including

the aminoglycosides (e.g., streptomycin), macrolides (e.g., erythromycin), and the tetracyclines. Endospore-forming bacillus species produce polypeptide antibiotics such as polymyxin and bacitracin.

ASEPSIS

Asepsis is the state of being free from disease-causing contaminants (such as bacteria, viruses, fungi, and parasites) or preventing contact with microorganisms. The term **asepsis** often refers to those practices used to promote or induce asepsis in surgery or medicine to prevent infection.

Asepsis is divided into the following two categories:

I. **Medical asepsis** consists of techniques that inhibit the growth and spread of pathogenic microorganisms. Medical asepsis is also known as clean technique and is used in many daily activities, such as hand hygiene and changing patients' bed linen. Principles of medical asepsis can be followed in the home, for instance, with the common practice of washing your hands before preparing food.

   Following are the principles of medical asepsis:

   Handwashing: Handwashing is the single most important means of preventing the spread of infection in the hospital. Hands should be washed.

   - Before beginning work
   - After using the bathroom
   - Before and after patient contact
   - Before eating and leaving work

   Using mechanical friction, all areas of the arms, lower than the elbows, should be well lathered and scrubbed. Special attention should be given to the nails and nail beds. Rings and jewelry should be removed from hands and wrists because these articles may shelter large numbers of microorganisms. Thoroughly rinse hands under running water.

   Dressing changes: Wash hands and use gloves as necessary. Remove dressings using no-touch technique and place them in a disposable bag. The physician will remove the sutures. Place the removed sutures in the disposable bag. If needed, apply a sterile dressing. Never touch the skin around a wound without sterile gloves being worn. Place tightly closed disposable bag

Table 5.1.2: Classes of antibiotics and their properties.

Chemical class	Examples	Biological source	Spectrum (effective against)	Mode of action
Beta-lactams (penicillins and cephalosporins)	Penicillin G, Cephalo-thin	*Penicillium notatum* and *Cephalosporium* species	Gram-positive bacteria	Inhibits steps in cell wall (peptidoglycan) synthesis and murein assembly
Semisynthetic penicillin	Ampicillin, Amoxycillin		Gram-positive and Gram-negative bacteria	Inhibits steps in cell wall (peptidoglycan) synthesis and murein assembly
Clavulanic acid	Clavamox is clavulanic acid plus amoxycillin	*Streptomyces clavuligerus*	Gram-positive and Gram-negative bacteria	Suicide inhibitor of beta-lactamases
Monobactams	Aztreonam	*Chromobacter violaceum*	Gram-positive and Gram-negative bacteria	Inhibits steps in cell wall (peptidoglycan) synthesis and murein assembly
Carboxypenems	Imipenem	*Streptomyces cattleya*	Gram-positive and Gram-negative bacteria	Inhibits steps in cell wall (peptidoglycan) synthesis and murein assembly

Contd...

Contd...

Chemical class	Examples	Biological source	Spectrum (effective against)	Mode of action
Aminoglycosides	Streptomycin	*Streptomyces griseus*	Gram-positive and Gram-negative bacteria	Inhibit translation (protein synthesis)
	Gentamicin	*Micromonospora species*	Gram-positive and Gram-negative bacteria esp. *Pseudomonas*	Inhibit translation (protein synthesis)
Glycopeptides	Vancomycin	*Streptomyces orientales*	Gram-positive bacteria, esp. *Staphylococcus aureus*	Inhibits steps in murein (peptidoglycan) biosynthesis and assembly
Lincomycins	Clindamycin	*Streptomyces lincolnensis*	Gram-positive and Gram-negative bacteria esp. anaerobic bacteroides	Inhibits translation (protein synthesis)
Macrolides	Erythromycin	*Streptomyces erythreus*	Gram-positive bacteria, Gram-negative bacteria not enterics, *Neisseria, Legionella, Mycoplasma*	Inhibits translation (protein synthesis)
Polypeptides	Polymyxin	*Bacillus polymyxa*	Gram-negative bacteria	Damages cytoplasmic membranes

Contd...

Contd...

Chemical class	Examples	Biological source	Spectrum (effective against)	Mode of action
	Bacitracin	*Bacillus subtilis*	Gram-positive bacteria	Inhibits steps in murein (peptidoglycan) biosynthesis and assembly
Polyenes	Amphotericin	*Streptomyces nodosus*	Fungi	Inactivate membranes containing sterols
	Nystatin	*Streptomyces noursei*	Fungi (Candida)	Inactivate membranes containing sterols
Rifamycins	Rifampicin	*Streptomyces mediterranei*	Gram-positive and Gram-negative bacteria, *Mycobacterium tuberculosis*	Inhibits transcription (eubacterial RNA polymerase)
Tetracyclines	Tetracycline	*Streptomyces species*	Gram-positive and Gram-negative bacteria, Rickettsias	Inhibit translation (protein synthesis)
Semisynthetic tetracycline	Doxycycline		Gram-positive and Gram-negative bacteria, *Rickettsias, Ehrlichia, Borrelia*	Inhibit translation (protein synthesis)
Chloramphenicol	Chloramphenicol	*Streptomyces venezuelae*	Gram-positive and Gram-negative bacteria	Inhibits translation (protein synthesis)

in the infectious waste receptacle in soiled utility room. Wash hands. The use of gloves does not negate the importance of hand washing before and after patient care.

Preoperative shave procedure: The purpose of preoperative shave is to cleanse, to remove hair from the operative site. It is important to be informed of the exact area to be prepared for any out of the ordinary aspects, i.e., rashes, lesions, warts or other skin eruptions. Nicking the skin during prepping increases the possibility of infection. Report any of these observations to your supervisor and the physician before continuing with the prep. If the skin is nicked, an incident report shall be completed. The physician shall be notified immediately. The preoperative preparation should be done as close to the time of surgery as practical as feasible. At times, clipping of hair or a depilatory agent will be used instead of shaving. This is also an acceptable practice.

Urinary catheter: Scrupulous aseptic technique in catheter insertion and daily cleaning at the point of insertion of the catheter with soap and water is utilized to reduce the incidence of infection.

Emptying urinary catheter bags: When a care provider is emptying a urinary catheter bag, this should be viewed as a single interaction for a single patient and the tasks for one patient should be completed before going to the next patient. Wearing gloves for emptying catheter bags is wise because it is difficult not to get urine on the hands. It is unacceptable to consider it a single task to empty the catheter bags for several patients in sequence without changing gloves and washing hands between patients. This is because of the real risk of transmitting organisms from the catheter bag drainage spout of one patient to the next patient's drainage spout on the hands of personnel.

Intravenous: Aseptic technique is mandatory in the preparation and administration of intravenous solutions. The longer the catheter remains in place, the greater the potential of infectious complications.

Care of the body after death from infectious disease: Infection control is of prime importance in the care of the body after death when the deceased patient has had an infectious disease. When taking care of a deceased patient who has had an airborne infectious disease, prescribed isolation technique should be followed and the patient's body labeled with "Airborne Precautions" before being transported to the morgue. All other patients are cared for under Standard Precautions Policy and Procedures.

Personal hygiene: All hospital personnel must be hygienic. If any employee is hygienically offensive, it is your responsibility to report the situation to the proper supervisor.

Employee rashes or skin lesions: Lesions on body such as boils, abscesses, impetigo, etc., must be reported to the employee's supervisor. The employee shall be referred to occupational health.

Patients with rashes or skin lesions: The most important intervention for rashes or skin lesions is to call it to the attention of the patient's physician and determine its cause promptly. In many cases, prompt recognition of the rash, identification of the cause, and prompt appropriate intervention can prevent transmission to the care provider and others. If a transmissible skin condition is identified, a "CONTACT PRECAUTIONS" sign shall be placed on the door of the patient's room so that ALL personnel can be advised of the protective barriers to be utilized.

Skin punctures/blood and body fluid exposure: If you break skin from a sharp object or sustain a blood or body fluid splash to the eyes, nose, or mouth or to open areas of your skin, you are required to report the incident to your supervisor for referral to occupational health services. An incident report is to be completed.

Equipment handling: Equipment used for patient care is contaminated after use whether visible soiled or not. Reusable equipment must be cleaned and disinfected before being used for another patient. Hands must be washed immediately after use of equipment for patient care.

Sterilized articles: Articles which have been sterilized must be carefully protected from contamination. Initial and expiration date shall be put on all packs and containers of sterile articles. If articles are not used within the specified period of time or if the packs become wet or damaged, the articles must be sterilized again. Consider all opened, wet or damaged packs as contaminated.

Work area sanitation: Work areas must be free from refuse, especially around refuse disposal units. Refuse in highrisk areas - Surgical Suites, Laboratory, Dietary, Emergency room, Isolation rooms and central sterile processing should be removed at least twice during the day shift.

Disposable equipment and supplies: Disposable equipment and supplies should be used whenever possible. Some of the used supplies become infectious waste if contaminated with large amounts of blood or body fluids or after use in high-risk areas.

Handling of all specimens: All specimens of blood or body fluids such as sputum, feces, urine or drainage from anybody site should be handled as if it were a source of infection. Disposable specimen containers are to be used and their disposal must be proper. Caution should be taken by persons who collect, transport and test specimens in order to prevent transmission of infection. All specimens should be transported to the laboratory in specimen transport bags.

Storage of clean equipment: All IV poles, weight scales, walkers, etc. should be stored in a clean storage area. These items should be wiped down with a disinfectant after patient use before storage.

Needle syringe disposal: Used needles and syringes are potential health hazards and should be treated with care. Contaminated needles and syringes must be discarded uncapped and unbroken into a needle and other sharps disposal boxes. Needle disposal boxes, when full, will be removed by building services.

Food: Food products are a major source of infectious microorganisms. The consumption of food by employees is forbidden in patient and/or work areas. Employees have designated areas for food consumption.

Various warm: Blooded animals are recognized as reservoirs of infectious disease agents of man. Because of this zoonosis, warm-blooded animals are forbidden in the hospital. A seeing-eye dog may be accompanied by a legally blind individual to certain areas of the hospital. Administrative policy may be seen. If rodents are observed, it is the responsibility of employee to report the incident to a supervisor.

Insects: Insects such as flies, cockroaches, etc. are main source for transmitting disease. All employees are to be instructed to report to their supervisor or any member of the Infection Control Committee when insects are observed.

Warning signs - All warning signs such as Biohazard, Isolation Precautions, Do Not Enter, Radioactivity, etc. are to be recognized and observed by all employees.

Refrigerators - Food is not to be stored in refrigerators containing medications, blood products, biohazard specimens or chemicals.

Smoking - Cigarettes are not sold in the hospital. Smoking is not allowed inside the hospital.

Preparation of medication sites - All patient skin sites utilized for intradermal, subcutaneous or intramuscular injections are to be cleaned prior to injecting with a disinfectant such as alcohol suitable for topical use. All intravenous injection ports are likewise to be cleaned prior to and after manipulation with alco-wipes.

II. **Surgical asepsis** destroys all microorganisms and their **spores** (the reproductive cells of some microorganisms, such as fungi or protozoa). Surgical asepsis is known as sterile technique and is used in specialized areas or skills, such as care of surgical wounds, urinary catheter insertion, invasive procedures and surgery.

Principles and Practices of Surgical Asepsis

Start with sterile equipment and set-up the sterile field.

- All objects used in a sterile field must be sterile.
- Confirm sterility of the package—Check expiration date and ensure package is clean and dry.
- Open the package—place in centre of table; top flap open away from you; touch only outside of wrapper; side flaps open with each hand; 4th flap toward you making sure it does not touch your uniform. If the inner surface touches any unsterile article it is contaminated.
- Opening a wrapped package while holding it: same as above.

- Using a drape to establish a field; with one hand pluck the corner of the drape that is folded back on the top.
  - Lift the drape out of the cover and allow it to open freely without touching any objects.
  - Lay the drape on a clean dry surface, placing the freely hanging side farthest from you (nurse should not lean over sterile field).
- If there is any doubt about the sterility of an object consider it unsterile, e.g. the package falls on the floor or has evidence of damage or moisture, even dried moisture.

Maintain the Sterile Field from Start to Finish

- The skin cannot be sterilized and is unsterile.
- Sterile persons and items contact only sterile areas, unsterile persons and items contact only unsterile areas.
- Sterile objects become unsterile when touched by unsterile objects.
- Sterile objects can become unsterile by prolonged exposure to airborne microorganisms. Do not cough, sneeze or talk excessively over a sterile field.
- Use a sterile package immediately once it has been opened. Leftover sterile solutions are no longer sterile and should be discarded.
- Sterile items that are out of vision or below the waist level of the nurse are considered unsterile. Sterile areas are continuously kept in view.
- Always face a sterile field. If you turn your back on a sterile field, you cannot guarantee its sterility.
- Movement within and around a sterile field must be such as not to cause contamination of that sterile field.
- Fluids flow in the direction of gravity. Moisture that passes through a sterile object draws microorganisms from unsterile surfaces above or below to the sterile surface by capillary action.
- The edges of sterile containers are not considered sterile once the package is open. The one inch margin around the edge of the sterile field is considered contaminated.
- Sterile gowns are considered sterile in front, shoulder to table level. The sleeves are also sterile.
- Tables are sterile only at table top level.
- Whenever bacterial barriers are permeated, contamination occur.

- Articles of doubtful sterility are considered unsterile.
- Conscientiousness, alertness and honesty are essential qualities in maintaining surgical asepsis.

Sterile Supplies

- Open each wrapped package as described above
- With free hand, grasp the corners of the wrapper and hold them against the wrist of the other hand (the unsterile hand is now covered by the sterile wrapper).
- Place the sterile item on the field by approaching from an angle rather than holding the arm over the field.
- **Commercially packaged supplies:** Hold the package above the field and allow contents to drop on center of the field.
- **Sterile solutions:** Read label to confirm solution. Outside of container is unsterile; inside sterile. Once it is opened, its sterility cannot be ensured for future use. Remove cap and inert before placing it on a table. Hold the bottle of fluid at a height of about 4-6" and to the side of the sterile field; discard a little solution before pouring; avoid splashing which will cause the field to be contaminated.
- **Use of sterile forceps:** Keep the tips of wet forceps lower than the wrist at all times. Hold sterile forceps above waist level and in sight.
- **Sterile gloves:** May be donned by open or closed method. Closed method requires a sterile gown so in the general care area, the open method is used. Gloves may be latex or vinyl and come in sizes.

The Surgical Team

- Team members are categorized as sterile or nonsterile in relation to the sterile surgical field.
- Sterile team members are those who scrub their hands and arms, don sterile attire, use sterile instruments and supplies and work in the sterile surgical field. This includes the surgeon, physician assistant and RN first assistant and the scrub person who may be a RN, a LVN or a surgical technician.
- The RNFA (Registered Nurse First Assistant) replaces an assisting surgeon and has had additional training. The duties include handling tissue and organs with instruments, providing exposure of the surgical site, suturing, etc.

- The scrub nurse (or surgical scrub technician) sets up and maintains the sterile field, hands supplies and instruments to the surgeon, keeps accurate count of instruments, sponges sharps and monitors aseptic technique.
- Nonsterile team members have responsibilities outside the sterile field and do not wear sterile attire.
  - The nonsterile team members include the anesthesiologists, the nurse anesthetist, and the circulating nurse.
  - The circulating nurse must be an RN and she coordinates the care of the client and manages activities outside the sterile field.

Medical Asepsis

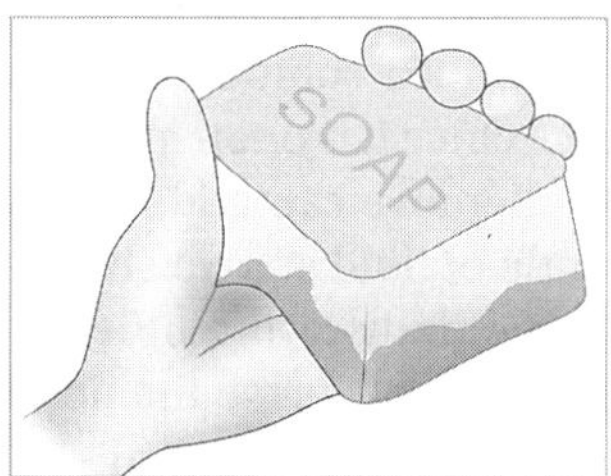

- Reduces number of pathogens
- Referred to as **"Clean techniques"**
- Used in administration of:
  - Medications
  - Enemas
  - Tube feedings
  - Daily hygiene
  - Handwashing is number

Surgical Asepsis

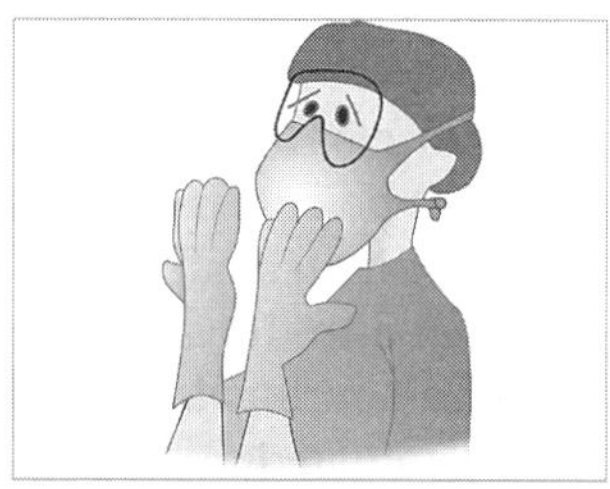

- Eliminates all pathogens
- Refered to as **"Sterile technique"**
- Used in:
  - Dressing changes
  - Catheterizations
  - Surgical procedures

Figure 5.1.4: Medical asepsis and surgical asepsis.

PRACTICAL PROCEDURES FOR HANDWASHING

Effective handwashing procedures can remove all transient bacteria. The adoption of this simple but effective technique has been demonstrated to significantly reduce rates of hospital acquired infection.

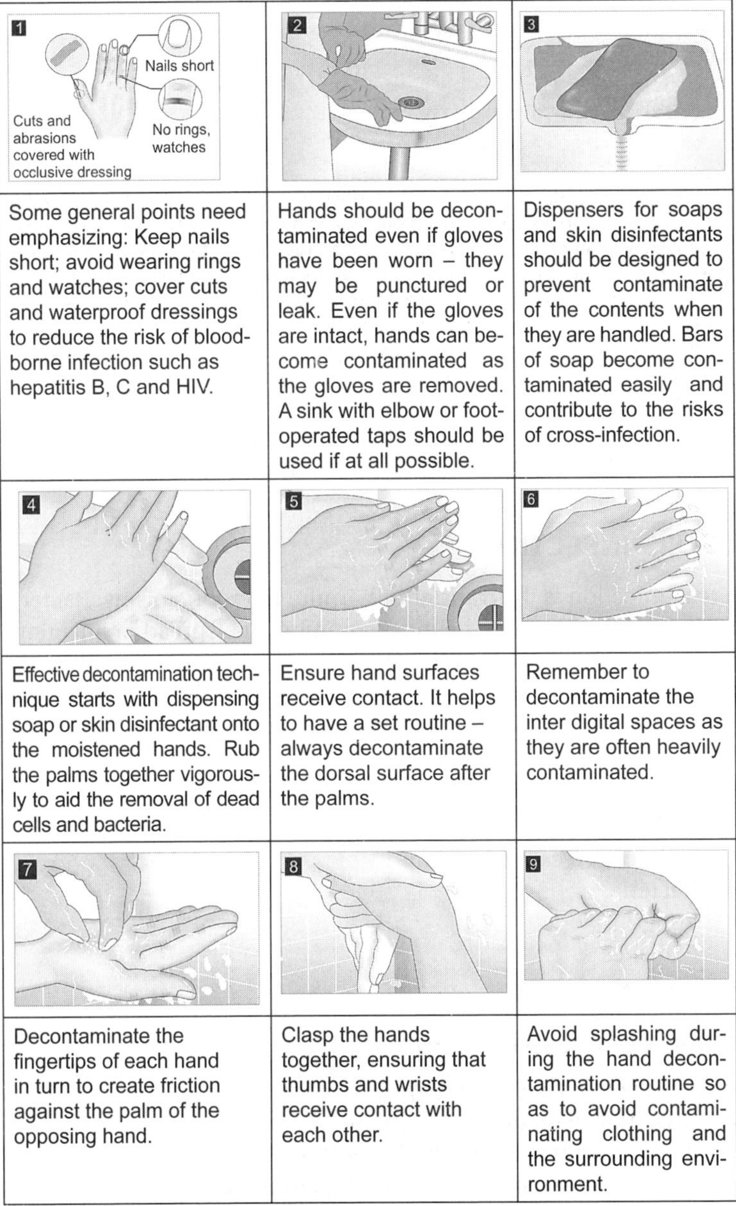

Figures 5.1.5(1 to 9): Technique of handwashing.

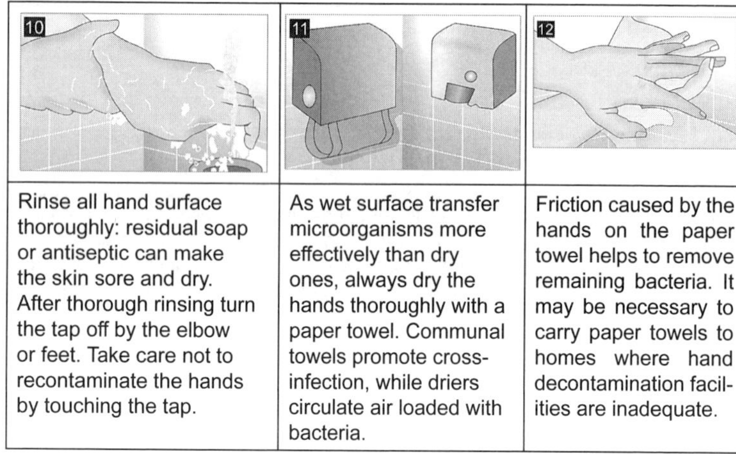

10	11	12
Rinse all hand surface thoroughly: residual soap or antiseptic can make the skin sore and dry. After thorough rinsing turn the tap off by the elbow or feet. Take care not to recontaminate the hands by touching the tap.	As wet surface transfer microorganisms more effectively than dry ones, always dry the hands thoroughly with a paper towel. Communal towels promote cross-infection, while driers circulate air loaded with bacteria.	Friction caused by the hands on the paper towel helps to remove remaining bacteria. It may be necessary to carry paper towels to homes where hand decontamination facilities are inadequate.

Figures 5.1.5(10 to 12): Technique of handwashing.

CROSS-INFECTION

Cross-infection is the transfer of harmful microorganisms. Bacteria and viruses are among the most common. The spread of infections can occur between people, pieces of equipment or within the body. These infections can cause many complications. Medical professionals work diligently to ensure equipment safety and a clean environment.

Types of Cross-infection

Cross-infection can stem from:

- Bacteria
- Fungi
- Parasites
- Viruses

Causes of Cross-infection

Cross-infections are caused by:

- Unsterilized medical equipment
- Bacteria from coughing and sneezing
- The transmission of viruses through human contact
- Touching contaminated objects
- Dirty bedding

Symptoms of Cross-infection

The exact symptoms of cross-infection depend on the source. For example, an infection caused by a catheter can result in a Urinary Tract Infection (UTI). The symptoms include pain in the kidneys, abdomen and groin. Infections spread through surgery may cause redness, swelling, and pus at the operation site. One of the first telling signs of a cross-infection is a fever. This is usually the body's first course of action to help to get rid of an infection.

Diagnosing Cross-infection

Doctors may use a combination of methods to diagnose cross-infection. These include:

- Physical examination
- Blood tests
- Culture tests
- Urine tests
- X-rays
- Health history review

Treating Cross-infection

Treating cross-infection depends on the condition. Antibiotics are often used for bacterial infections. These medicines don't treat viruses. The problem with antibiotics is that bacteria can learn to adapt and potentially become resistant to medications overtime. This not only leads to individual resistance, but can lead to the evolution of "superbugs." These are strains of bacteria immune to antibiotics, which make the risk for related complications high.

Prescription of anti-viral drugs are used to treat specific types of viruses. Anti-fungal medications can be used to treat fungal infections, either in topical or oral form. Parasites transferred through cross-infection may be treated with antibiotics as well as dietary changes.

Cross-infection Complications

Untreated bacterial and viral infections can lead to:

- Diarrhea
- Pneumonia
- Meningitis
- Death

Preventing Cross-infection

Cross-infection is the best treated at the source. Medical professionals use techniques to help preventing infections at facilities as well as during and after surgical procedures. Aseptic technique is a common process used to properly sterilize equipment so that harmful microorganisms can't spread from patient to patient.

CONTROL OF SPREAD OF INFECTION

Infection control in a health care facility is the prevention of spreading of microorganisms from:

- Patient to patient
- Patient to hospital staff member
- Hospital staff member to patient

Who does Infection Control?
Every health care facility should have a nominated person or team to ensure infection control policies and procedures are in place. However, all employees who have contact with patients or items used in the care of patients must adhere to infection control policies and procedures.

Why is Infection Controls important in Health care facilities?
In most health care facilities many sick people are treated or cared for in confined spaces. This means there are many microorganisms present. Patients will come into contact with many members of staff who can potentially spread the microorganisms and infections between patients. Large amounts of waste contaminated with blood and body substances are handled and processed in health care settings increasing the risk of infection.

The following medical procedures also increase the risk of infection:

- Inserting a tube into the body to drain or deliver fluids provides a pathway through which bacteria can enter.
- Surgery requires cutting the skin which is one of the body's most important defences against infection.
- The over-use of antibiotics have caused the development of some drug resistant bacteria that are harder to destroy. Controlling the spread of infections in a health care facility is, therefore, very important.

Note that the risk of people working in health care facilities getting infections from patients is very low if all staff members follow good hygiene principles and other standard precautions.

General Infection Control Measures

Implementation and adherence to infection control practices are the keys to prevent transmission of healthcare associated infections including respiratory diseases spread by droplet or airborne routes. Recommended infection control practices include the following:

- Hand hygiene
- Standard precautions/transmission-based precautions (Contact, Droplet, Airborne) and
- Respiratory hygiene
- **Hand Hygiene**

Proper hand hygiene is the most effective way to prevent the spread of infection.

- Wash hands with soap and water when they are visibly dirty or soiled with blood or other body fluids.
  - When washing hands with soap and water, wet hands with water, apply soap to hands and rub them together vigorously for at least 15 seconds covering all surfaces of the hands and fingers.
  - Rinse hands with water and dry thoroughly with a disposable towel. Use towel to turn off the faucet.
- If hands are not visibly soiled, an alcohol-based hand rub or gel may be used in place of soap and water.
  - When using an alcohol-based hand rub or gel, apply product to the palm of one hand and rub hands together covering all surfaces of hands and fingers until the hands are dry.
  - Avoid wearing artificial fingernails when caring for patients at high-risk for infection and keep natural nail tips less than 1/4-inch long.
  - Wear gloves when contact with blood, mucous membranes, non-intact skin or other potentially infectious materials could occur.
  - Remove gloves after caring for a patient. Always perform hand hygiene after removing gloves. Never wear the same pair of gloves for the care of more than one patient.
  - Change gloves during patient care if moving from a contaminated body site to a clean body site.

Standard Precautions

Standard precautions and transmission-based precautions are designed to prevent transmission of infectious microorganisms. They require the use of work practice controls and protective apparel for all contacts with blood and body substances and airborne infection isolation, droplet and contact precautions for patients with diseases known to be transmitted in whole or in part by those routes. Standard precautions include consistent and prudent preventive measures to be used at all times, regardless of a patient's infection status.

Standard precautions include the following:

Hand hygiene: Practice hand hygiene after touching blood, body fluids, secretions, excretions or contaminated items, whether or not gloves are worn. Wash hands immediately after gloves are removed between patient contacts and when otherwise indicated to avoid transfer of microorganisms to other patients or environment.

Gloves: Wear gloves (clean, nonsterile gloves are adequate) when touching blood, body fluids, secretion, excretion, or contaminated items. Put on clean gloves just before touching mucous membranes and nonintact skin. Change gloves between tasks and procedures. Practice hand hygiene whenever gloves are removed.

Mask, eye protection/face shield: Wear a mask and adequate eye protection (eyeglasses are not acceptable), or a face shield to protect mucous membranes of the eyes, nose and mouth during procedures and patient care activities that are likely to generate splashes or sprays of blood, body fluids, secretion, or excretion.

Gown: Wear a gown (a clean, nonsterile gown is adequate) to protect skin and to prevent soiling of clothing during procedure and patient care activities that are likely to generate splashes or sprays of blood, body fluids, secretion or excretion. Remove a soiled gown as promptly as possible, with care to avoid contamination of clothing, and wash hands.

Patient care Equipment: Handle used patient care equipment soiled with blood, body fluids, secretion, or excretion in a manner that prevents skin and mucous membrane exposures, contamination of clothing and transfer of microorganisms to one's self, other patients and environment. Ensure that reusable equipment is not used for the care of another patient until it has been cleaned and sanitized appropriately. Ensure that single-used items are discarded properly.

Droplet Precautions

In addition to standard precautions, use droplet precautions for a patient known or suspected to be infected with microorganisms transmitted by droplets (large-particle, wet droplets [larger than 5mμ in size]) that can be generated by the patient during coughing, sneezing, talking or in the course of procedure.

Droplet precautions include the following:

Patient placement: Place the patient in a private room. When a private room is not available, place the patient in a room with a patient who has active infection with the same microorganism but with no other infection (cohorting). When a private room is not available and cohorting is not achievable, maintain spatial separation of at least six feet between the infected patient and other patients and visitors. Special air handling and ventilation are not necessary and the door may remain open.

Mask: In addition to standard precautions, wear a mask or respirator when working within three to six feet of the patient. (Hospitals may want to implement the practice of wearing a mask to enter the room.)

Patient transport: Limit the movement and transport of the patient from the room to essential purposes only. If transport or movement is necessary, minimize patient dispersal of droplets by masking the patient, if possible.

Contact Precautions

In addition to standard precautions, contact precautions should be used for the care of patients known or suspected to have illnesses that can be spread by usual contact with an infected person or the surfaces or patient care items in the room.

Contact precautions include the following:

- **Gloves and hand hygiene:** Wear gloves when entering the room. During the course of providing care for a patient, change gloves after having contact with infectious material. Remove gloves before leaving the patient's room and wash hands immediately with an antimicrobial agent or use a waterless antiseptic agent. After glove removal and hand- washing, ensure that hands do not touch potentially contaminated surfaces or items in the patient's room.
- **Gown:** Wear a gown when entering the room. Remove the gown before leaving the patient's environment. After gown removal, ensure that clothing does not contact potentially contaminated environmental surfaces. Wash or decontaminate hands.

- **Patient transport:** Limit the movement of the patient from the room to essential purposes only. During transport, ensure that all precautions are maintained.
- **Patient care equipment:** When possible, dedicate the use of noncritical patient care equipment to a single patient (or cohort of patients infected or colonized with the pathogen requiring precautions) to avoid sharing between patients. If use of common equipment or items is unavoidable, then adequately clean and disinfect them before use for another patient.
- **Patient placement (private room):** Place the patient in a private room. If a private room is not available, place the patient in a room with other patients with the same illness (cohorting). Apply appropriate cleaning and decontamination of the room after the patient has vacated it.

Airborne Infection Isolation

In addition to standard precautions, airborne infection isolation measures are designed to reduce the risk of transmission of infectious microorganisms that may be suspended in the air either in small particle aerosols or dust. Patients requiring airborne infection isolation must be given a private room with special air handling and ventilation (negative pressure). Respiratory protection for healthcare workers is necessary when entering the patient's room.

Respiratory Hygiene/Cough Etiquette

"Respiratory hygiene" includes the measures that can be taken to decrease the risk of spreading respiratory pathogens. A universal "respiratory hygiene/cough etiquette" strategy for a healthcare facility should include the following:

- Place signs at the entrances of all outpatient facilities requesting that patients and visitors inform healthcare personnel of respiratory symptoms upon registration.
- Provide masks (e.g., surgical) for all patients presenting with respiratory symptoms (especially cough) and provide instructions on the proper use and disposal of masks.
- If a patient cannot wear a mask, provide tissues and instructions on when to use them (i.e., when coughing, sneezing or controlling nasal secretions), how and where to dispose of them and the importance of hand hygiene after handling this material.

- Provide hand hygiene materials in waiting room areas and encourage patients with respiratory symptoms to wash their hands.
- If possible, designate an area in waiting rooms where patients with respiratory symptoms can be segregated (ideally by more than three feet) from other patients without respiratory symptoms.
- Place patients with respiratory symptoms in a private room or cubicle as soon as possible for further evaluation.
- Healthcare workers evaluating patients with respiratory symptoms should wear a surgical or procedure mask.
- Consider the installation of Plexiglas barriers at the point of triage or registration to protect healthcare workers.
- If a physical barrier is not possible, instruct registration and triage staff to remain at least three to six feet from unmasked patients. Staff should consider wearing a surgical mask during registration and triage.
- Continue to use droplet precautions to manage patients with respiratory symptoms until it is determined that the cause of symptoms is not an infectious agent that requires precautions beyond standard precautions.

POSSIBLE QUESTIONS

1. Define sterilization and explain briefly the methods of sterilization.
2. What are the roles of nurses in preventing cross-infections?
3. Give a detail account of chemical agents used for controlling microorganisms.
4. What are the various physical methods of sterilization? What are its advantages and disadvantages?
5. Write an essay on chemotherapy and antibiotics.
6. What is asepsis? Differentiate between medical and surgical asepsis?
7. Write Short Notes:
   a. Medical and surgical asepsis
   b. Pasteurization
   c. Autoclave
   d. Chemical sterilization
   e. Sterilization
   f. Radiation sterilization
   g. Chemotherapy
   h. Antibiotics
   i. Principles of surgical asepsiss
   j. Cross-infection

k. Technique of handwashing
l. Surgical team
m. Personal hygiene
n. Asepsis dry heat and moist heat

MULTIPLE CHOICE QUESTIONS

1. The primary reasons to control and destroy microbes are:
   a. To prevent transmission of disease and infection
   b. To prevent decomposition and spoilage
   c. To prevent contamination
   d. All of the above
2. Which of the following best describes the process of 'Disinfection'?
   a. The elimination of all forms of microorganisms and bacterial spores
   b. The elimination of all forms of bacterial spores
   c. The reduction or elimination of microorganisms and bacterial spores
   d. The reduction or elimination of many microorganisms and some bacterial spores
3. Name the sterilization agent that is most frequently used in hospitals and clinical laboratories for the heat-labile liquid substances or antibiotics:
   a. Dry heat b. Radiation
   c. Filtration d. Formaldehyde
4. Which of the following is the correct definition for the **'pasteurization'** process of milk and fermented products?
   a. The sterilization method that uses heat at a boiling temperature of 100°C
   b. The sterilization method that uses heat at 100 to 120°C
   c. The sterilization method that uses moist heat below 100°C
   d. The sterilization method that uses moist heat above 100°C
5. Which of the following rays lead to formation of Thymine-Thymine dimers?
   a. X-ray b. Gamma-ray
   c. UV-ray d. None of the above
6. Name the ionizing radiation:
   a. Infrared b. X-rays and gamma rays
   c. Halogens d. Ethylene oxide
7. The biological source of Rifampicin is:
   a. Streptomyces mediteranei b. *Streptomyces nodosus*
   c. *Streptomyces erythreus* d. None of the above
8. Handwashing is an example of:
   a. Sterility b. Safety
   c. Medical asepsis d. Surgical asepsis
9. The absence of disease producing pathogens or microorganisms:
   a. Antisepsis b. Clean
   c. Disinfection d. Asepsis

10. The level of aseptic control which kills all microorganisms, including spores and viruses is:
    a. Antisepsis b. Disinfection
    c. Sterilization d. None of the above
11. Which of these is not considered as a cleaning agent for handwashing?
    a. Water b. Alcohol
    c. Soap d. None of the above
12. How long hands should be washed for after wetting hands and applying soap?
    a. 5 seconds b. 15 seconds
    c. 20 seconds d. 30 seconds
13. When a person suffers from droplet infection which of the following is essential precaution material for use?
    a. Gloves b. Gowns
    c. Masks d. Goggles
14. Beta-propiolactone (BPL) is a:
    a. Alkylating agent b. Sweetener
    c. Potential life inhibitor d. None of the above

Answers

1. d	2. d	3. c	4. c	5. c
6. b	7. a	8. c	9. d	10. c
11. b	12. c	13. c	14. a	

Biosafety and Waste Management

BIOSAFETY

Biosafety means efforts done by us to ensure safety while using, transporting, transferring, releasing and disposing parts or whole of organisms.

Many countries proposed strict laws and regulations to avoid any harm that happen due to lack of biosafety. However, even few other countries lack biosafety awareness and thus they create problems to the as well as to the environment.

NEED FOR BIOSAFETY

Coming in contact with human blood or blood products or with certain harmful chemicals used in laboratories is potentially dangerous (technically called hazardous). Biosafety involves taking precautions to protect you and co-workers against infection, injury or even poisoning.

Most policy and regulatory activities under Biosafety are local limited to Nations. However, International agreements are found essential to make all Nations equal and to standardize the rules of Biosafety throughout the earth. Certain Organizations deal with different rule sets of Biosafety. For instance, FAO deals with risks associated with environment and food under Biosafety. The organization also helps in providing Sanitary and Phytosanitary (meaning sanitation through plants) measures (SPS). It develops methods for analyzing risks in food and agriculture industry, fisheries and forestry as well.

TERMS USED IN BIOSAFETY

Stability: The ability of chemical to stay strong without getting decomposed.

Incompatibility: Certain chemicals should not be mixed or even stored together which may create dangerous consequences.

Hazardous Decomposition Products: Harmful chemical products formed when chemicals decomposes of burns.

Hazardous Polymerization: Accumulation of more likely harmful substances is called hazardous polymerization. This enhances the severity of consequences. It causes more heat to be released which might explode the containers.

Accessibility: Ensured sites are secure to limit unauthorized or unintentional access.

Clear Access: If the waste collection point is inside the work area, access to the area shall be kept clean. A dedicated chemical waste storage area should be considered.

Signage: Signage should be erected advising the location of collection point.

Conditions: Collection points and storage areas shall be cool, dry and free from contamination.

Cleaning: Floors shall be smooth and impervious for easy cleaning. A water supply shall be in close proximity for cleaning purposes.

Ventilation: Natural or mechanical ventilation shall be provided to prevent build-up of fumes and vapors.

Location: Shall be sited away from food preparation, smoking or storage areas.

Drainage: Drainage systems shall not allow run-off from spills, etc., to enter storm-water drains.

Security: Collection points must be secured at all time when not in use. **Arrangement** shall be established to provide waste contractors with accessibility for collection of waste.

SPILL, LEAK AND DISPOSAL PROCEDURES

When accidental spills, leaks or disposal of harmful chemicals happen while you work in laboratory, there are certain procedures which need to be followed. These procedures include appropriate waste disposal methods required for safety and environmental protection.

Eye protection: Recommendations are dependent upon the irritancy, corrosivity and special handling procedures.

Skin protection: Describes the particular types of protective garments and appropriate glove materials to provide personnel protection.

Respiratory protection: Appropriate respirators for conditions exceeding the recommended occupational exposure limits.

BIOSAFETY CABINETS AND OTHER SAFETY EQUIPMENT (FIGURES 5.2.1 AND 5.2.2)

Biological Safety Cabinets (BSC) prevents the contamination of harmful microorganisms in air while working with highly infectious materials inside the Laminar flow chamber. Among various types of classes available for Biological Safety Cabinets, only Class II BSC is mostly preferred. The followings are instruments used for providing additional protection through Biosafety.

Chemical Fume Hoods: Protect the environment from vapors and gases.

Biological Safety Cabinets (Figure 5.2.1): Protect the environment from small particles.

Clean Benches: For doing work comfortably with maximum sterility.

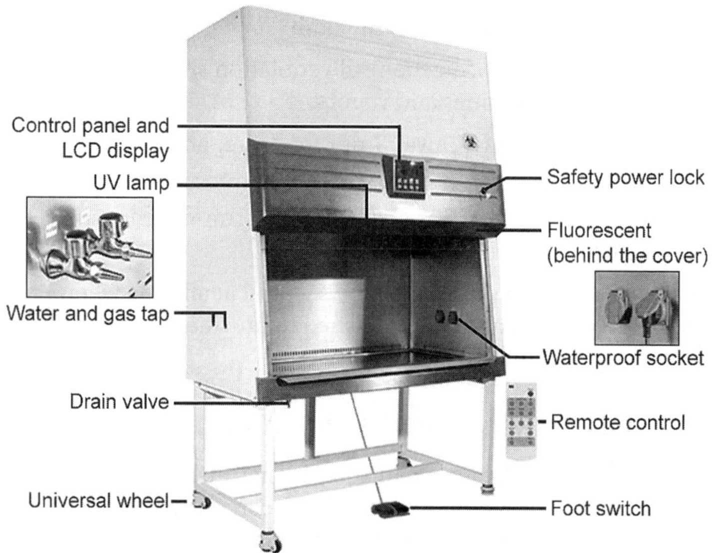

Figure 5.2.1: Biosafety cabinet (BSC).

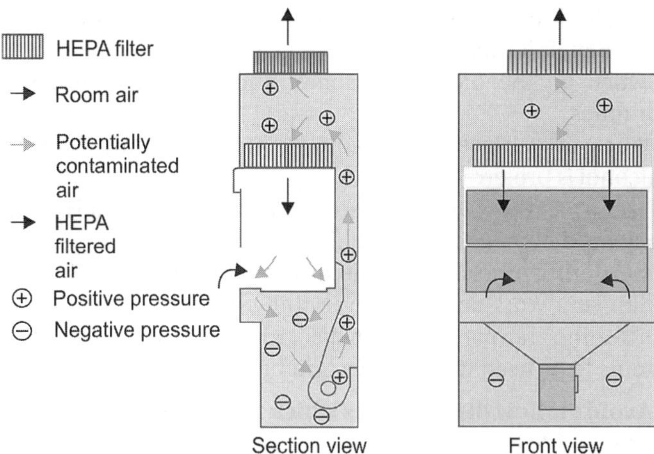

Figure 5.2.2: Internal view of biological safety cabinet (BSC).

BIOSAFETY CABINET ALARMS

Try not to work with Biosafety Cabinets connected to Alarming System. This Alarming system is necessary for those laboratories where biosafety is not practised absolutely. When alarm rings, it says that there are certain spills, leakages or even contamination happened. Make sure that you get out of the laboratory to protect yourself from infections.

OTHER SAFETY EQUIPMENT

The use of some devices like blenders, homogenizers, sonicators produce aerosols. "Aerosols" means small particles mixed in air. These aerosols might contaminate the BSC. To reduce exposure to aerosols, these devices should be used in BSC only when it is really necessary.

SAFE AND EFFECTIVE USE OF THE BIOSAFETY CABINET (BSC)

I. Before starting the work in laboratory:

- Check Biosafety Cabinet Alarms, pressure gauges, flow indicators for any changes.

- Switch off the UV-light otherwise, you might get skin cancer as UV- light is a carcinogen.
- Switch on the Biosafety Cabinet and allow it to run for 3-5 minutes.
- Wipe work surface with an appropriate disinfectant. Mostly 90% alcohol is preferred.
- Place a pan filled with disinfectant or lined with a small biohazard bag inside the BSC to collect discards. Avoid reaching outside of BSC during procedures to discard waste in floor containers.
- Plan your work and place everything needed for the procedure including the pan for your discards inside the BSC. Wipe all items to be used with disinfectant before placing them in BSC.

II. Avoid air flow disturbances which might affect the protection level in BSC:

- Keep the BSC free of clutter like extra unwanted equipment and supplies. Keep all necessary items only in the BSC.
- Do not place objects over the front air intake grille.
- Do not block the rear air intake grille.
- Do not allow more people to be near BSC when it is in use.
- Always check whether laboratory door is closed. Try to avoid opening and closing door if the door is near BSC.
- Work slowly.
- Do not operate a Bunsen Burner inside the BSC.

III. While working:

Work as far as possible to the back of BSC workspace as possible. Do not use BSC for preparing media and all. Try to finish majority of your steps outside BSC.

Separate contaminated and clean items. Work from "Clean to dirty". Clean up all spills in the cabinet immediately then and there when it happens. Allow cabinet to run for 3–5 minutes before resuming work when there is any spill.

IV. After completing the work:

Wipe down all items with an appropriate disinfectant before removing. Remove all materials and wipe the interior surfaces with the same.

Check for the decontaminates in regular intervals under work grilles.

GENERAL LABORATORY SAFETY (FIGURE 5.2.3)

- Laboratory employees must notify immediately to the laboratory manager or PI in case of an accident, injury, illness, or overt exposure associated with laboratory activities.
- No eating, drinking, smoking, handling contact lenses or applying cosmetics in the laboratory at any time.
- No animals or minors (persons under the age of 18), or Immunocompromised persons will be allowed to enter the laboratory at any time.
- Food, medications or cosmetics should not be brought into the laboratory for storage or later use. Food is stored outside in areas designated specifically for that purpose.
- No open-toed shoes or sandals are allowed in the laboratory.
- Personal Protective Equipment (PPE) includes gloves, lab coat and eye protection.
- All skin defects such as cuts, abrasions, ulcers, areas of dermatitis, etc., should be covered with an air tight and water proof bandage.
- Pipetting out solutions by mouth is prohibited; mechanical pipetting devices are to be used at all times.
- All procedures are to be performed carefully to minimize the creation of splashes or aerosols.
- Follow all manufacturer's instructions and Standard Operating Procedures (SOPs) when using any of the laboratory equipment.
- Wash hands: After removing gloves and before leaving the laboratory.
- Razor blades, scalpels, and hypodermic needles ("sharps") should be discarded into the "sharps" container in the biosafety cabinet. Needles should not be recapped.
- Work surfaces will be decontaminated as needed with. Follow manufacturer instructions for contact time.
- All cultures, stocks and other regulated wastes are decontaminated by autoclaving before disposal. Liquids (non-organic) can be decontaminated with bleach, bringing the solution to 10% bleach, and discarded in the sink. No other chemicals can be discarded in the sink.

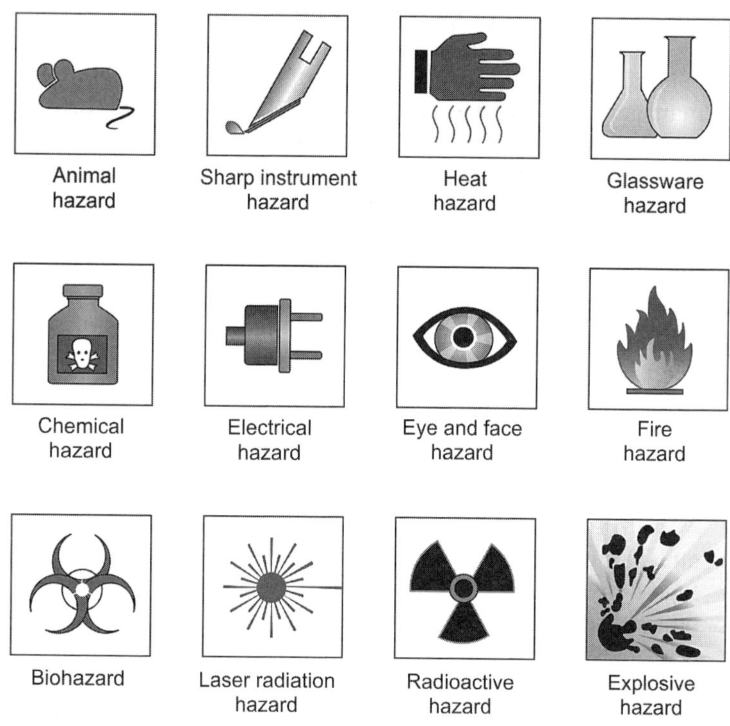

Figure 5.2.3: Laboratory safety symbols for warning labels.

WASTE DISPOSAL

Waste is anything that is not required for us and must be discarded. Decontamination of wastes and their ultimate disposal are closely interrelated. Most glassware, instruments and laboratory clothing will be reused or recycled. The overriding principle is that all infectious materials should be decontaminated (meaning: removed with harmful microorganisms or organisms or harmful chemicals), autoclaved (meaning: heated to high temperature about 121°C for 15 minutes at 15 lbs) or incinerated (meaning: burnt in high temperature to ash) within the laboratory. The principal question that hints our mind before discharge of any objects or materials by laboratory workers who deal with highly infectious microorganisms or animal tissues:

- Have the objects or materials been effectively decontaminated or disinfected by an approved procedure?
- If not, have they been packaged in an approved manner for immediate on-site incineration or transfer to another facility with incineration capacity?
- Does the disposal of the decontaminated objects or materials involve any additional potential hazards, biological or otherwise, to those who carry out the immediate disposal procedures or who might come into contact with discarded items outside the facility?

PROPER DISPOSAL OF SHARPS AND WASTES

- Take precautions to avoid needl-estick injury which can be caused due to several reasons including lack of focus, inexperience, lack of concern for others, improper disposal of sharps, etc.
- Always drop used sharps in special containers.
- Do not break, bend, re-sheath or reuse lancets, syringes or needles.
- Do not shake sharps containers to create space.
- Never place needles or sharps in Office waste containers.
- Sharps containers must be placed near workspace closed when not in use. Usually, these sharps containers should be sealed three quarters to avoid injuries.

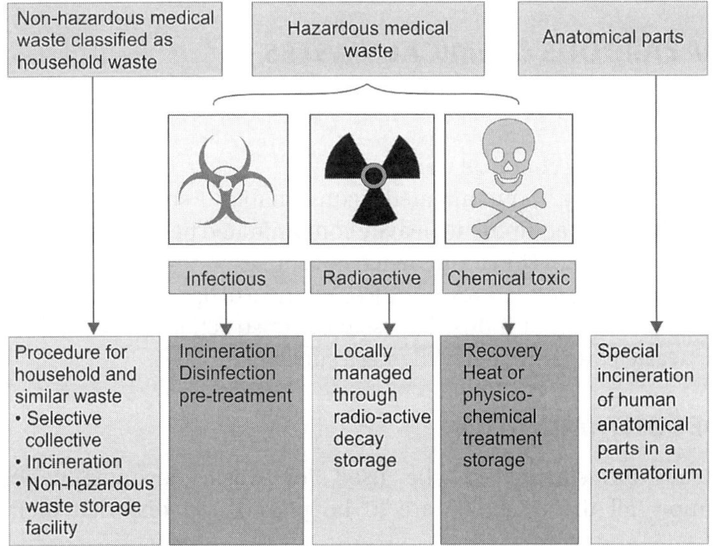

POLICY FOR HANDLING SHARPS

- User is responsible for disposal of sharps.
- Must dispose of sharps after each test.
- Must place sharps in sharps boxes.
- Do not drop sharps on the floor or in the Office waste bin.
- Place sharps container near your workspace.
- Seal and remove when box is three quarters full.
- Incinerate all waste.

Handling Chemicals

Chemicals are sometimes ignitable, corrosive, reactive or toxic. Therefore, they should be handled properly. In case there is any spill of chemicals then do the following: Paper towels are to be applied to absorb the spill, and then paper towels are soaked with any of the disinfectants. For spills outside the bio-safety hood, alert others in the area. Use N95 mask if there is a possibility of harmful aerosols. All aspects of the emergency SOPs are followed without exception.

DISINFECTION

- Always disinfectants are used to kill germs and pathogens to keep the work surface clean.
- Disinfection prevents cross contamination and reduces risk of infection.

HAZARDOUS CHEMICAL WASTES

Hazardous chemical wastes may be in liquid, solid or gaseous form and include:

- Laboratory chemical waste
- Chemically contaminated consumables such as broken laboratory equipment, heavily contaminated personal protective environment (PPE) and bench covers
- Other by-products resulting from the use of hazardous chemicals
- Commercial or industrial waste or construction and demolition waste contaminated with or is a substance.

DECONTAMINATION

Steam autoclaving can be used for waste decontamination. Simply all the materials are to be placed and disposed in the containers. These are then placed in autoclave. There are certain commercially available plastic bags which can be used for carrying all the above mentioned materials for autoclaving. This method kills microorganisms, however not spores. Some laboratories choose incineration method (burning things to ash) for waste disposal.

There are some materials and equipment which cannot be autoclaved. For these materials and equipment you can use chemical disinfectants for removing harmful organisms or harmful chemicals. Depending on the resistance of harmful organisms contained in wastes the disinfectant can be choosen. Using chemical disinfectants can easily kill vegetative bacteria, fungi and enveloped viruses while Mycobacteria and non-enveloped viruses are killed slowly. Other organisms like bacterial spores and protozoan cysts cannot be killed by disinfectants.

Gamma irradiation is another method of killing harmful organisms and also decontaminating heat sensitive materials. Depending on the density of waste materials and strength of gamma irradiation source, the efficiency of treatment can be determined.

Finally, incineration has traditionally been the chosen method for destroying anatomical biomedical waste and animal carcasses. In most cases, wastes to be incinerated have to be packaged and transported off-site in accordance with provincial or territorial legislation. Steam autoclaving of materials should be done initially, only then followed by incineration.

THE HANDLING AND DISPOSAL OF CONTAMINATED MATERIALS AND WASTES

There should be identification and separation system for infectious materials and their containers. Since there are no stringent national regulations; international regulations best practices must be followed. Categories should include:

- Non-contaminated (non-infectious) waste that can be reused or recycled or disposed of as general, "household" waste.
- Contaminated (infectious) "sharps" – hypodermic needles, scalpels, knives and broken glass; should always be collected

in puncture-proof containers fitted with covers and treated as infectious.
- Contaminated material for decontamination by autoclaving and thereafter washing and reuse or recycling.
- Contaminated material for autoclaving and disposal.
- Contaminated material for direct incineration.

SHARPS

After use, hypodermic needles should not be recapped, clipped removed from disposable syringes. The complete assembly should be placed in a sharps disposal container. Disposable syringes, used alone or with needles, should be placed in sharps disposal containers and incinerated with prior autoclaving if required. Sharps disposal containers must be puncture-proof-resistant and must not be filled to capacity. When they are three-quarters full they should be placed in "infectious waste" containers and incinerated with prior autoclaving. Sharps disposal containers must not be discarded in landfills.

CONTAMINATED (POTENTIALLY INFECTIOUS) MATERIALS FOR AUTOCLAVING AND REUSE

No pre-cleaning should be attempted if any contaminated or potentially infectious materials are to be autoclaved and reused. Any necessary cleaning or repair must be done only after autoclaving or disinfection.

CONTAMINATED MATERIALS FOR DISPOSAL

Apart from sharps, all contaminated materials should be autoclaved in leak-proof containers, example autoclavable, color-coded plastic bags, before disposal. After autoclaving, the material may be placed in transfer containers for transport to the incinerator. If possible, materials deriving from healthcare activities should not be discarded in landfills even after decontamination.

PROCESS FOR HAZARDOUS CHEMICALS WASTE MANAGEMENT (TABLE 5.2.1)

Table 5.2.1: Different types of wastes including hazardous wastes.

Term	Definition/ Explanation/ Details	Term	Definition/ Explanation/Details
Clinical Waste	Waste that has the potential to cause disease, including for example animal waste, discarded sharps, human tissue waste, laboratory waste, etc. Note: Clinical waste does not include waste from laboratories that do not conduct testing of blood, body fluids or tissues from humans or animals	Hazardous Chemical	Means 'a substance, mixture or article that satisfied the criteria for a hazard class in the Globally Harmonized System (GHS)' and may include radioactive and waste chemicals or other material contaminated with hazardous chemicals.
Cytotoxic Waste	Material that is, or may be, contaminated by a cytotoxic medication	Hazardous Chemical Waste	Waste generated from the use of hazardous chemicals in workplace procedures. This includes procedures undertaken in laboratories, workshops, oral health and clinical services and other functional areas.
Dangerous Goods	Goods are dangerous goods if they are defined under the Australian Dangerous Goods (ADG) Code as dangerous goods; or goods too dangerous to be transported.	Sharps	Objects or devices having sharp points or protuberances or cutting edges, capable of cutting or piercing the skin. Includes hypodermic, intravenous or other medical needles, Pasteur pipettes, scalpel blades, lancets, scissors, glass slides, broken glass such as vials, bottles and laboratory glass

Contd...

Contd...

Term	Definition/ Explanation/ Details	Term	Definition/ Explanation/Details
Environmental Harm	Any adverse effect, or potential adverse effect (whether temporary or permanent and of whatever magnitude, duration or frequency) on an environmental value, and includes environmental nuisance. Note: Material and serious environmental harm denote varying degrees of environmental harm.	Related waste	Waste that constitutes, or is contaminated with, chemicals, cytotoxic drugs, human body parts, pharmaceutical products or radioactive substances.
General Waste	Waste other than regulated waste	Regulated Waste	Means waste that is or contains a substance, or residues of a substance
Industrial Waste	Is interceptor waste or waste other than commercial waste; domestic cleanup and domestic waste; green waste; recyclable interceptor waste; recyclable waste; waste discharged to sewer.	Laboratory Waste	A specimen or culture discarded in the course of dental, medical or veterinary practice or research, including material that is, or has been contaminated by, genetically manipulated material or imported biological material.

Waste Characterization

- Dangerous by-products may result when mixing incompatible waste categories.
- To ensure safe storage, handling and disposal of hazardous chemical waste, work area managers shall ensure producing

chemical waste mixtures record ingredient information and properties of the waste (e.g., corrosive, flammable or other specif ic hazards).

- This information should be followed by workers, waste contractors and others who likely to work with any of the hazardous chemical wastes.

Waste Segregation

- Hazardous chemical waste shall be segregated according to hazard class and waste category.
- Mixed hazard classes include chemical wastes of differing hazard classes which shall not be mixed. For instance, concentrated acids or alkalis shall not be mixed with other chemicals.
- Mixed waste categories - where the chemical waste may belong to more than one waste category the following guide shall be used:
  - Radioactive and chemical waste - treat as radioactive waste in the first instance.
  - Clinical and chemical waste - if grossly contaminated with biological material treat as clinical in the first instance.

On-site Collection, Transport and Storage

- Chemical waste, and in particular flammable or combustible liquid waste, shall not be allowed to accumulate and regular collections shall be established.
- When establishing regular waste collections consideration shall be given to
  - Appropriateness of waste receptacles and containers
  - Frequency of collection
  - Collection points and storage sitting
  - Container management
  - Containment of spills and leaks
  - On-site transport
  - Accessibility of SDS
- Where practicable, transportation shall be scheduled for non-peak traffic times and consideration given to the following:
  - Route and method of transport
  - Use trolleys or carts that are easy to load, unload and clean
  - Transport equipment shall be free of sharp edges or protrusions that may puncture container

- Equipment shall regularly be cleaned to remove any chemical residues and reduce exposure risks
- Containment of smaller drums/bottles within plastic tubs (for fume and spill containment)
- Use of original packaging or specific packaging to limit damage during transport (e.g. Glass Winchesters used in laboratories).

Container Management

Containers utilized as part of waste management shall:

- be maintained in good condition at all times
- be securely closed at all times unless adding or removing waste
- only be filled to three quarters full to allow for contraction or expansion of the contents
- be appropriate for the type of waste to be collected
- Khall, if practicable, be legibly labelled with the following:
  - Product identifier
  - Name, Address and Telephone number of the manufacturer or importer
  - Hazard classification (e.g., oxidizing liquid)
  - A hazard pictogram and hazard statement consistent with the classification of the chemical.
  - Glass containers shall be packaged to minimize risk of breakage.

Empty Containers

- Empty waste containers that cannot safely be decontaminated shall be treated as chemical waste and stored at a secured collection point.
- Labels shall be left on containers which are unable to be properly decontaminated.
- Empty gas cylinders shall be returned to the vendor for reuse or disposal.
- Option for dealing with empty containers are:
  - Option 1 – return to the vendor for re-use or disposal
  - Option 2 – disposal to general or recycling waste.

If option 2 is adopted, the container shall be completely empty and triple rinsed with water to remove residual material and vapors. The rinse water used for cleaning may need to be contained for treatment or packaged as chemical waste for collection and disposal.

POSSIBLE QUESTIONS

1. Define biosafety and explain its needs.
2. Why mouth pipetting is strictly prohibited?
3. Using disinfectants to clean your work surface is highly helpful to keep you healthy. Justify the statement.
4. What is hazardous waste? In which form, you can see hazardous waste?
5. Mention the steps involved in the process of hazardous waste management.
6. Enumerate different types of waste and its management.
7. Write Short Notes:
   a. Biosafety
   b. Biological safety cabinet (BSC)
   c. General laboratory safety
   d. Hospital waste disposal
   e. Types of medical waste
   f. Disinfection
   g. Decontamination
   h. Container management

MULTIPLE CHOICE QUESTIONS

1. The application of combinations of laboratory practices and procedures, laboratory facilities, safety equipment when working with potentially infectious microbes is called:
   a. Containment b. Biosafety
   c. Risk assessment d. Decontamination
2. The ability of a chemical to stay strong without getting decomposed is known as:
   a. Stability b. Incompatibility
   c. Susceptibility d. None of the above
3. What is the function of biosafety cabinet?
   a. A work space to culture and sub-culture the bacteria
   b. A designed space to prevent the cross-contamination due to air-borne contaminant during transfer of the bacteria
   c. A primary barrier to reduce the spreading of disease caused by microorganisms into the laboratory environment.
   d. All of the above
4. What is the minimum age of a person to be entered into the laboratory:
   a. 14 b. 16
   c. 18 d. 20
5. PPE is:
   a. Protective physical equipment
   b. Personal protective equipment
   c. Possible protective equipment
   d. Personal protection enhancements

6. Which of the following practices should be utilized when working in a BSC?
   a. Disinfect all equipment which go into and come out of the BSC
   b. Do not store any items in the BSC
   c. Disinfect the work surface of the BSC before and after the work
   d. All of the above
7. Which of the following practices are allowed in the laboratory?
   a. Handling contact lenses
   b. Applying cosmetics
   c. Eating and drinking
   d. None of the above
8. Personal Protective equipment for each task is:
   a. Not required for students
   b. Not necessary until the task is of High risk
   c. Designated by the supervisor and specified by the exposure control plan or by Standard operating procedures
   d. None of the above
9. Mouth pipetting is allowed:
   a. When working with well characterized agents
   b. Never
   c. If trained properly
   d. Both a and c
10. Which of the following procedures can generate aerosols?
    a. Sonicating tissue culture cells
    b. Cell sorters
    c. Pipetting
    d. All of the above
11. Which of the following is not a waste disposal method?
    a. Incineration b. Decontamination
    c. Autoclaving d. Sieving
12. Which of the following is a Suitable or chosen method for destroying anatomical biomedical wastes?
    a. Incineration b. Decontamination
    c. Autoclaving d. None of the above
13. GHS refers to:
    a. Globally harmonized systems
    b. Governing high school
    c. Global human service
    d. All of the above

Answers

1. b	2. a	3. c	4. c	5. b
6. d	7. d	8. c	9. b	10. d
11. d	12. a	13. a		

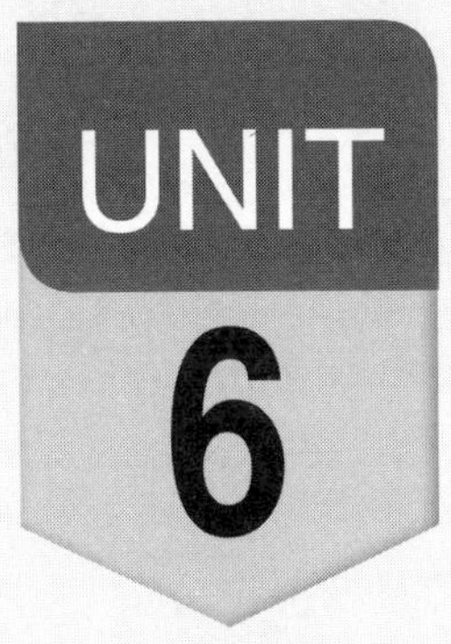

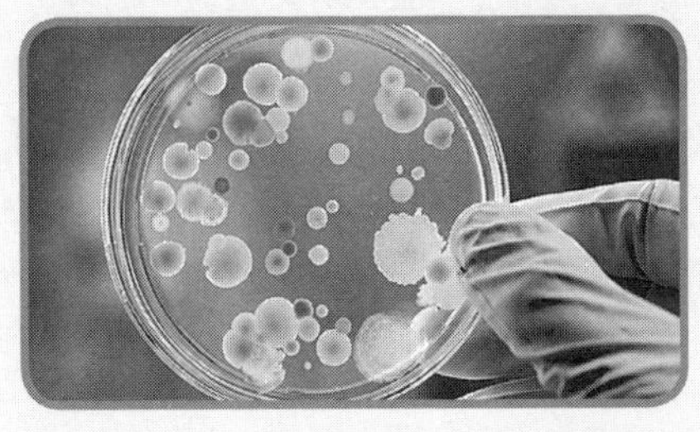

Practical Microbiology

Learning Objectives

- Microscope–parts, uses, handling and care of microscope
- Observation of staining procedure, preparation and examination of slides and smears
- Identification of common microbes under the microscope for morphology of different microbes

Introduction to Laboratory Techniques

INTRODUCTION

Microorganisms are present everywhere in nature. They are seen in soil, air, water, food, sewage and on body surfaces. The main aim of every microbiologists is to separate these mixtures of different microorganism populations into individual group of species for their studies. A culture containing only a single species of microorganism is referred to as pure culture. For isolation and studies on microorganisms as pure culture, the microbiologists need various basic laboratory equipment and techniques as shown in the following.

Table 6.1.1: Different laboratory apparatus and techniques used in microbiology laboratory.

Laboratory Apparatus	Techniques Used
Media	For isolation of pure cultures: Streak plate Pour plate-loop dilution Spread plate
Autoclave	
Bunsen burner	
Culture tubes	
Petri dishes	Staining methods: Simple staining-negative staining Differential staining-gram staining and acid fast staining
Pipettes	
Water baths	
Incubators	
Refrigerators	
Wood Chamber	
Inoculation tube	
Culture flasks	
Wire loops and needles	

APPARATUS IN MICROBIOLOGY LABORATORY

Media

- Growing bacteria under artificial conditions in the laboratory is called as culturing.
- To culture bacteria we provide them nutrients through media called as growth media or culture media.
- There are various reasons why we have to culture bacteria in the laboratory on artificial culture media.
- One of the most important reasons being its utility in diagnosing infectious diseases.

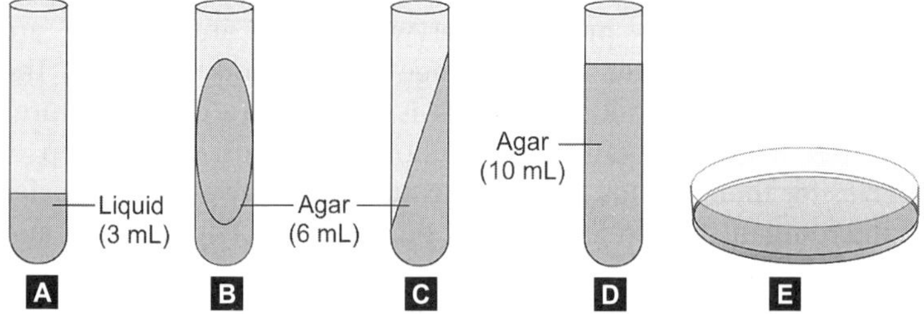

Figures 6.1.1A to E: Different forms of media: (A) Broth medium; (B) Agar slant–front view; (C) Agar slant–side view; (D) Agar deep tube; (E) Agar plate or petri dish.

Culture Tubes and Petri Dishes

- Glass test tubes and glass based or even plastic based Petri dishes are widely used for cultivating microorganisms.
- Glass tubes are found to be suitable for both solid and liquid forms of nutrient medium while Petri dishes are suitable only for solid medium.
- There are different closures available to maintain sterility in these medium tubes and Petri dishes.
- Schroder and von Dusch was the first person to develop a very good closure type called cotton plug.
- Cotton plug is used to cover the test tube in avoiding contamination. Microorganisms grown in the test tube also need oxygen. Cotton plug allows oxygen to pass through and so, microorganism grows better.
- However, preparing sterile cotton plugs is difficult which should be done inside the laminar hood.

- Commercially available sleeve-like caps are helpful in replacing cotton plugs.
- Most laboratories prefer sleeve-like caps than cotton plugs.
- Petri dish is the apparatus which has two parts. One is the top portion which is bigger in size and the other is the bottom portion which is smaller in size.
- As both parts are not matching perfectly, there is a gap between these two parts when closed. Through this gap the air can enter the Petri dish and microorganism can grow better.

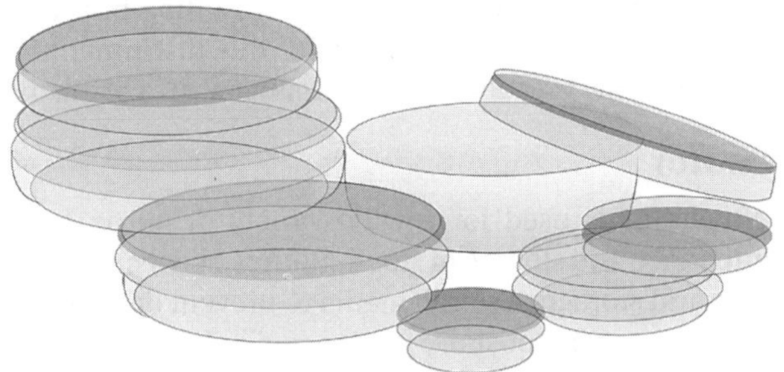

Figure 6.1.2: Petri dishes.

Transfer Instruments

- Microorganisms must be transferred from one vessel to another for maintenance and study.
- Such a transfer is called as **subculturing** and must be carried out under sterile conditions to prevent possible combination.
- Wire loops and needles are made from inert metals such as Nichrome or Platinum and are inserted into metal shafts that serve as handles.
- They are extremely durable instruments and are easily sterilized by incineration in the blue (hottest) portion of the Bunsen burner flame.
- A pipette is another instrument used for sterile transfers.
- Pipettes are similar in function to straws; that is, they draw up liquids. They are made up of glass or plastic drawn out to a tip at one end and with a mouthpiece forming the other end.

Cultivation Chambers

- The most important requirement for the cultivation of microorganisms is that they can be grown at their optimum temperature. An incubator is used to maintain optimum temperature during the necessary growth period.

- Most incubators use dry heat. Moisture is supplied by placing a beaker of water in the incubator during the growth period. A moist environment retards dehydration of the medium and thereby avoids spurious experimental results.
- A heat controlled shaking water bath is another piece of apparatus used to cultivate microorganisms. Its advantage is that it provides a rapid and uniform transfer of heat to the culture vessel and its agitation provides increased aeration, resulting in acceleration of growth. The single disadvantage of this instrument is that it can be used only for cultivation of organisms in a broth medium.

Refrigerator

- A refrigerator is used for a wide variety of purposes such as maintenance and storage of stock cultures between subculturing periods and storage of sterile media to prevent dehydration.
- It is also used as a repository for thermolabile (destroyed by high heat) solutions, antibiotics, serums and biochemical reagents.

ISOLATION OF MICROORGANISMS

In nature, at any place, various microorganisms co-exist as a group. In the laboratory, these microorganisms can be separated into pure cultures. These cultures contain only one type of organism and are suitable for the study of their cultural, morphological and biochemical properties.

The followings are techniques that can be used to accomplish this necessary dilution:

Streak Plate Method

The streak plate method is a rapid qualitative isolation method. It is essentially a dilution technique that involves spreading a loopful of culture over the surface of an agar plate. Although many types of procedures are performed, the four-way or quadrant, streak is explained as follows:

(Ensure to follow all these steps inside the Laminar Air Flow Hood)

- Take the inoculation loop. Hold it upright. Show the loop in the flame of Bunsen burner until it turns red hot. Allow it to cool by keeping it in your right hand for few seconds (10-20 preferably).
- Hold the culture tube in your left hand. Using smaller finger and palm of your right hand open the cotton plug from the culture tube.

- Insert the cooled loop into the culture tube to collect the sample.
- Swipe the loop onto the surface of culture tube. Now you will get a loopful of culture.
- Then, close the culture tube with cotton plug using the same smaller finger and palm.
- Then, take Petri dish containing only media on your left hand and open it slowly.
- Now gently place the loopful of culture at one end of the media. 'A' as shown in the following figure.
- Spread the culture perpendicularly like lines in two directions using the same loop continuously.
- Repeat "step a" to sterilize inoculation loop.
- From the end of lines in A, you have to spread the culture again perpendicularly like lines in two directions using the same loop continuously. This is referred to as "B".
- Repeat "step a" to sterilize inoculation loop.
- From the end of lines in B, you have to spread the culture again perpendicularly like lines in two directions using the same loop continuously. This is referred to as "C".
- Repeat "step a" to sterilize inoculation loop.
- From the end of lines in C, you have to spread the culture again perpendicularly like lines in two directions using the same loop continuously. This is referred to as "D".
- Repeat "step a" to sterilize inoculation loop.
- From the end of lines in D, you have to spread the culture again perpendicularly like lines in two directions using the same loop continuously. This is referred to as "E".
- Repeat "step a" to sterilize inoculation loop. Keep the inoculation loop aside.
- Now, individual colonies of microorganisms are separated in E.

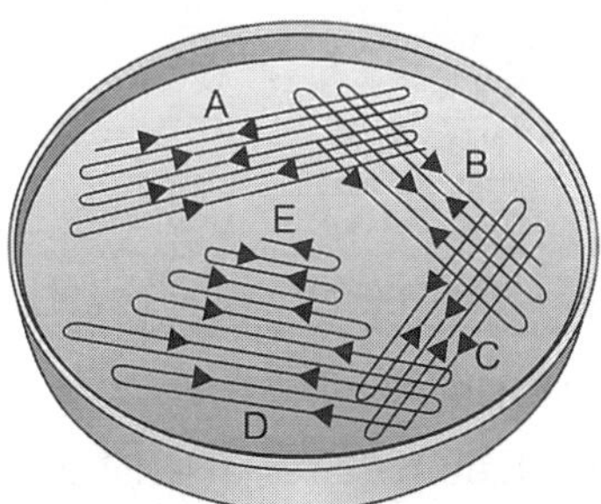

Figure 6.1.3: Streak plate method for isolation of pure culture.

Spread Plate Technique

The spread plate technique requires that a previously diluted mixture of microorganisms be used. During inoculation, the cells are spread over the surface of a solid agar medium with a sterile, L-shaped bent rod while the Petri dish is spun on a "Lazy-Susan" turntable. The step by step procedure for this technique includes:
(Make sure you do all these steps inside the Laminar Air Flow Hood)

- Take the sterile beaker containing nutrient broth with single colony of microorganism on your left hand.
- Using smaller finger and palm of your right hand open the cotton plug from the sterile beaker.
- Insert the sterile pipette into the nutrient broth containing beaker to pipette out the sample culture. (You should not pipette out the sample culture by mouth. Using pointing finger of your right hand try pipetting out sample culture)
- Then using smaller finger and palm of your right hand close the cotton plug over the sterile beaker.
- Take sterile Petri dish containing agar media and pour the sample culture over the agar surface.
- Using sterile glass spreader spread the culture evenly all over the Petri plate by rotating the spreader at 360°.

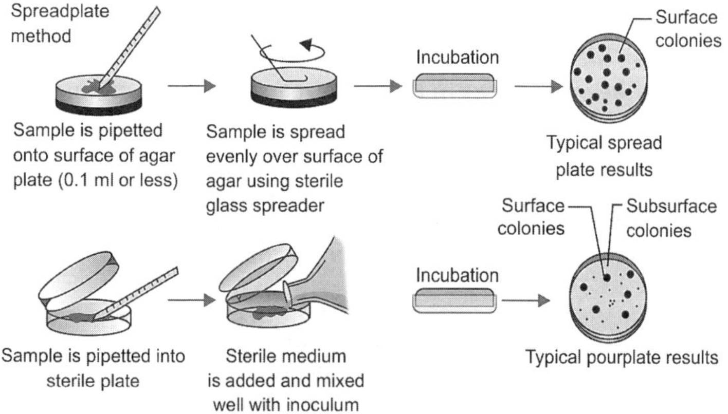

Figure 6.1.4: Spread plate and pour plate method of isolating pure culture.

Pour Plate Technique

The pour plate technique requires a serial dilution of the mixed culture by means of a loop or pipette. The diluted inoculums are then added to a molten agar medium in a Petri dish, mixed and allowed to solidify. It is well demonstrated in the picture.

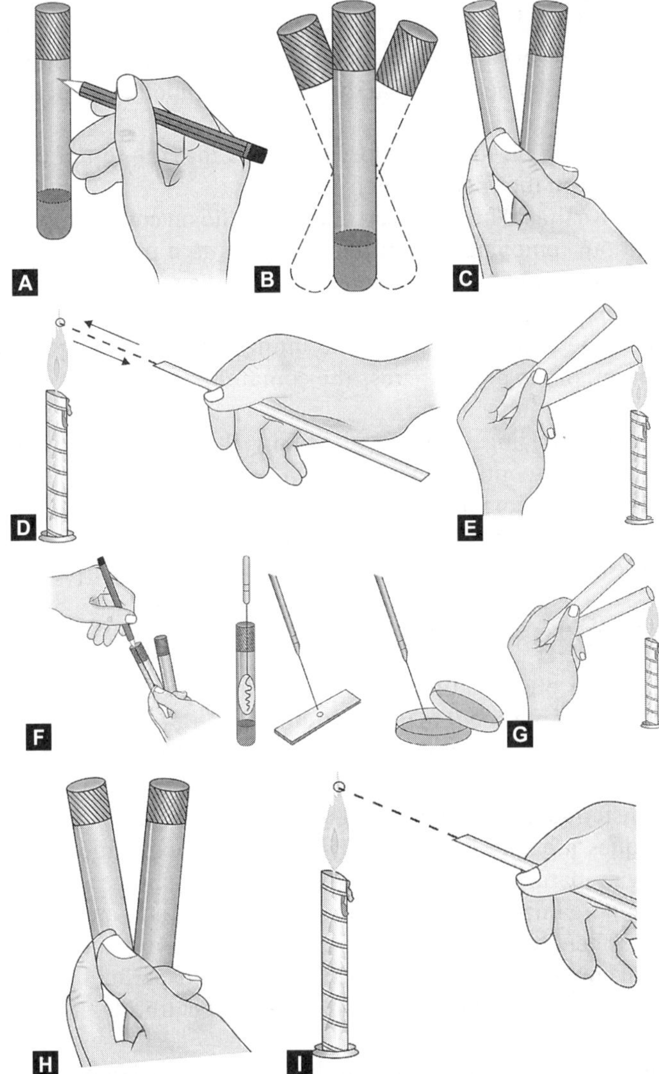

Figures 6.1.5A to I: Method of subculturing: (A) With a wax pencil label the medium to be inoculated; (B) Shake the primary culture tube to suspend the bacteria; (C) Place both tubes in the palm of one hand to form aV; (D) Place both tubes in the palm of one hand to form aV; (E) Remove the caps from the tubes and flame the necks of the tubes; (F) Cool the loop or needle and pick up bacteria or streak the surface of a slant or place the bacteria on slide or streak the bacteria on plate; (G) Remove the necks of the tubes; (H) Flip the tubes; (I) Remove the loop or needle.

Pipette Transfer

The procedure for carrying out pipette transfer includes the following:

- Tilt a can of pipettes so that the tops of the pipettes are at the top of can.
- Set the can on the laboratory bench so that the top of the can extends off the edge of bench.
- Remove the lid from the can and set the lid on countertop.
- Without removing it from the can, pick up a pipette with your non-dominant hand. Use your dominant hand to place a pipette aid on the pipette.
- Slide the pipette from the can, lifting it to avoid dragging the bottom of the pipette across the contaminated surfaces of other pipettes.
- Use the little finger of the hand holding the pipette to remove the lid from the container containing your sample.
- Touch the tip of pipette to the side of container.
- Measure the sample into the container.
- Place the pipette into a discard container and remove the pipette aid.

PURE CULTURE TECHNIQUES

After getting pure culture from any of the three methods as seen above, the culture needs to be sub-cultured by transferring them into a new medium. This would ensure continuous growth and division of microorganisms. Also, you can have the live culture. Microorganisms are transferred from one medium to another by subculturing. These techniques are very basic for all microbiology experiments which include preparation of stock cultures and their maintenance.

Microorganisms are always present in the air and on laboratory surfaces, benches and equipment. They can serve as a source of external contamination and thus interfere with experimental results unless proper techniques are used during subculturing. It includes the following:

- Sterilize the inoculation loop by holding it in the flame of Bunsen burner until it turns red hot. This is the very basic step used more frequently. While doing this, caution must be taken in order to sterilize the inoculation loop. Then, the inoculation loop should be placed in your hand for 10-20 seconds to cool. The stock culture tube and the tube to be inoculated need to be placed in the same hand. It would look like V in hand which represents two test tubes: one with culture tube and another tube to be inoculated.

- Using the little finger to grasp the first cap tightly for uncapping and with the next finger try to remove the cap of another tube. Insert the sterile inoculation loop into the cultured tube to collect the sample and then insert the same loop into the test tube which contains only media. Then, close the caps one by one.
- After completing this step, again sterilize the inoculation loop by holding it in the flame of Bunsen burner. This is to kill any organisms that are left in the loop.

CULTURE MEDIA

Need for Culture Media

It is usually essential to obtain a culture by growing the organism in an artificial medium. If more than one species or type of organism is present, each requires to be separated carefully or isolated as pure culture. Several organisms need the determination of antibiotic sensitivity pattern for optimal antibiotic selection.

Types of Culture Media

Table 6.1.2: Description of raw materials used in culture media with its nutritional value.

Raw Material	Characteristic	Nutritional Value
Beef extract	An aqueous extract of lean beef tissue concentrated to a paste	Contains the water-soluble substances of animal tissue, which include carbohydrates, organic nitrogen compounds, water-soluble vitamins and salts
Peptone	The product resulting from the digestion of proteinaceous materials example, meat, casein and gelatin; digestion of the protein material is accomplished with acids or enzymes; many different peptones (depending upon the protein used and the method of digestion) are available for use in bacteriological media; peptones differ in their ability to support growth of bacteria	Principal source of organic nitrogen; may also contain some vitamins and sometimes carbohydrates, depending upon the kind of proteinaceous material digested

Contd...

Contd...

Raw Material	Characteristic	Nutritional Value
Agar	A complex carbohydrate obtained from certain marine algae; processed to remove extraneous substances	Used as a solidification agent for media; agar, dissolved in aqueous solutions, gels when the temperature is reduced below 45°C; agar not considered a source of nutrient to the bacteria
Yeast extract	An aqueous extract of yeast cells, commercially available as a powder	A very rich source of the B vitamins; also contains organic nitrogen and carbon compounds

Table 6.1.3: Composition of nutrient broth and nutrient agar.

Nutrient broth	Beef extract – 3 g Peptone – 5 g Water – 1000 mL
Nutrient agar	Beef extract – 3 g Peptone – 5 g Agar – 15 g Water – 1000 mL

Table 6.1.4: Types of culture media.

Based on their consistency	Solid medium Liquid medium Semi solid medium
Based on the constituents or ingredients	Simple medium Complex medium Synthetic or defined medium Special medium (includes enriched media, enrichment media, selective media, indicator media, differential media, transport media)
Based on oxygen requirement	Aerobic media Anaerobic media

Based on Their Consistency

Solid media: Solid media has agar in concentration of 1.5 to 2%, e.g., nutrient agar.

Liquid media: Liquid media does not have agar e.g., example: nutrient broth.

Semisolid media: Semisolid media has agar in concentration less than 0.5%. The media looks very soft like jelly, e.g., Fluid thioglycollate media.

Based on the Constituents or Ingredients

Basal media/simple media: Such are basically simple media that supports non-fastidious bacteria. Peptone water, nutrient broth and nutrient agar are considered as basal media. These media are generally used for the primary isolation of microorganisms, e.g., peptone water, nutrient broth, nutrient agar, etc.

Synthetic or chemically defined media: A chemically defined medium is one prepared from purified ingredients and therefore whose exact composition is known, e.g., minimal media for *Bacillus megaterium.*

Complex media: Non-synthetic medium contains at least one component that is neither purified nor completely known. Often these are partially digested proteins from various organism sources, e.g., Nutrient Broth.

Enriched media (Added Growth Factors): When basal media contains special ingredients like blood, serum, egg yolk, etc., then the medium is considered as enriched media, e.g., chocolate agar, blood agar, etc.

Selective and Enrichment Media

These are designed to inhibit unwanted commensal or contaminating bacteria and help to recover pathogen from a mixture of bacteria. While selective media are agar based and enrichment media are liquid in consistency. Both these media serve the same purpose. Any agar media can be made selective by addition of certain inhibitory agents that don't affect the pathogen. Various approaches to make a medium selective include addition of antibiotics, dyes, chemicals, alteration of pH or a combination of these.

Selective media: Selective medium is designed to suppress the growth of some microorganisms while allowing the growth of others (i.e., they select for certain microbes). Solid medium is employed with selective medium so that individual colonies may be isolated. Examples of selective media include: Thayer-Martin Agar used to recover *N. gonorrhoeae* contains Vancomycin, Colistin and Nystatin.

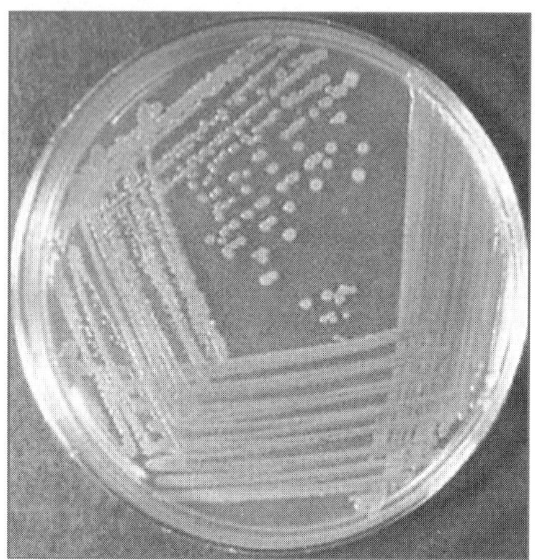

Figure 6.1.6: Bacteria grown on simple media (Nutrient agar).

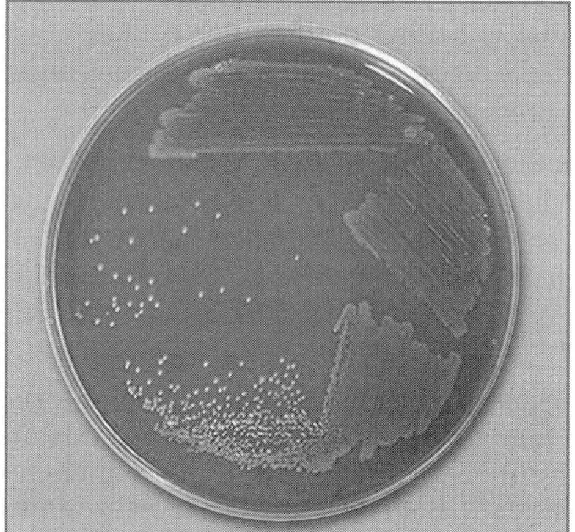

Figure 6.1.7: Enriched media (Blood agar).

Enrichment media: Enrichment medium is used to increase the relative concentration of certain microorganisms in the culture prior to plating on solid selective medium. Unlike selective media, enrichment culture is typically used as broth medium. Enrichment media are liquid media that also serves to inhibit commensals in the clinical specimen. For example, Selenite F broth, Tetrathionate broth

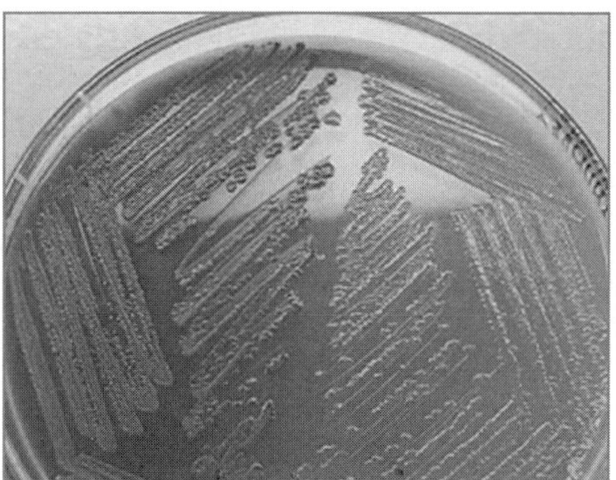

Figure 6.1.8: Thayer-Martin agar.

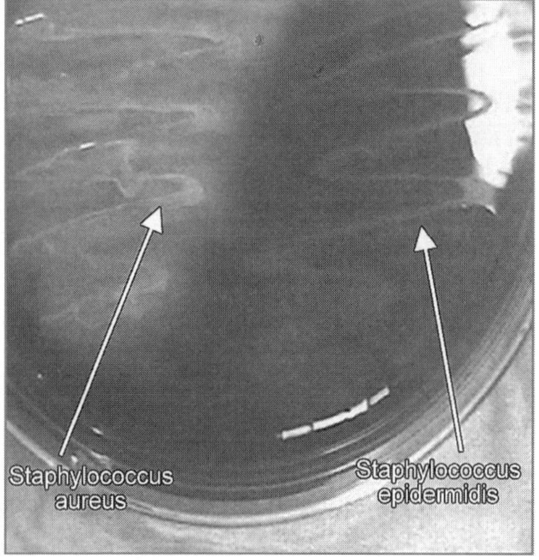

Figure 6.1.9: Differential medium–MacConkey agar.

and Alkaline peptone water are used to recover pathogens from fecal specimens.

Differential media: Special type of media used for differentiating two varieties of bacteria or other microorganisms is called differential media. Differentiation of two bacterial colonies can be identified through various methods including dye absorption, metabolism, etc. Example - MacConkey agar.

Transport media: Clinical specimens must be transported to the laboratory immediately after collection to prevent overgrowth of contaminating organisms or commensals. This can be achieved by

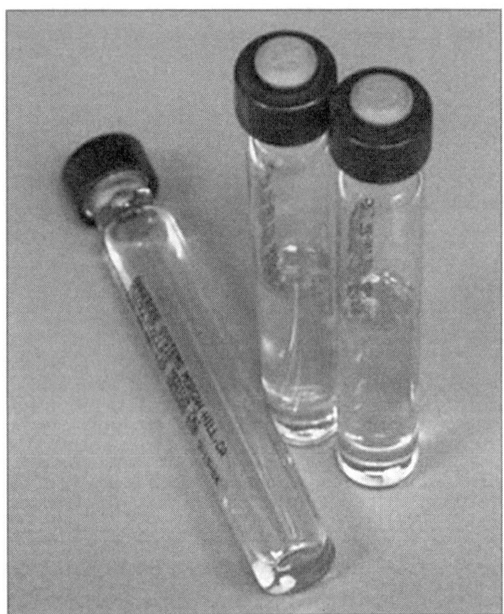

Figure 6.1.10: Anaerobic media.

using transport media. Transport media should fulfill the following criteria:

- Temporary storage of specimens being transported to the laboratory for cultivation.
- Maintain the viability of all organisms in the specimen without altering their concentration.
- Contain only buffers and salts.
- Lack of carbon, nitrogen and organic growth factors so as to prevent microbial multiplication.
- Transport media used in the isolation of anaerobes much be free of molecular oxygen.

Examples: Cary Blair Media for *Campylobacter*

Assay media: These media are used for the assay of vitamins, amino acids and antibiotics, e.g., antibiotic assay media are used for determining antibiotic potency by the microbiological assay technique.

Other types of media include media for enumeration of bacteria, media for characterization of bacteria, maintenance media, etc.

Based on the Oxygen Requirement

Aerobic media: Media which contains oxygen are called aerobic media. All the above seen media fall under this group.

Anaerobic media: Anaerobic bacteria need special media for growth because they need low oxygen content, reduced oxidation-reduction potential and extra nutrients. Media for anaerobes may have to be supplemented with nutrients like hemin and vitamin K. Such media may also have to be reduced by physical or chemical means.

INOCULATION OF CULTURE MEDIA

For all microbiological experiments, we need good techniques for separating our desired sample from culture media. This is very important to study the characteristics of sample organism. Several modified techniques are available depending on the needs of the microbiologists. All commercially available culture media should be checked whether they are pure or contaminated along with the details of their expiry date. This is also very important as contaminated culture media might facilitate the growth of unwanted organism when sample organisms are grown. After expiry date when the culture media is used that might affect the growth of the sample organisms. It is very easy to identify the plates which exceed expiry date or even contaminated plates as the media might become turbid.

Inoculation loops can be sterilized by holding the loop end shown in the flame of Bunsen burner until the loop turns red hot. Then the inoculation loop is kept on the rack for cooling before being used. If the inoculation loop in red hot is used, then the microorganisms would die in hotness. For every plate different disposable inoculation loops can be used. When transfer of colonies between test tubes happen, every time the loop should be sterilized by showing it to the flame of Bunsen burner.

Aseptic Transfer

Specific Transfer Methods

There are two basic stages in transfers: (1) obtaining the sample to be transferred and (2) transferring to the sterile culture medium. These may be combined in various ways. The following descriptions are organized to reflect that flexibility.

- Materials are neatly positioned and not in the way. To prevent spills, culture tubes are stored upright in a test tube rack. They are never laid on the table. The microbiologist is relaxed and ready for work. He should hold the loop like a pencil, not gripping it like a dagger.
- Incineration of an inoculating loop's wire is done by passing it through the tip of the flame's inner cone. Begin at the wire's base and continue to the end making sure that all parts are heated to a uniform orange color. Allow the wire to cool before touching it or placing it on/in a culture. The former will burn and latter will cause aerosols of microorganisms.
- Remove the tube's cap with your little finger by pulling the tube away with the other hand; the loop hand is kept still. The cap should be hold with little finger during the transfer. When replacing the cap, always move the tube back to the cap in order to keep your loop hand still. The replaced cap doesn't need to be on firmly yet - just enough to cover the tube.
- The open tube should be hold on an angle to minimize the chance that airborne microbes will drop into it. The tube's mouth will quickly be passed through the flame a couple of times. The tube's cap being held in the loop hand is to be noticed.

TRANSFERS USING AN INOCULATING LOOP OR NEEDLE

Inoculating loops and needles are the most commonly used instruments for transferring microbes between all media types—broths, slants, or plates can be the source and any can be the destination. Since loops and needles are handled in the same way, we refer only to loops in the following instructions for ease of reading.

Obtaining a Sample with an Inoculating Loop or Needle

i. **From a Broth**

- Suspend bacteria in the broth with a vortex mixer or by agitating the tube with your fingers.
- Flame the loop.
- Remove and hold the tube's cap with little finger of your loop hand.

- Flame the open end of the tube by passing it through a flame two or three times.
- Hold the open tube at an angle to prevent airborne contamination.
- Holding the loop hand still, move the tube up the wire until the tip is in the broth. Continuing to hold the loop hand still, remove the tube from the wire. There should be a film of broth in the loop. Be especially careful not to catch the loop tip on the tube lip. This springing action of the loop creates bacterial aerosols.
- Flame the tube lip as before. Keep your loop hand still.
- Keeping the loop hand still (remember, it has growth on it), move the tube to replace its cap.
- What you do next depends on the medium to which you are transferring the growth. Please continue with appropriate inoculation section.

ii. **From a Slant**

- Flame the loop.
- Remove and hold the culture tube's cap with the little finger of your loop hand.
- Flame the open end of the tube by passing it through a flame two or three times.
- With the agar surface facing upward, hold the open tube at an angle to prevent airborne contamination.
- Holding the loop hand still, move the tube up the wire until the wire tip is over the desired growth. Touch the loop to the growth and obtain the smallest visible mass of bacteria. Then, holding the loop hand still, remove the tube from the wire. Be especially careful not to catch the loop tip on the tube lip. This springing action of the loop creates bacterial aerosols.
- **The Vortex Mixer:** Bacteria are suspended in a broth with a vortex mixer. Caution must be used to prevent broth from getting into the cap or losing control of the tube and causing a spill.
- **Mixing by Hand:** A broth culture should always be mixed prior to transfer. Tapping the tube with your fingers gets the job done safely and without special equipment.
- **Use the Lid as a Shield:** When transferring bacteria to or from a Petri dish, keep the agar surface covered with the lid to minimize airborne contamination.
- **A Loop and Broth:** Hold the open tube on an angle to minimize airborne contamination. When placing a loop into a broth tube or removing it, keep the loop hand still and move the tube. Be

careful not to catch the loop on the tube's lip when removing it. This produces aerosols that can be dangerous or produce contamination.

- Flame the tube lip as before. Keep your loop hand still.
- Keeping the loop hand still (remember, it has growth on it), move the tube to replace its cap.
- What you do next depends on the medium to which you are transferring the growth. Please continue with the appropriate inoculation section.

iii. **From an Agar Plate**

- Flame the loop
- Lift the lid of agar plate, but continue to use it as a cover to prevent contamination from above.
- Touch the loop to an uninoculated portion of the plate to cool it. (Placing a hot wire on growth may cause spattering of the growth and create aerosols.) Obtain a small amount of bacterial growth by gently touching a colony with the wire tip.
- Carefully remove the loop from the plate and hold it still as you replace the lid.
- What you do next depends on the medium to which you are transferring the growth. Please continue with the appropriate inoculation section. Inoculation of media with an inoculating loop or needle.
- **Fishtail Inoculation of Agar Slants.**
- Agar slants are generally used for growing stock cultures that can be refrigerated after incubation and maintained for several weeks. Many differential media used in identification of microbes are also slants.
- Remove the cap of the sterile medium with little finger of your loop hand and hold it there.
- Flame the tube by quickly passing it through the flame a couple of times. Keep your loop hand still.
- Hold the open tube on an angle to minimize airborne contamination. Keep your loop hand still.
- With the agar surface facing upward, carefully move the tube over the wire. Gently touch the loop to the agar surface near the base.
- Beginning at the bottom of the exposed agar surface, drag the loop in a zigzag pattern as the tube is withdrawn. Be careful not

to cut the agar surface and be especially careful not to catch the loop tip on the tube lip as you remove it. This springing action of the loop creates bacterial aerosols.

- Flame the tube mouth as before. Keep your loop hand still.
- Keeping the loop hand still (remember, it has growth on it), move the tube to replace its cap.
- **Replacing the Cap:** Keeping the loop hand still (remember it has growth on it), move the tube to replace the cap. The cap doesn't have to be on firmly at this point-just enough to cover the tube.
- **A Loop and an Agar Slant:** When placing a loop into a slant tube or removing it, keep the loop hand still and move the tube. Hold the tube so the agar is facing upwards.
- **Fishtail Inoculation of a Slant:** Begin at the base of the slant surface and gently move the loop back and forth as you withdraw the tube. Be careful not to cut the agar. Sterilize the loop upon completion of the transfer.
- Sterilize the loop as before by incinerating it in the Bunsen burner flame. It is especially important to flame it from base to tip now because the loop has lots of bacteria on it.
- Label the tube with your name, date and organism. Incubate at the appropriate temperature for the assigned time.

Inoculation of Broth Tubes

Broth cultures are often used to grow cultures for use when fresh cultures or large numbers of cells are desired. Many differential media are also broths.

- Remove the cap of sterile medium with little finger of your loop hand and hold it there.
- Sterilize the tube by quickly passing it through the flame a couple of times. Keep your loop hand still.
- Hold the open tube on an angle to minimize airborne contamination. Keep your loop hand still.
- Carefully move the broth tube over the wire. Gently swirl the loop in the broth to dislodge microbes.
- Withdraw the tube from over the loop. Before completely removing it, touch the loop tip to the glass to remove any excess broth. Then be especially careful not to catch the loop tip on the tube lip when withdrawing it. This springing action of the wire creates bacterial aerosols.

- **Inoculation of a Broth:** When entering or leaving the tube, move the tube keep the loop hand still. Gently swirl the loop in the broth to transfer the organisms.
- **Remove excess broth from loop:** Before removing it from the tube, touch the loop to the glass to remove excess broth. Failure to do so will result in splattering and aerosols when sterilizing the loop in a flame.
- Flame the tube lip as before. Keep your loop hand still.
- Keeping the loop hand still (remember, it has growth on it), move the tube to replace its cap.
- Sterilize the loop as before by incinerating it in the Bunsen burner flame. It is especially important to flame it from base to tip now because the loop and wire have lots of bacteria on them.
- Label the tube with your name, date and organism. Incubate at the appropriate temperature for the assigned time.

STAINING

Because microbial cytoplasm is usually transparent, it is necessary to stain microorganisms before they can be viewed with light microscope. In some cases, staining is unnecessary, for example, when microorganisms are very large or when motility is to be studied and a drop of the microorganisms can be placed directly on the slide and observed. A preparation like this is called a wet mount.

In preparation for staining, a small sample of microorganism is placed on a slide and permitted to air dry. The smear is heat fixed by quickly passing it over a flame. Heat fixing kills the organisms, makes them adhere to the slide and permits them to accept the stain.

Simple Stain Techniques

Staining can be performed with basic dyes such as crystal violet or methylene blue, positively charged dyes that are attracted to the negatively charged materials of the microbial cytoplasm. Such a procedure is the simple stain procedure. An alternative is to use a dye such as Nigrosin or Congo red, acidic, negatively charged dyes. They are repelled by negatively charged cytoplasm and gather around the cells, leaving the cells clear and unstained. This technique is called the negative stain technique.

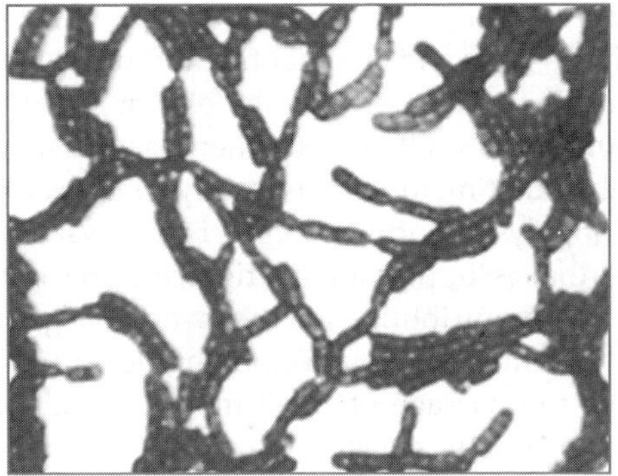

Bacillus megaterium simple stained with methylene blue (1,000 x)

Figure 6.1.11: Simple stained *Bacillus megaterium* with methylene blue.

Differential Staining Techniques

Differential staining techniques help to differentiate two different types of organisms, e.g., Gram Staining Technique. This technique helps to separate bacteria into two groups, such as Gram positive bacteria and Gram-negative bacteria.

Gram Staining Technique

Although simple stains are useful, they do not reveal details about the bacteria other than morphology and arrangement. The Gram stain is a differential stain commonly used in the microbiology laboratory that differentiates bacteria on the basis of their cell wall structure. Most bacteria can be divided into two groups based on the composition of their cell wall: gram-positive and gram-negative.

Principle

- Gram-positive cell walls have a thick peptidoglycan layer beyond the plasma membrane. Characteristic polymers called Teichoic and Lipoteichoic acids stick out above the peptidoglycan and it is because of their negative charge that the cell wall is overall negative. These acids are also very important in the body's ability to recognize foreign bacteria. Gram-positive cell walls stain blue/purple with the Gram stain.

- Gram-negative cell walls are more complex. They have a thin peptidoglycan layer and an outer membrane beyond the plasma membrane. The space between the plasma membrane and the outer membrane is called as the periplasmic space. The outer leaflet of the outer membrane is largely composed of a molecule called Lipopolysaccharide (LPS). Lipopolysaccharide is an endotoxin that is important in triggering the body's immune response and contributing to the overall negative charge of the cell. Spanning the outer membrane are porin proteins that enable the passage of small molecules. Lipoproteins join the outer membrane and the thin peptidoglycan layer. Gram-negative cells will stain pink with the Gram stain. This is the most important staining technique in bacteriology.

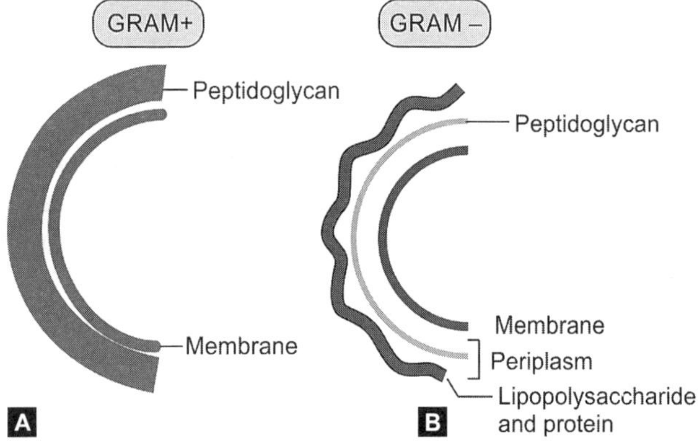

Figures 6.1.12A and B: The cell wall of: (A) Gram-positive bacteria showing peptidoglycan layer; (B) Gram-negative bacteria showing lipopolysaccharide layer over peptidoglycan layer.

Steps of Gram Staining

- Place a slide with a bacterial smear on a staining rack.
- **STAIN** the slide with Crystal Violet for 1-2 min.
- Pour off the stain.
- Note: Fingers stain Gram-positive - use forceps!
- Flood slide with Gram's iodine for 1-2 min.
- Pour off the Iodine.
- Decolourize by washing the slide briefly with acetone for (2–3 seconds).

- Wash slide thoroughly with water to remove the acetone - do not delay this step.
- Flood slide with Safranin counterstain for 2 min.
- Wash with water.
- Blot excess water and dry in hand over bunsen flame.

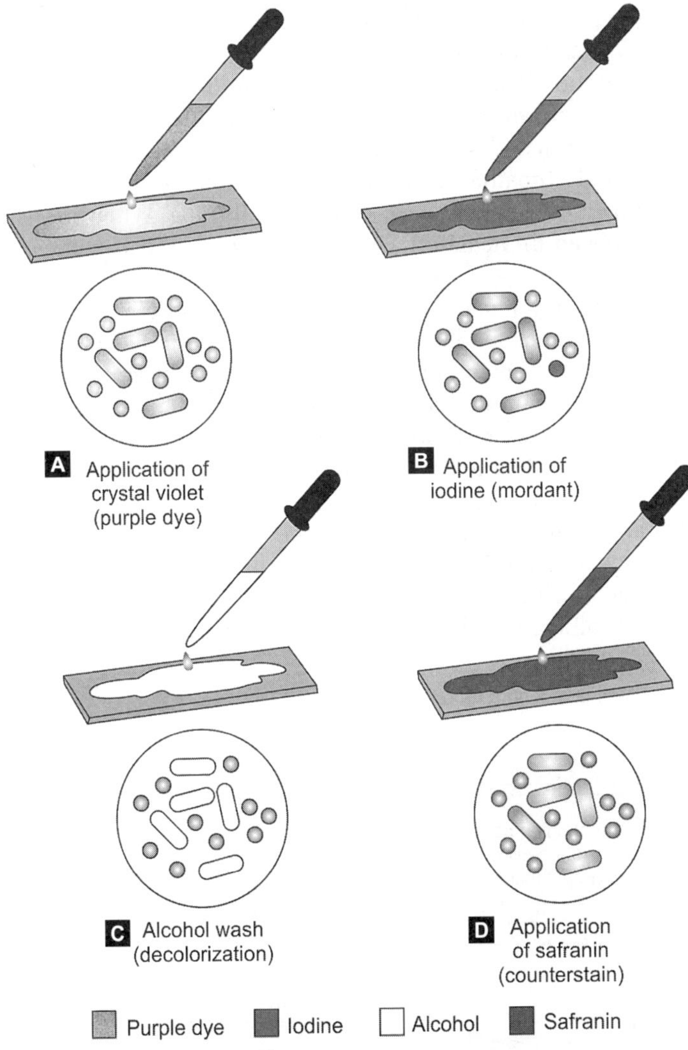

Figures 6.1.13A to D: Gram staining.

PREPARATION OF SLIDE

A properly prepared smear accomplishes two things. It causes bacteria to adhere to a slide so that they can be stained and observed. It also kills them, rendering pathogenic bacteria safe to handle. An objective in preparing smears is to learn to recognize the correct density of bacteria to place on the slide. Too much of overlapping gives false positives or crowd each other to make a mess. A few of it cannot be located on the slide.

- A circle should be marked on the underside of a slide with a glass etching tool. Several circles can be located on the same slide.
- The slide must be grease-free. A good way to clean a slide is to repeatedly breathe on it followed by rubbing vigorously with a Kimwipe or paper towel to remove the fog. When the slide is defogged immediately after breathing on it, it is sufficiently cleaned.
- To prepare a smear from a dry culture, a very small drop of distilled water should be placed over the circled area. After aseptically removing material from a culture it is them mixed with the drop or placed directly on the slide if it is a dilute broth culture. It takes very little material to produce a successful smear.
- The drop is air-dried completely which takes a short time if a small drop is prepared.
- While holding the slide with a clothes pin it is quickly passed it through a flame. Three quick passes are usually sufficient to kill the bacteria and cause them to adhere.
- After cooling the slide, the staining procedure is conducted.

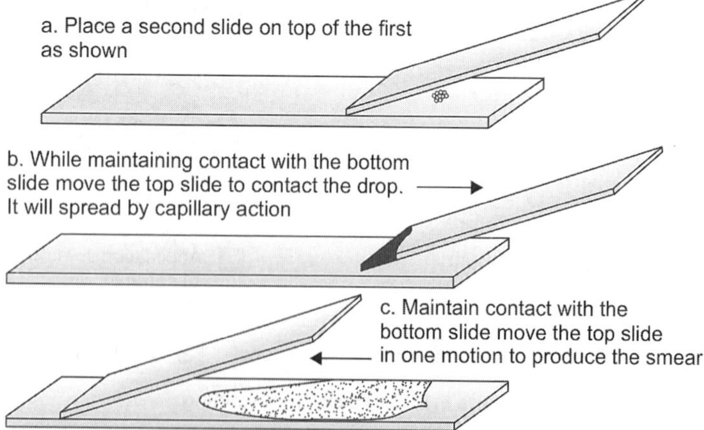

Figure 6.1.14: Preparation of smear.

Direct Stain

Microbial cells are small and transparent. Stains are often used to increase contrast between the cells and the background, making them easier to see under the microscope. Since many of the cell components are negatively charged, stains with positively charged chromophores (the colored ion of the dye) will attach to the cells. Examples of such stains include Methylene blue, Crystal violet and Carbon Fuschin.

- Make a heat-fixed smear, taking care not to use too much culture if working from an agar culture.
- Place the slide on a staining rack over a sink or catch basin.
- Add a drop of dye to the smear. You need enough stain to just cover the smear, not the whole slide.
- Allow the dye to act. (One minute is generally adequate.)
- Gently rinse the dye from the slide with water from a squirt bottle.
- Gently blot the slide and observe under the microscope.

Fixation

The process by which the internal and external structures of microorganisms are preserved and fixed in place is called fixation.

- **Heat fixation:** Fixation by means of application of heat. The prepared smear of microorganisms is gently heated and dried.
- **Chemical fixation:** It involves the use of chemicals such as ethanol and formaldehyde.

EXAMINATION OF SLIDE

Methods by which you can examine culture slides which include the following:

- Staining
- Microscopy

Staining

Because microbial cytoplasm is usually transparent, it is necessary to stain microorganisms before they can be viewed with light microscope. In some cases, staining is unnecessary, for example when microorganisms are very large or when motility is to be studied and a drop of microorganisms can be placed directly on the slide and observed. A preparation such as this is called a wet mount. A wet mount can also be prepared by placing a drop of culture on a cover slip (a glass cover for a slide) and then inverting it over a hollowed out slide. This procedure is called the hanging drop.

In preparation for staining, a small sample of microorganisms is placed on a slide and permitted to air dry. The smear is heat fixed by quickly passing it over a flame. Heat fixing kills the organisms, makes them adhere to the slide and permits them to accept the stain.

Applications of Staining

1. Used to increase visibility of microorganisms being studied.
2. Used to identify the shape of bacteria.
3. Used to determine the morphological features of microorganisms.
4. Used to detect contamination.
5. Used to differentiate and classify microorganisms (differential stains).
6. Used to detect bacterial parts, such as capsule, spores, flagella or inclusion bodies (special stains).

Microscopy

What is a Microscope?

To view microscopic organisms, their magnification is essential. The microscope is the instrument used to magnify microscopic images. Its function and some aspects of design are similar to those of telescopes although the microscope is designed to visualize very small close objects while telescope magnifies distant objects.

Types of Microscope

Depending on the working principle, construction and mode of functioning microscope is of two types:

1. **Light microscope**—which functions in the presence of light rays. It is of following types:
   a. Bright-field microscope,
   b. Dark-field microscope,
   c. Phase-contrast microscope,
   d. Differential interference contrast (DIC) microscope and
   e. Fluorescence microscope.
2. **Electron microscope**—which functions in the presence of beam of electrons. It is of following types:
   a. Scanning electron microscope, and
   b. Transmission electron microscope.

The Light Microscope

The bright-field microscope is the most common type of light microscope found in the microbiology diagnostic laboratories. We will discuss that in detail.

Working Principle

Basically, a light microscope magnifies small objects and makes them visible. The science of microscopy is based on the following concepts and principles:

Magnification is simply the enlargement of the specimen. In a compound lens system, each lens sequentially enlarges or magnifies the specimen. The **objective lens** magnifies the specimen, producing a **real image** that is then magnified by the **occular lens** resulting in the final image. The **total magnification** can be calculated by multiplying the objective lens value by the occular lens value.

Resolving power is the ability of a lens to show two adjacent objects as discrete entities.

Limit of resolution is the ability to see two closely placed dots as two separate dots. If the distance between the two points is lessened, it would appear as a single point. It is expressed quantitatively as limit of resolution. The resolution of human unaided eye is 200 mμ.

Numerical aperture of the lens decides the angle at which the light enters it. The light-gathering ability of a microscope objective lens is quantitatively expressed in terms of numerical aperture.

Contrast is the ability to distinguish an object from its background. Since most microbes are relatively transparent when viewed under a standard light microscope they are difficult to identify. Using a stain that will bind to the microorganism and not the glass slide, enhances their contrast enabling them to be observed more clearly.

Depth-of-focus is the "thickness" of the sample that appears in focus at a particular magnification. As the magnification increases the depth-of-focus decreases or the "slice" of the sample that appears in focus gets thinner.

Field-of-view is the area of the slide that you are observing through the microscope. As you increase the magnification the actual area of the slide that you are looking at is getting smaller.

Working distance is the distance between the objective and the slide. As you increase magnification (by using more powerful objective lenses) the working distance decreases.

Construction

Eyepiece—contains the ocular lens, which provides a magnification power of 10 to 15, usually. This is where you look through.

Nosepiece—holds the objective lenses and can be rotated easily to change magnification.

Objective lenses—usually, there are three or four objective lenses on a microscope, consisting of 4 x 10 x 40 x and 100 x magnification powers. In order to obtain the total magnification of an image, you need to multiply the eyepiece lens power by the objective lens power. So, if you couple a 10 eyepiece lens with a 40 x objective lens, the total magnification is of $10 \times 40 = 400$ times.

Stage clips—hold the slide in place.

Stage—it is a flat platform that supports the slide being analyzed.

Diaphragm—it controls the intensity and size of the cone light projected on the specimen. As a rule of thumb, the more transparent the specimen, less light is required.

Light source—it projects light upwards through the diaphragm, slide and lenses.

Base—supports the microscope.

Condenser lens—it helps to focus the light onto the sample analyzed. They are particularly helpful when coupled with the highest objective lens.

Arm—supports the microscope when carried.

Coarse adjustment knob—when the knob is turned, the stage moves up or down, in order to coarse adjust the focus.

Fine adjustment knob—used fine adjust the focus.

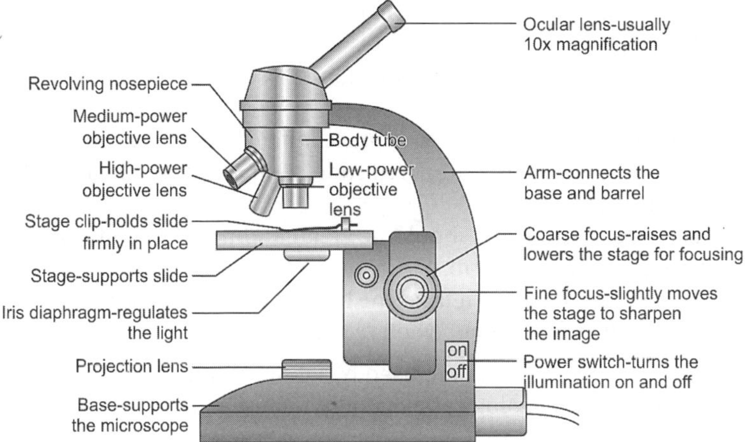

Figure 6.1.15: Parts of a bright-field compound microscope used in microbiology laboratories.

Handling and Care

- Use two hands when carrying a microscope, be gentle, these are sensitive and expensive instruments. Keep the microscope upright, oculars are removable and could fall out.
- Clean or dry lenses with grit-free lens paper only. Booklets of it are on your table's tray.
- Never use anything but lens paper. Other papers, tissues, or cloth will scratch lenses.
- Keep eyepiece (s) in the microscope at all times to keep dust out of the tube.
- Do not unscrew or otherwise tamper with lenses unless instructed to do so.
- At the start, do not look into the microscope. Begin by raising the stage as high as it can go by turning the coarse focal knob. You can now look through the ocular and focus on the specimen by turning the focus knob very slowly, in one direction.
- To change the magnification, grasp the ring of the revolving nosepiece and rotate until the desired objective clicks into place. Do not use the objectives to turn the nosepiece.
- Each time you complete work, particularly with oil immersion, clean the lenses with lens paper. Clean oil and other liquids from the stage and table as well.

- When you have finished with the microscope.
- The lowest power objective (it is also the shortest one) or none, should be returned to the position of use, before removing the slide.
- The slide is removed from stage and cleaned by rinsing in ethanol, unless it is a prepared slide, then it should go back onto a slide tray.
- The lenses and stage should be clean and dry. The cord loosely wrapped about the arm.
- The ocular rotated so it faces the back of the scope. (As not hit the back wall of the cabinet when returned to the shelf.)

Uses: These microscopes are used by laboratories, universities and hospitals to look at biological specimens for research and diagnostics.

Advantages

- Bright-field microscopy is very simple to use with fewer adjustments needed to be made to view specimens.
- Some specimens can be viewed without staining and the technology used in the bright-field technique don't alter the color of the specimen.

Limitations

- Bright-field microscopy can't be used to observe living specimens of bacteria, although when using fixed specimens, bacteria have an optimum viewing magnification of 1000x.
- Bright-field microscopy has very low contrast and most cells absolutely have to be stained to be seen. Staining may introduce extra details into the specimen that should not be present.
- This method requires a strong light source for high magnification applications and intense lighting can produce heat that will damage specimens or kill living microorganisms.

POSSIBLE QUESTIONS

1. Describe the methods of isolating pure cultures with necessary diagrams.
2. Write in detail about the culture media with its classification.
3. What are the types of culture media?
4. What are the different methods of preparing culture slides? Explain fixation.
5. What are the different staining methods? Explain each of them with necessary examples.

6. What is a microscope? Describe its structure with diagram.
7. Describe the types of microscopes in detail.
8. Explain the following:
   a. Aseptic transfer
   b. Inoculation from a broth
   c. Inoculation from a slant
   d. Negative staining
   e. Gram staining
   f. Method of inoculation
   g. Inoculation of culture media
   h. Culture media
   i. Subculturing
   j. Isolation of microorganisms
   k. Streak plate and pour plate
   l. Selective and enrichment media
   m. Differential media

MULTIPLE CHOICE QUESTIONS

1. The growth of microbes under artificial condition using laboratory techniques is known as:
   a. Heritage
   b. Biological media
   c. Culture
   d. All of the above
2. Separation of a single bacterial colony is called:
   a. Isolation
   b. Separation
   c. Pure culturing
   d. All of these
3. During staining, placing a drop of microorganisms directly on the slide and observing it is called:
   a. Whole mount
   b. Dry mount
   c. Wet mount
   d. None of the above
4. What is the correct order of staining reagents in Gram-Staining?
   a. Crystal violet, alcohol, iodine solution, safranin
   b. Crystal violet, iodine solution, alcohol, safranin
   c. Crystal violet, safranin, alcohol, iodine solution
   d. Iodine solution, crystal violet, alcohol, safranin
5. Which bacteria appears purple-blue color after staining?
   a. Gram-positive
   b. Gram-negative
   c. Both Gram-positive and Gram-negative
   d. Neither Gram-positive nor Gram-negative
6. Which of the following is used as a solidifying agent for media?
   a. Beef extract
   b. Peptone
   c. Agar
   d. Yeast extract

7. The isolation of gonorrhea-causing organism, *Neisseria gonorrhoeae* by the use of certain antibiotics in media is an example of which of the following?
   a. Selective media b. Differential media
   c. Enriched media d. Assay media
8. Peptone water and nutrient broth, both are:
   a. Enriched media b. Basal media
   c. Differential media d. None of the above
9. For obtaining a specific or desired bacteria from a mixture of pathogens which culture method is used?
   a. Nutrient broth b. Selective media
   c. Differential media d. Enriched media
10. The concentration of agar in solid media is:
    a. 1.5 to 2% b. 2 to 5%
    c. 0.5 to 1 d. None of the above
11. Which part of the light microscope controls the intensity of light entering the viewing area?
    a. Coarse adjustment knob b. Fine adjustment knob
    c. Diaphragm d. Condenser lens
12. The resolving power of human unaided eye is:
    a. 300 mμ. b. 100 mμ.
    c. 360 mμ. d. 200 mμ.
13. Lysozyme is effective against:
    a. Gram-negative bacteria b. Gram-positive bacteria
    c. Protozoa d. Helminthes
14. Lyophilization means:
    a. Sterilization b. Freeze-drying
    c. Burning to ashes d. Exposure to formation
15. What is the function of the diaphragm in a microscope?
    a. Diaphragm controls the angle of the light cone reaching the specimen.
    b. Controls only the width of the bundle of light rays reaching the condenser.
    c. Both of these
    d. None of these

Answers

1. c	2. a	3. c	4. b	5. a
6. c	7. a	8. b	9. b	10. a
11. c	12. d	13. b	14. b	15. c

Model Questions and Answers

1. Give a detail account of the bacterial cell.

Answer

- **Introduction:** Bacteria are microscopic, prokaryotic, unicellular organisms which are found everywhere.
- **Ultrastructure of bacterial cell:** Following are the parts of a bacterial cell:

(a) Capsule and Slime Layer

- **Location:** Outermost covering of the bacterial cell.
- **Structure:** Polysaccharide layers can be thick and stable like capsule or loosely attached to cell wall like slime layer.
- **Function:** Assist cells in adhesion to solid surface, and also protect pathogenic bacteria from the attack of the host's immune system.

(b) Cell Wall

- **Location:** It is present next to the capsule or slime layer.
- **Structure:** It is mostly composed of Peptidoglycan. In Gram-positive bacteria, the peptidoglcan layer is thicker and contains techoic acid, whereas in Gram-negative bacteria, the peptidoglycan layer is thinner and contains lipopolysaccharide.
- **Function:** It protects the cell from osmotic shock and physical damage. It also provides rigidity and shape to bacterial cells.

(c) Cell Membrane

- **Location:** Next to cell wall.
- **Structure:** The cell membrane is made up of Phospholipid bilayer, having thickness of 6-8 nm. A phospholipid molecule consists of one hydrophilic phosphate group and two

hydrophobic fatty acid chains. Hydrophillic heads are exposed to the external environments or the cytoplasm. The fatty acid chains direct inward, facing each other due to hydrophobic effects.

- **Function:** Regulates the specific transport of substances between the cells and the outer environment.

(d) Cytoplasm

- **Location:** Present inside the cell.
- **Composition:** It is a semifluid substance enclosed by the cell membrane. It appears granular due to the presence of large number of ribosomes. Different structures such as chromosomes, plasmids as well as cytoplasmic organelles are found in the cytoplasm.
- **Function:** It is the site for various biochemical reactions and contains genetic material of the cell.

(e) Chromosome

This is also called as nucleoid.

- **Location:** Found to float freely in the cytoplasm.
- **Number:** One chromosome in each cell.
- **Size:** In *E. coli,* the size of chromosome is 4640 kilo base pairs (kbp).
- **Structure and Composition:** It is made up of circular DNA attached at a point to the plasma membrane. The DNA in bacterial cell is not associated with histone protein. The DNA molecule is composed of Nitrogen Bases (A,T,G,C), deoxyribose sugar and phosphate molecules.
- **Function:** It is the storehouse of genetic information.

Note: Apart from the nucleoid, some bacterial cells also contain plasmids.

(f) Ribosomes

- **Location:** It is evenly distributed in the cytoplasm.
- **Structure and Composition:** Bacteria contain 70S Ribosome made up of ribosomal RNA (rRNA) and proteins. 70S Ribosome has two subunits (30S and 50S).
- **Function:** They are involved in bacterial protein synthesis.

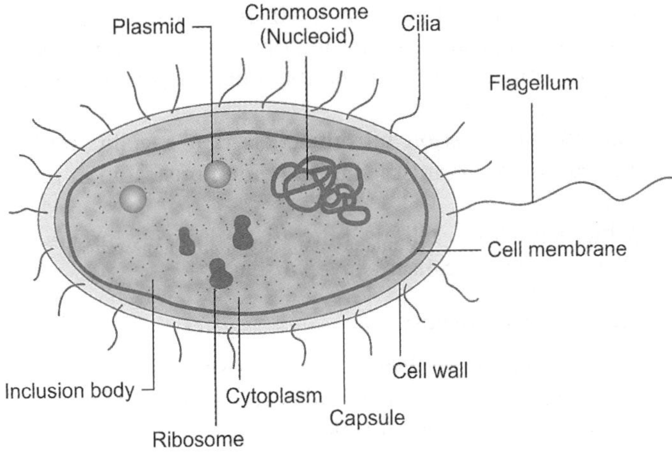

Figure 1: Ultra structure of a bacterial cell.

(g) Locomotory Organs

They are of two types—Flagella and Cilia.

- **Location:** Outermost part of the cell.
- **Structure:** Flagella are made of flagellin proteins.
- **Function:** The primary function of flagella is to make the bacteria move.

(h) Inclusion Bodies

- **Location:** Distributed in the cytoplasm.
- They are the non-living components present in the cell which do not possess metabolic activity. The most common inclusion bodies are glycogen, lipid droplets, crystals, pigments, volutin granules and metachromatic granules.

2. Write short notes

(a) Koch's Postulates

Answer: Koch's postulates are criteria designed to establish a relationship between a microbe and a disease. The postulates were published by Koch in 1890. Following are the Koch's postulates:

- A specific organism should be found constantly in association with the disease.
- The organism should be isolated and grown in a pure culture in the laboratory.

- The pure culture when inoculated into a healthy susceptible animal should produce symptoms/lesions of the same disease.
- From the inoculated animal, the microorganism should be isolated in pure culture.
- An additional criterion introduced is that specific antibodies to the causative organism should be demonstrable in patient's serum.
- **Significance:** They tell us how to definitively prove that a particular microbe causes a given disease.

(b) Structure of Antibody

- It is a "Y"-shaped molecule that consists of four polypeptide chains; two identical heavy chains (H) and two identical light chains (L) connected by disulfide bonds.
- Each heavy and light chain are made up of a number of domains.
- Each domain is about 110 amino acids in length and contains an interchain disulfide bond.

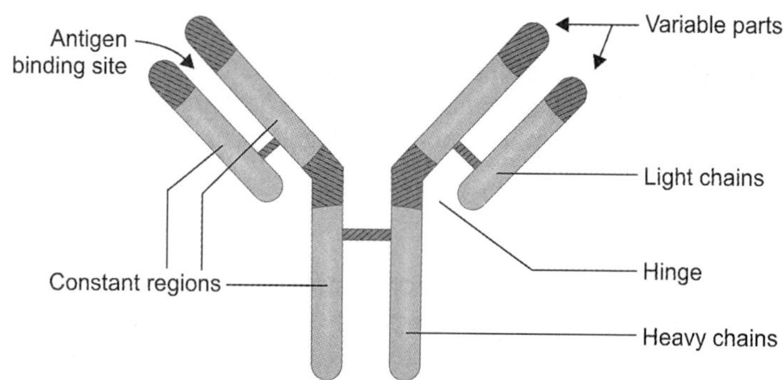

Figure 2: Structure of antibody.

- Each chain in antibody consists of two regions—Constant (C) and Variable (V) region. Amino acid sequence in the C-terminal regions of the H and L chains is the same whereas the amino acid sequence in the variable region of H and L chains is different.
- The regions of the variable domains actually contact the antigen and hence make up the antigen-binding site.
- Some parts of an antibody have unique functions. The arms of the Y, for example, contain the sites that can bind two antigens (in general identical) and therefore, recognize specific foreign objects. This region of the antibody is called the Fab (fragment,

antigen binding) region. It is composed of one constant and one variable domain from each heavy and light chain of the antibody.

- The variable domain is referred to as the FV region and is the most important region for binding to antigens.
- Fc region of the antibody is the region that trigger complement fixation reaction.

(c) Pasteurization

- This is a special technique of heat sterilization developed by Louis Pasteur.
- Originally, it was used to kill undesirable microorganisms that cause souring of wine.
- This process was originally employed by Louis Pasteur.
- Currently, this procedure is employed in food and dairy industry.
- There are three methods of pasteurization:
  - Holder method—Heated at 63°C for 30 minutes
  - Flash method—Heated at 72°C for 15 seconds followed by quickly cooling to 13°C
  - Ultra-High Temperature (UHT)—140°C for 15 sec and 149°C for 0.5 sec.
- This method is suitable to destroy most milk borne pathogens like *Salmonella, Mycobacteria, Streptococci, Staphylococci* and *Brucella.*
- However, *Coxiella* may survive pasteurization.

(d) Gram Staining

Objective: To differentiate between Gram-positive and Gram-negative bacteria.

Requirements: Glass slide, microbial culture, inoculation loop, Bunsen burner, Crystal violet, Ethanol, Safranin, Distilled water, Blotting paper, Light microscope.

Methodology:

- Place a slide with a bacterial smear on a staining rack.
- Stain the slide with Crystal Violet for 1-2 min.
- Pour off the stain.
- Flood slide with Gram's iodine for 1-2 min.
- Pour off the iodine.
- Decolorize by washing the slide briefly with acetone for 2-3 seconds.

- Wash slide thoroughly with water to remove the acetone—do not delay this step.
- Flood slide with Safranin counter stain for 2 min.
- Wash with water.
- Blot excess water and dry in hand over bunsen flame.
- Observe it under the microscope.

Inference: Bacteria with blue stain are Gram-positive where as bacteria with red stain are Gram-negative.

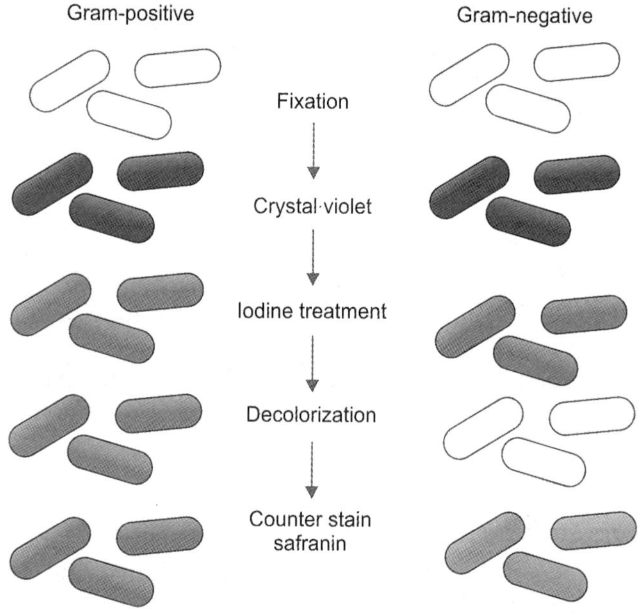

Figure 3: Steps of gram staining.

Glossary

1. **AB Toxins:** The structure and activity of many exotoxins are based on the AB model. In this model, the B portion of the toxin is responsible for toxin binding to a cell but does not directly harm it. The A portion enters the cell and disrupts its function.

2. **Accessory Pigments:** Photosynthetic pigments such as carotenoids and phycobiliproteins that aid chlorophyll in trapping light energy.

3. **Acid Fast:** Refers to bacteria like the mycobacteria that cannot be easily decolorized with acid alcohol after being stained with dyes such as basic fuchsin.

4. **Acid-Fast Staining:** A staining procedure that differentiates between bacteria based on their ability to retain a dye when washed with an acid alcohol solution.

5. **Acidophile:** A microorganism that has its growth optimum between about pH 0 and 5.5.

6. **Acquired Immune Deficiency Syndrome (AIDS):** An infectious disease syndrome caused by the human immunodeficiency virus and is characterized by the loss of a normal immune response, followed by increased susceptibility to opportunistic infections and an increased risk of some cancers.

7. **Acquired Immune Tolerance:** The ability to produce antibodies against nonself antigens while "tolerating" (not producing antibodies against) self-antigens.

8. **Acquired Immunity:** Refers to the type of specific (adaptive) immunity that develops after exposure to a suitable antigen or is produced after antibodies are transferred from one individual to another.

9. **Actinobacteria:** A group of Gram-positive bacteria containing the actinomycetes and their high G + C relatives.

10. Actinomycete: An aerobic, Gram-positive bacterium that forms branching filaments (hyphae) and asexual spores.

11. Actinorhizae: Associations between actinomycetes and plant roots.

12. Activated Sludge: Solid matter or sediment composed of actively growing microorganisms that participate in the aerobic portion of a biological sewage treatment process. The microbes readily use dissolved organic substrates and transform them into additional microbial cells and carbon dioxide.

13. Active Immunization: The induction of active immunity by natural exposure to a pathogen or by vaccination.

14. Acute Infections: Virus infections with a fairly rapid onset that last for a relatively short time.

15. Acute Viral Gastroenteritis: An inflammation of the stomach and intestines, normally caused by Norwalk and Norwalk-like viruses, other caliciviruses, rotaviruses and astroviruses.

16. Adenine: A purine derivative, 6-aminopurine, found in nucleosides, nucleotides, coenzymes and nucleic acids.

17. Adenosine Diphosphate (ADP): The nucleoside diphosphate usually formed upon the breakdown of ATP when it provides enregy for work.

18. Adenosine 5′-triphosphate (ATP): The triphosphate of the nucleoside adenosine, which is a high energy molecule or has high phosphate group transfer potential and serves as the cell's major form of energy currency.

19. Adhesin: A molecular component on the surface of a microorganism that is involved in adhesion to a substratum or cell. Adhesion to a specific host issue usually is a preliminary stage in pathogenesis, and adhesins are important virulence factors.

20. Adjuvant: Material added to an antigen to increase its immunogenicity. Common examples are alum, killed *Bordetella pertussis,* and an oil emulsion of the antigen, either alone (Freund's incomplete adjuvant) or with killed mycobacteria (Freund's complete adjuvant).

21. Aerobe: An organism that grows in the presence of atmospheric oxygen.

22. Aerobic Anoxygenic Photosynthesis: Photosynthetic process in which electron donors such as organic matter or sulfide, which do not result in oxygen evolution, are used under aerobic conditions.

23. Aerobic Respiration: A metabolic process in which molecules, often organic, are oxidized with oxygen as the final electron acceptor.

24. Aerotolerant Anaerobes: Microbes that grow equally well whether or not oxygen is present.

25. Aflatoxin: A polyketide secondary fungal metabolite that can cause cancer.

26. Agar: A complex sulfated polysaccharide, usually from red algae, that is used as a solidifying agent in the preparation of culture media.

27. Agglutinates: The visible aggregates or clumps formed by an agglutination reaction.

28. Agglutination Reaction: The formation of an insoluble immune complex by the cross-linking of cells or particles.

29. Airborne Transmission: The type of infectious organism transmission in which the pathogen is truly suspended in the air and travels over a meter or more from the source to the host.

30. Alkinetes: Specialized, nonmotile, dormant, thick-walled resting cells formed by some cyanobacteria.

31. Alga: A common term for a series of unrelated groups of photosynthetic eucaryotic microorganisms lacking multicellular sex organs (except for the charophytes) and conducting vessels.

32. Algicide: An agent that kills algae.

33. Alkalophile: A microorganism that grows best at pHs from about 8.5 to 11.5.

34. Allergen: A substance capable of inducing allergy or specific susceptibility.

35. Alpha Hemolysis: A greenish zone of partial clearing around a bacteria colony growing on blood agar.

36. Alpha-proteobacteria: One of the five subgroups of proteobacteria, each with distinctive 16S rRNA sequences. This group contains most of the oligotrophic proteobacteria; some have unusual metabolic modes such as methylotrophy, chemolithotrophy, and nitrogen fixing ability.

Many have distinctive morphological features.

37. Alveolar Macrophage: A vigorously phagocytic macrophage located on the epithelial surface of the lung alveoli where it ingests inhaled particulate matter and microorganisms.

38. Amensalism: A relationship in which the product of one organism has a negative effect on another organism.

39. Ames Test: A test that uses a special Salmonella strain to test chemicals for mutagenicity and potential carcinogenicity.

40. Amino Acid Activation: The initial stage of protein synthesis in which amino acids are attached to transfer RNA molecules.

41. Aminoglycoside Antibiotics: A group of antibiotics synthesized by *Streptomyces* and *Micromonospora,* which contain a cyclohexane ring and amino sugars; all aminoglycoside antibiotics bind to the small ribosomal subunit and inhibit protein synthesis.

42. Amphibolic Pathways: Metabolic pathways that function both catabolically and anabolically.

43. Amphitrichous: A cell with a single flagellum at each end.

44. Amphotericin B: An antibiotic from a strain of *Streptomyces nodosus* that is used to treat systemic fungal infections; it also is used topically to treat candidiasis.

45. Anaerobe: An organism that grows in the absence of free oxygen.

46. Anaerobic Digestion: The microbiological treatment of sewage wastes under anaerobic conditions to produce methane.

47. Anaerobic Respiration: An erergy-yielding process in which the electron transport chain acceptor is an inorganic molecule other than oxygen.

48. Anammox Process: The coupled use of nitrite as an electron acceptor and ammonium ion as a donor under anaerobic conditions to yield nitrogen gas.

49. Anaphylaxis: An immediate (type I) hypersensitivity reaction following exposure of a sensitized individual to the appropriate antigen. Mediated by reagin antibodies, chiefly IgE.

50. Anthrax: An infectious disease of animals caused by ingesting Bacillus anthracis spores. Can also occur in humans and is sometimes called woolsorter's disease.

51. Antibiotic: A microbial product or its derivative that kills susceptible microorganisms or inhibits their growth.

52. Antimetabolite: A compound that blocks metabolic pathways function by competitively inhibiting a key enzyme's use of a metabolite because it closely resembles the normal enzyme substrate.

53. Antimicrobial Agent: An agent that kills microorganisms or inhibits their growth.

54. Antisepsis: The prevention of infection or sepsis.

55. Antiseptic: Chemical agents applied to tissue to prevent infection by killing or inhibiting pathogens.

56. Antitoxin: An antibody to a microbial toxin, usually a bacterial exotoxin, that combines specifically with the toxin, in vivo and in vitro, neutralizing the toxin.

57. Apoptosis: Programmed cell death. The fragmentation of a cell into membrane-bound particles that are eliminated by phagocytosis. Apoptosis is a physiological suicide mechanism that preserves homeostasis and occurs during normal tissue turnover. It causes cell death in pathological circumstances, such as exposure to low concentrations of xenobiotics and infections by HIV and various other viruses.

58. Artificially Acquired Active Immunity: The type of immunity that results from immunizing an animal with a vaccine. The immunized animal now produces its own antibodies and activated lymphocytes.

59. Artificially Acquired Passive Immunity: The type of immunity that results from introducing into an animal antibodies that have been produced either in another animal or by in vitro methods. Immunity is only temporary.

60. Ascocarp: A multicellular structure in ascomycetes lined with specialized cells called asci in which nuclear fusion and meiosis produce ascospores. An ascocarp can be opened or closed and may be referred to as a fruiting body.

61. Ascogenous Hypha: A specialized hypha that gives rise to one or more asci.

62. Ascomycetes: A division of fungi that form ascospores.

63. Ascus: A specialized cell, characteristic of the ascomycetes, in which two haploid nuclei fuse to produce a zygote, which immediately divides by meiosis; at maturity an ascus will contain ascospores.

64. Aspergillosis: A fungal disease caused by species of *Aspergillus*.

65. Atomic Force Microscope: A type of scanning probe microscope that images a surface by moving a sharp probe over the surface at a constant distance : a very small amount of force is exerted on the tip and probe movement is followed with a laser.

66. Attenuation: (1) A mechanism for the regulation of transcription of some bacterial operons by aminoacyl-tRNAs. (2) A procedure that reduces or abolishes the virulence of a pathogen without altering its immunogenicity.

67. Attenuator: A rho-independent termination site in the leader sequence that is involved in attenuation.

68. Autoclave: An apparatus for sterilizing objects by the use of steam under pressure. Its development tremendously stimulated the growth of microbiology.

69. Autogenous Infection: An infection that results from a patient's own microbiota, regardless of whether the infecting organism became part of the patient's microbiota subsequent to admission to a clinical care facility.

70. Autoimmune Disease: A disease produced by the immune system attacking self-antigens. Autoimmune disease results from the activation of self-reactive T and B cells that damage tissues after stimulation by genetic or environmental triggers.

71. Autoimmunity: Autoimmunity is a condition characterized by the presence of serum autoantibodies and self-reactive lymphocytes. It may be benign or pathogenic. Autoimmunity is a normal consequence of aging; is readily inducible by infectious agents, organisms, or drugs; and is potentially reversible in that it disappears when the offending "agent" is removed or eradicated.

72. Autotroph: An organism that uses CO_2 as its sole or principal source of carbon.

73. Auxotroph: A mutated prototroph that lacks the ability to synthesize an essential nutrient and therefore, must obtain it or a precursor from its surroundings.

74. Axenic: Not contaminated by any foreign organisms; the term is used in reference to pure microbial cultures or to germfree animals.

75. Bacillus: A rod-shaped bacterium.

76. Bacteremia: The presence of viable bacteria in the blood.

77. Bacteria: The domain that contains procaryotic cells with primarily diacyl glycerol diesters in their membranes and with bacterial rRNA. Bacteria also is a general term for organisms that are composed of procaryotic cells and are not multicellular.

78. Bacterial Artificial Chromosome (BAC): A cloning vector constructed from the *E. coli* F-factor plasmid that is used to clone foreign DNA fragments in *E. coli.*

79. Bacterial Vaginosis: Bacterial vaginosis is a sexually trasmitted disease caused by Gardnerella vaginalis, *Mobiluncus* spp., *Mycoplasma hominis,* and various anaerobic bacteria. Although a mild disease it is a risk factor for obstetric infections and pelvic inflammatory disease.

80. Bactericide: An agent that kills bacteria.

81. Bacteriochlorophyll: A modified chlorophyll that serves as the primary light-trapping pigment in purple and green photosynthetic bacteria.

82. Bacteriocin: A protein produced by a bacterial strain that kills other closely related strains.

83. Bacteriophage: A virus that uses bacteria as its host; often called a phage.

84. Bacteriophage (phage) Typing: A technique in which strains of bacteria are identified based on their susceptibility to bacteriophages.

85. Bacteriostatic: Inhibiting the growth and reproduction of bacteria.

86. Bacteroid: A modified, often pleomorphic, bacterial cell within the root nodule cells of legumes; after transformation into a symbiosome it carries out nitrogen fixation.

87. Baeocytes: Small, spherical, reproductive cells produced by pleurocapsalean cyanobacteria through multiple fission.

88. Balanced Growth: Microbial growth in which all cellular constituents are synthesized at constant rates relative to each other.

89. Balanitis: Inflammation of the glans penis usually associated with *Candida* fungi; a sexually transmitted disease.

90. Barophilic or Barophile: Organisms that prefer or require high pressures for growth and reproduction.

91. Barotolerant: Organisms that can grow and reproduce at high pressures but do not require them.

92. Basal Body: The cylindrical structure at the base of procaryotic and eucaryotic flagella that attaches them to the cell.

93. Batch Culture: A culture of microorganisms produced by inoculating a closed culture vessel containing a single batch of medium.

94. B-cell Antigen Receptor (BCR): A transmembrane immunoglobulin complex on the surface of a B cell that binds an antigen and stimulates the B cell. It is composed of a membrane-bound immunoglobulin, usually IgD or a modified IgM, complexed with another membrane protein (the Ig-α/Ig-β heterodimer).

95. Beta Hemolysis: A zone of complete clearing around a bacterial colony growing on blood agar. The zone does not change significantly in color.

96. β-Oxidation Pathway: The major pathway of fatty acid oxidation to produce NADH, FADH2 and acetyl coenzyme A.

97. Beta-proteobacteria: One of the five subgroups of proteobacteria, each with distinctive 16S rRNA sequences. Members of this subgroup are similar to the alpha-proteobacteria metabolically, but tend to use substances that diffuse from organic matter decomposition in anaerobic zones.

98. Binal Symmetry: The symmetry of some virus capsids (e.g., those of complex phages) that is a combination of icosahedral and helical symmetry.

99. Binary Fission: Asexual reproduction in which a cell or an organism separates into two cells.

100. Bioaugmentation: Addition of pregrown microbial cultures to an environment to perform a specific task.

101. Biochemical Oxygen Demand (BOD): The amount of oxygen used by organisms in water under certain standard conditions; it provides an index of the amount of microbially oxidizable organic matter present.

102. Biodegradation: The breakdown of a complex chemical through biological processes that can result in minor loss of functional groups, fragmentation into larger constituents, or complete breakdown to carbon dioxide and minerals. Often the term refers to the undesired microbial-mediated destruction of materials such as paper, paint, and textiles.

103. Biofilms: Organized microbial systems consisting of layers of microbial cells associated with surfaces, often with complex structural and functional characteristics. Biofilms have physical/chemical gradients that influence microbial metabolic processes. They can form on inanimate devices (catheters, medical prosthetic devices) and also cause fouling (e.g., of ships' hulls, water pipes, cooling towers).

104. Biogeochemical Cycling: The oxidation and reduction of substances carried out by living organisms and/or abiotic processes that results in the cycling of elements within and between different parts of the ecosystem (the soil, aquatic environment and atomshpere).

105. Bioinsecticide: A pathogen that is used to kill or disable unwanted insect pests. Bacteria, fungi, or viruses are used, either directly or after manipulation, to control insect populations.

106. Biologic Transmission: A type of vector-borne transmission in which a pathogen goes through some morphological or physiological change within the vector.

107. Bioluminescence: The production of light by living cells, often through the oxidation of molecules by the enzyme luciferase.

108. Biopesticide: The use of a microorganism or another biological agent to control a specific pest.

109. Bioremediation: The use of biologically mediated processes to remove or degrade pollutants from specific environments. Bioremediation can be carried out by modification of the environment to accelerate biological processes, either with or without the addition of specific microorganisms.

110. Biosensor: The coupling of a biological process with production of an electrical signal or light to detect the presence of particular substances.

111. Bioterrorism: The intentional or threatened use of viruses, bacteria, fungi, or toxins from living organisms to produce death or disease in humans, animals, and plants.

112. Biotransformation or Microbial Transformation: The use of living organisms to modify substances that are not normally used for growth.

113. Black Piedra: A fungal infection caused by Piedraia hortae that forms hard black nodules on the hairs of the scalp.

114. Blastomycosis: A systemic fungal infection caused by Blastomyces dermatitidis and marked by suppurating tumors in the skin or by lesions in the lungs.

115. Botulism: A form of food poisoning caused by a neurotoxin (botulin) produced by *Clostridium botulinum* serotypes A-G; sometimes found in improperly canned or preserved food.

116. Bright-field Microscope: A microscope that illuminates the specimen directly with bright ıight and forms a dark image on a brighter background.

117. Broad-spectrum Drugs: Chemotherapeutic agents that are effective against many different kinds of pathogens.

118. Budding: A vegetative outgrowth of yeast and some bacteria as a means of asexual reproduction; the daughter cell is smaller than the parent.

119. Bulking Sludge: Sludges produced in sewage treatment that do not settle properly, usually due to the development of filamentous microorganisms.

120. Butanediol Fermentation: A type of fermentation most often found in the family Enterobacteriaceae in which 2, 3-butanediol is a major product; acetoin is an intermediate in the pathway and may be detected by the Voges-Proskauer test.

121. Candidiasis: An infection caused by *Candida* species of dimorphic fungi, commonly involving the skin.

122. Capsule: A layer of well-organized material, not easily washed off, lying outside the bacterial cell wall.

123. Carboxysomes: Polyhedral inclusion bodies that contain the CO_2 fixation enzyme ribulose 1, 5-bisphosphate carboxylase; found in cyanobacteria, nitrifying bacteria and thiobacilli.

124. Carrier: An infected individual who is a potential source of infection for others and plays an important role in the epidemiology of a disease.

125. Caseous Lesion: A lesion resembling cheese or curd; cheesy. Most caseous lesions are caused by *M. tuberculosis*.

126. Casual Carrier: An individual who harbors an infectious organism for only a short period.

127. Cathelicidins: Antimicrobial peptides that are produced by skin cells and kill bacterial pathogens. They destroy invaders by either punching holes in their membranes or solubilizing membranes through detergent-like action.

128. Cellulitis. A diffuse spreading infection of subcutaneous skin tissue caused by streptococci, staphylococci, or other organisms. The tissue is inflamed with edema, redness, pain, and interference with function.

129. Cell Wall: The strong layer or structure that lies outside the plasma membrane; it supports and protects the membrane and gives the cell shape.

130. Cephalosporin: A group of β-lactam antibiotics derived from the fungus Cephalosporium, which share the 7-aminocephalosporanic acid nucleus.

131. Chancroid: A sexually transmitted disease caused by the Gram-negative bacterium *Haemophilus ducreyi*. Worldwide, chancroid is an important cofactor in the transmission of the AIDS virus. Also known as genital ulcer disease due to the painful circumscribed ulcers that form on the penis or entrance to the vagina.

132. Chemical Oxygen Demand (COD): The amount of chemical oxidation required to convert organic matter in water and waste water to CO_2.

133. Chemolithotropic Autotrophs: Microorganisms that oxidize reduced inorganic compounds to derive both energy and electrons; CO_2 is their carbon source. Also called chemolithoautotrophs.

134. Chemoorganotrophic Heterotrophs: Organisms that use organic compounds as sources of energy, hydrogen, electrons, and carbon for biosynthesis.

135. Chemostat: A continuous culture apparatus that feeds medium into the culture vessel at the same rate as medium containing microorganisms is removed; the medium in a chemostat contains one essential nutrient in a limiting quantity.

136. Chemotaxis: The pattern of microbial behavior in which the microorganism moves toward chemical attractants and/or away from repellents.

137. Chemotherapeutic Agents: Compounds used in the treatment of disease that destroy pathogens or inhibit their growth at concentrations low enough to avoid doing undesirable damage to the host.

138. Chemotrophs: Organisms that obtain energy from the oxidation of chemical compounds.

139. Chickenpox (varicella): A highly contagious skin disease, usually affecting 2- to 7- year-old children; it is caused by the varicella-zoster virus, which is acquired by droplet inhalation into the respiratory system.

140. Chlamydiae: Members of the genus *Chlamydia*: gram-negative, coccoid cells that reproduce only within the cytoplasmic vesicles of host cells using a life cycle that alternates between elementary bodies and reticulate bodies.

141. Chlamydial Pneumonia: A penumonia caused by *Chlamydia pneumoniae*. Clinically, infections are mild and 50% of adults have antibodies to the chlamydiae.

142. Cholera: An acute infectious enteritis, endemic and epidemic in Asia, which periodically spreads to the Middle East, Africa, Southern Europe, and South America; caused by *Vibrio cholerae*.

143. Choleragen: The cholera toxin; an extremely potent protein molecule elaborated by strains of *Vibrio cholerae* in the small intestine after ingestion of feces-contaminated water or food. It acts on epithelial cells to cause hypersecretion of chloride and bicarbonate and an outpouring of large quantities of fluid from the mucosal surface.

144. Chromoblastomycosis: A chronic fungal skin infection, producing wart-like nodules that may ulcerate. It is caused by the black molds Phialophora verrucosa or Fonsecaea pedrosoi.

145. Cilia: Thread-like appendages extending from the surface of some protozoa that beat rhythmically to propel them; cilia are membrane-bound cylinders with a complex internal array of microtubules, usually in a 9 + 2 pattern.

146. Classical Complement Pathway: The antibody-dependent pathway of complement activation; it leads to the lysis of pathogens and stimulates phagocytosis and other host defenses.

147. Classification: The arrangement of organisms into groups based on mutual similarity or evolutionary relatedness.

148. Clone: A group of genetically identical cells or organisms derived by asexual reproduction from a single parent.

149. Coaggregation: The collection of a variety of bacteria on a surface such as a tooth surface because of cell-to-cell recognition of genetically distinct bacterial types. Many of these interactions appear to be mediated by a lectin on one bacterium that interacts with a complementary carbohydrate receptor on another bacterium.

150. Coagulase: An enzyme that induces blood clotting; it is characteristically produced by pathogenic staphylococci.

151. Coccidioidomycosis: A fungal disease caused by *Coccidioides immitis* that exists in dry, highly alkaline soils. Also known as valley fever, San Joaquin fever, or desert rheumatism.

152. Coccus: A roughly spherical bacterial cell.

153. Cold Sore: A lesion caused by the herpes simplex virus; usually occurs on the border of the lips or nares. Also known as a fever blister or herpes labialis.

154. Colicin: A plasmid-encoded protein that is produced by enteric bacteria and binds to specific receptors on the cell envelope of sensitive target bacteria, where it may cause lysis or attack specific intracellular sites such as ribosomes.

155. Coliform: A Gram-negative, non-sporing, facultative rod that ferments lactose with gas formation within 48 hours at 35°C.

156. Colonization: The establishment of a site of microbial reproduction on an inanimate surface or organism without necessarily resulting in tissue invasion or damage.

157. Colony: An assemblage of microorganisms growing on a solid surface such as the surface of an agar culture medium; the assemblage often is directly visible, but also may be seen only microscopically.

158. Colony Forming Units (CFU): The number of microorganisms that form colonies when cultured using spread plates or pour plates, an indication of the number of viable microorganisms in a sample.

159. Colorless Sulphur Bacteria: A diverse group of non-photosynthetic proteobacteria that can oxidize reduced sulfur compounds such as hydrogen sulfide. Many are lithotrophs and derive energy from sulfur oxidation. Some are unicellular, whereas others are filamentous gliding bacteria.

160. Combinatorial Biology: Introduction of genes from one microorganism into another microorganism to synthesize a new product or a modified product, especially in relation to antibiotic synthesis.

161. Cometabolism: The modification of a compound not used for growth by a microorganism, which occurs in the presence of another organic material that serves as a carbon and energy source.

162. Commensal: Living on or within another organism without injuring or benefiting the other organism.

163. Common Vehicle Transmission: The transmission of a pathogen to a host by means of an inanimate medium or vehicle.

164. Communicable Disease: A disease associated with a pathogen that can be transmitted from one host to another.

165. Competent: A bacterial cell that can take up free DNA fragments and incorporate them into its genome during transformation.

166. Competition: An interaction between two organisms attempting to use the same resource (nutrients, space, etc.).

167. Competitive Exclusion Principle: Two competing organisms overlap in resource use, which leads to the exclusion of one of the organisms.

168. Complex Medium: Culture medium that contains some ingredients of unknown chemical composition.

169. Complex Viruses: Viruses with capsids having a complex symmetry that is neither icosahedral nor helical.

170. Composting: The microbial processing of fresh organic matter under moist, aerobic conditions, resulting in the accumulation of a stable humified product, which is suitable for soil improvement and stimulation of plant growth.

171. Confocal Scanning Laser Microscope (CSLM): A light microscope in which monochromatic laser-derived light scans across the specimen at a specific level and illuminates one area at a time to form an image. Stray light from other parts of the specimen is blocked out to give an image with excellent contrast and resolution.

172. Congenital (neonatal) Herpes: An infection of a newbown caused by transmission of the herpesvirus during vaginal delivery.

173. Conjugation: 1. The form of gene transfer and recombination in bacteria that requires direct cell-to-cell contact. 2. A complex form of sexual reproduction commonly employed by protozoa.

174. Conjugative Plasmid: A plasmid that carries the genes for sex pili and can transfer copies of itself to other bacteria during conjugation.

175. Conoid: A hollow cone of spirally coiled filaments in the anterior tip of certain apicomplexan protozoa.

176. Constitutive Mutant: A strain that produces as inducible enzyme continually, regardless of need, because of a mutation in either the operator or regulator gene.

177. Constructed Wetlands: Intentional creation of marshland plant communities and their associated microorganisms for environmental restoration or to purify water by the removal of bacteria, organic matter, and chemicals as the water passes through the aquatic plant communities.

178. Consumer: An organism that feeds directly on living or dead animals, by ingestion or by phagocytosis.

179. Contact Transmission: Transmission of the pathogen by contact of the source or reservoir of the pathogen with the host.

180. Continuous Culture System: A culture system with constant environmental conditions maintained through continual provision of nutrients and removal of wastes.

181. Convalescent Carrier: An individual who has recovered from an infectious disease but continues to harbor large numbers of the pathogen.

182. Cooperation: A positive but not obiligatory interaction between two different organisms. Also called protocooperation.

183. Cortex: The layer of a bacterial endospore that is thought to be particularly important in conferring heat resistance on the endospore.

184. Cryptococcosis: An infection caused by the basidiomycete. *Cryptococcus neoformans*, which may involve the skin, lungs, brain, or meninges.

185. Cryptosporidiosis: Infection with protozoa of the genus Cryptosporidium. The most common symptoms are prolonged diarrhea, weight loss, fever, and abdominal pain.

186. Cutaneous Diphtheria: A skin disease caused by *Corynebacterium diphtheriae* that infects wound or skin lesions, causing a slow-healing ulceration.

187. Cyanobacteria: A large group of bacteria that carry out oxygenic photosynthesis using a system like that present in photosynthetic eucaryotes.

188. Cyst: A general term used for a specialized microbial cell enclosed in a wall. Cysts are formed by protozoa and a few bacteria. They may be dormant, resistant structures formed in response to adverse conditions or reproductive cysts that are a normal stage in the life cycle.

189. Cytopathic Effect: The observable change that occurs in cells as a result of viral replication. Examples include ballooning, binding together, clustering, or ever death of the cultured cells.

190. Cytoplasmic Matrix: The protoplasm of a cell that lies within the plasma membrane and outside any other organelles. In bacteria it is the substance between the cell membrane and the nucleoid.

191. Cytotoxin. A toxin or antibody that has a specific toxic action upto cells; cytotoxins are named according to the cell for which they are specific (e.g., nephrotoxin).

192. Dane Particle: A 42 nm spherical particle that is one of three that are seen in hepatitis B virus infections. The Dane particle is the complete virion.

193. Dark-Field Microscopy: Microscopy in which the specimen is brightly illuminated while the background is dark.

194. Death Phase: The decrease in viable microorganisms that occurs after the completion of growth in a batch culture.

195. Decimal Reduction Time (D or D value): The time required to kill 90% of the microorganisms or spores in a sample at a specified temperature.

196. Decomposer: An organism that breaks down complex materials into simpler ones, including the release of simple inorganic products. Often a decomposer, such as an insect or earthworm physically reduces the size of substrate particles.

197. Defensin: Specific peptides produced by neutrophils that permeabilize the outer and inner membranes of certain microorganisms, thus killing them.

198. Defined Medium: Culture medium made with components of known composition.

199. Delta-proteobacteria: One of the five subgroups of proteobacteria. Chemoorganotrophic bacteria that usually are either predators on other bacteria or anaerobes that generate sulfide from sulfate and sulfite.

200. Dendrogram: A tree-like diagram that is used to graphically summarize mutual similarities and relationships between organisms.

201. Denitrification: The reduction of nitrate to gaseous products, primarily nitrogen gas, during anaerobic respiration.

202. Dental Plaque: A thin film on the surface of teeth consisting of bacteria embedded in a matrix of bacterial polysaccharides, salivary glycoproteins, and other substances.

203. Deoxyribonucleic Acid (DNA): The nucleic acid that constitutes the genetic material of all cellular organisms. It is a polynucleotide composed of deoxyribonucleotides connected by phosphodiester bonds.

204. Dermatomycosis: A fungal infection of the skin; the term is a general term that comprises the various forms of tinea, and it is sometimes used to specifically refer to athlete's foot (tinea pedis).

205. Desert Crust: A crust formed by microbial binding of sand grains in the surface zone of desert soil; crust formation primarily involves cyanobacteria.

206. Detergent: An organic molecule, other than a soap, that serves as a wetting agent and emulsifier; it is normally used as cleanser. But some may be used as antimicrobial agents.

207. Deuteromycetes: In some classification systems, the deuteromycetes or Fungi Imperfecti are a class of fungi. These organisms either lack a sexual stage or it has not yet been discovered.

208. Diauxic Growth: A biphasic growth pattern or response in which a microorganism, when exposed to two nutrients, initially uses one of them for growth and then alters its metabolism to make use of the second.

209. Differential Interference Contrast (DIC) Microscope: A light microscope that employs two beams of plane polarized light. The beams are combined after passing through the specimen and their interference is used to create the image.

210. Differential Media: Culture media that distinguish between groups of microorganisms based on differences in their growth and metabolic products.

211. Differential Staining Procedures: Staining procedures that divide bacteria into separate groups based on staining properties.

212. Diffusely Adhering *E. coli* (DAEC): DAEC strains of *E. coli* adhere over the entire surface of epithelial cells and usually cause diarrheal disease in immunologically naive and malnourished children.

213. Dikaryotic Stage: In fungi, having pairs of nuclei within cells or compartments. Each cell contains two separate haploid nuclei, one from each parent.

214. Dinoflagellate: An algal protist characterized by two flagella used in swimming in a spinning pattern. Many are bioluminescent and an important part of marine phytoplankton, some also are important marine pathogens.

215. Diphtheria: An acute, highly contagious childhood disease that generally affects the membranes of the throat and less frequently the nose. It is caused by *Corynebacterium diphtheriae.*

216. Dipicolinic Acid: A substance present at high concentrations in the bacterial endspore. It is thought to contribute to the endospore's heat resistance.

217. Diplococcus: A pair of cocci.

218. Directed or Adaptive Mutation: A mutation that seems to be chosen so the organism can better adapt to its surroundings.

219. Disinfectant: An agent, usually chemical, that disinfects; normally, it is employed only with inanimate objects.

220. Disinfection: The killing, inhibition, or removal of microorganisms that may cause disease. It usually refers to the treatment of inanimate objects with chemicals.

221. Disinfection By-products (DBPs): Chlorinated organic compounds such as trihalomethanes formed during chlorine use for water disinfection. Many are carcinogens.

222. Dissimilatory Nitrate Reduction: The process in which some bacteria use nitrate as the electron acceptor at the end of their electron transport chain to produce ATP. The nitrate is reduced to nitrite or nitrogen gas.

223. Dissimilatory Reduction: The use of a substance as an electron acceptor in energy generation. The acceptor (e.g., sulfate or nitrate) is reduced but not incorporated into organic matter during biosynthetic processes.

224. DNA Vaccine: A vaccine that contains DNA which encodes antigenic proteins. It is injected directly into the muscle; the DNA is taken up by the muscle cells and encoded protein antigens are synthesized. This produces both humoral and cell-mediated responses.

225. Eclipse Period: The initial part of the latent period in which infected host bacteria do not contain any complete virions.

226. Effacing Lesion: The type of lesion caused by enteropathogenic strains of *E. coli* (EPEC) when the bacteria destroy the brush border of intestinal epithelial cells. The term AE (attaching-effacing) *E. coli* is now used to designate true EPEC strains that are an important cause of diarrhea in children from developing countries and in traveller's diarrhea.

227. Ehrlichiosis: A tick-borne (*Dermacentor andersoni, Amblyomma americanum*) rickettsial disease caused by Ehrlichia chaffeensis. Once inside leukocytes, a nonspecific illness develops that resembles Rocky Mountain spotted fever.

228. Endogenous Infection: An infection by a member of an individual's own normal body microbiota.

229. Endosymbiont: An organism that lives within the body of another organism in a symbiotic association.

230. Endosymbiosis: A type of symbiosis in which one organism is found within another organism.

231. Endosymbiotic Theory or Hypothesis: The theory that eucaryotic organelles such as mitochondria and chloroplasts arose when bacteria established an endosymbiotic relationship with the eucaryotic ancestor and then evolved into organelles.

232. Enteric Bacteria (enterobacteria): Members of the family Enterobacteriaceae (Gram-negative, peritrichous or nonmotile, facultatively anaerobic, straight rods with simple nutritional requirements); also used for bacteria that live in the intestinal tract.

233. Enterohemorrhagic *E. coli* (EHEC): EHEC strains of *E. coli* (O157:H7) produce several cytotoxins that provoke fluids secretion in traveller's diarrhea; however, their mode of action is unknown.

234. Enteroinvasive *E. coli* (EIEC): EIEC strains of *E. coli* cause traveller's diarrhea by penetrating and binding to the intestinal epithelial cells, EIEC may also produce a cytotoxin and enterotoxin.

235. Enteropathogenic *E. coli* (EPEC): EPEC strains of *E. coli* attach to the brush border of intestinal epithelial cells and cause a specific type of cell damage called effacing lesions that lead to traveller's diarrhea.

236. Enterotoxigenic *E. coli* (ETEC): ETEC strains of *E. coli* produce two plasmid-encoded enterotoxins (which are responsible for traveller's diarrhea) and the distinguished by their heat stability: heat-stable enterotoxin (ST) and heat-labile enterotoxin (LT).

237. Epidemic (louse-borne) Typhus: A disease caused by *Rickettsia prowazekii* that is transmitted from person to person by the body louse.

238. Epsilon-proteobacteria: One of the five subgroups of proteobacteria, each with distinctive 16S rRNA sequences. Slender Gram-negative rods, some of which are medically important (*Campylobacter* and *Helicobacter*).

239. Ergot: The dried sclerotium of *Claviceps purpurea*. Also, an ascomycete that parasitizes rye and other higher plants causing the disease called ergotism.

240. Ergotism: The disease or toxic condition caused by eating grain infected with ergot; it is often accompanied by gangrene, psychotic delusions, nervous spasms, abortion, and convulsions in humans and in animals.

241. Eucarya: The domain that contains organisms composed of eucaryotic cells with primarily glycerol fatty acyl diesters in their membranes and eucaryotic rRNA.

242. Excystation: The escape of one or more cells or organisms from a cyst.

243. Exergonic Reaction: A reaction that spontaneously goes to completion as written; the standard free energy change is negative, and the equilibrium constant is greater than one.

244. Exogenote: The piece of donor DNA that enters a bacterial cell during gene exchange and recombination.

245. Exotoxin: A heat-labile, toxic protein produced by a bacterium as a result of its normal metabolism or because of the acquisition of a plasmid or prophage. It is usually released into the bacterium's surroundings.

246. Exponential Phase: The phase of the growth curve during which the microbial population is growing at a constant and maximum rate, dividing and doubling at regular intervals.

247. Extracutaneous Sporotrichosis: An infection by the fungus *Sporothrix schenckii* that spreads throughout the body.

248. Extreme Barophilic Bacteria: Bacteria that require a high-pressure environment to function.

249. Extreme Environment: An environment in which physical factors such as temperature, pH, salinity, and pressure are outside of the normal range for growth of most microorganisms; these conditions allow unique organisms to survive and function.

250. Extremophiles: Microorganisms that grow under harsh or extreme environmental conditions such as very high temperatures or low pHs.

251. Extrinsic Factor: An environmental factor such as temperature that influences microbial growth in food.

252. Facultative Anaerobes: Microorganisms that do not require oxygen for growth, but do grow better in its presence.

253. Fecal Coliform: Coliforms whose normal habitat is the intestinal tract and that can grow at 44.5°C.

254. Fecal Enterococci: Enterococci found in the intestine of humans and other warm-blooded animals.

They are used as indicators of the fecal pollution of water.

255. Fimbria (Fimbriae): A fine, hair-like protein appendage on some gram-negative bacteria that helps attach them to surfaces.

256. Flagellin: The protein used to construct the filament of a bacterial flagellum.

257. Flagellum (Flagella): A thin, thread-like appendage on many prokaryotic and eukaryotic cells that is responsible for their motility.

258. Fluorescence Microscope: A microscope that exposes a specimen to light of a specific wavelength and then forms an image from the fluorescent light produced. Usually the specimen is stained with a fluorescent dye or fluorochrome.

259. Fomite (Fomites): An object that is not in itself harmful but is able to harbor and transmit pathogenic organisms. Also called fomes.

260. Food-borne Infection: Gastrointestinal illness caused by ingestion of microorganisms, followed by their growth within the host. Symptoms arise from tissue invasion and/or toxin production.

261. Food Web: A network of many interlinked food chains, encompassing primary producers, consumers, decomposers and detritivores.

262. Gamma-proteobacteria: One of the five sub-groups of proteobacteria, each with distinctive 16S rRNA sequences. This is the largest subgroup and is very diverse physiologically; many important genera are facultatively anaerobic chemoorganotrophs.

263. Gas Gangrene: A type of gangrene that arises from dirty, lacerated wounds infected by anaerobic bacteria, especially species of *Clostridium*. As the bacteria grow, they release toxins and ferment carbohydrates to produce carbon dioxide and hydrogen gas.

264. Gastroenteritis: An acute inflammation of the lining of the stomach and intestines, characterized by anorexia, nausea, diarrhea, abdominal pain, and weakness. It has various causes including food poisoning due to such organisms as *E. coli, S. aureus, Campylobacter* (campy-lobacteriosis) and *Salmonella* species; consumption of irritating food or drink; or psychological factors such as anger, stress, and fear. Also called enterogastritis.

265. Gas Vacuole: A gas-filled vacuole found in cyanobacteria and some other aquatic bacteria that provides flotation. It is composed of gas vesicles, which are made of protein.

266. Generalized Transduction: The transfer of any part of a bacterial genome when the DNA fragment is packaged within a phage capsid by mistake.

267. General Recombination: Recombination involving a reciprocal exchange of a pair of homologous DNA sequences; it can occur any place on the chromosome.

268. Generation Time: The time required for a microbial population to double in number.

269. Genetic Engineering: The deliberate modification of an organism's genetic information by directly changing its nucleic acid genome.

270. Genital Herpes: A sexually transmitted disease caused by the herpes simplex virus type 2.

271. Germicide: An agent that kills pathogens and many nonpathogens but not necessarily bacterial endospores.

272. Giardiasis: A common intestinal disease caused by the parasitic protozoan *Giardia lamblia.*

273. Glycocalyx: A network of polysaccharides extending from the surface of bacteria and other cells.

274. Gnotobiotic: Animals that are germfree (microorganisms free) or live in association with one or more known microorganisms.

275. Gonococci: Bacteria of the species *Neisseria gonorrhoeae*—the organism causing gonorrhea.

276. Gonorrhea: An acute infectious sexually transmitted disease of the mucous membranes of the genitourinary tract, eye, rectum, and throat. It is caused by *Neisseria gonorrhoeae.*

277. Gram Stain: A differential staining procedure that divides bacteria into Gram-positive and Gram-negative groups based on their ability to retain crystal violet when decolorized with an organic solvent such as ethanol.

278. Greenhouse Gases: Gases released from the Earth's surface through chemical and biological processes that interact with the chemicals in the stratosphere to decrease the release of radiation from the Earth. It is believed that this leads to global warming.

279. Guillain-Barré Syndrome: A relatively rare disease affecting the peripheral nervous system, especially the spinal nerves, but also the cranial nerves. The cause is unknown, but it most often occurs after an influenza infection or flu vaccination. Also called French Polio.

280. Halophile: A microorganism that requires high levels of sodium chloride for growth.

281. Harborage Transmission: The mode of transmission in which an infectious organism does not undergo morphological or physiological changes within the vector.

282. Healthy Carrier: An individual who harbors a pathogen, but is not ill.

283. Hemolysis: The disruption of red blood cells and release of their hemoglobin. There are several types of hemolysis when bacteria such as streptococci and staphylococci, grow on blood agar. In α-hemolysis, a narrow greenish zone of incomplete hemolysis forms around the colony. A clear zone of complete hemolysis without any obvious color change is formed during β-hemolysis.

284. Hemolytic Uremic Syndrome: A kidney disease characterized by blood in the urine and often by kidney failure. It is caused by enterohemorrhagic strains of *Escherichia coli* O157 : H7 that produce a Shiga-like toxin, which attacks the kidneys.

285. Hepatitis A (formerly infectious hepatitis): A type of hepatitis that is transmitted by fecal-oral contamination; it primarily affects children and young adults, especially in environments where there is poor sanitation and overcrowding. It is caused by the hepatitis A virus, a single-stranded RNA virus.

286. Hepatitis B (formerly serum hepatitis): This form of hepatitis is caused by a double-stranded DNA virus (HBV) formerly called the "DNA particle". The virus is transmitted by body fluids.

287. Hepatitis C: About 90% of all cases of viral hepatitis can be traced to either HAV or HBV. The remaining 10% is believed to be caused by one and possibly several other types of viruses. At least one of these is hepatitis C (formerly non-A, non-B).

288. Hepatitis D (formerly delta hepatitis): The liver diseases caused by the hepatitis D virus in those individuals already infected with the hepatitis B virus.

289. Hepatitis E (formerly enteric-transmitted NANB hepatitis): The liver disease caused by the hepatitis E virus. Usually, a subclinical, acute infection results, however, there is a high mortality in women in their last trimester of pregnancy.

290. Heterolactic Fermenters: Microorganisms that ferment sugars to form lactate and also other products such as ethanol and CO_2.

291. Heterotroph: An organism that uses reduced, preformed organic molecules as its principal carbon source.

292. Heterotrophic Nitrification: Nitrification carried out bychemoheterotrophic microorganisms.

293. Hfr Strain: A bacterial strain that denotes its genes with high frequency to a recipient cell during conjugation because the F factor is integrated into the bacterial chromosome.

294. High Oxygen Diffusion Environment: A microbial environment in close contact with air and through which oxygen can move at a rapid rate (in comparison with the slow diffusion rate of oxygen through water).

295. Holdfast: A structure produced by some bacteria and algae that attaches them to a solid object.

296. Holozoic Nutrition: In this type of nutrition, nutrients (such as bacteria) are acquired by phagocytosis and the subsequent formation of a food vacuole or phagosome.

297. Homolactic Fermenters: Organisms that ferment sugars almost completely to lactic acid.

298. Host: The body of an organism that harbors another organism. It can be viewed as a microenvironment that shelters and supports the growth and multiplication of a parasitic organism.

299. Host Restriction: The degradation of foreign genetic material by nucleases after the genetic material enters a host cell.

300. Human Immunodeficiency Virus (HIV): A lentivirus of the family, Retroviridae that is associated with the onset of AIDS.

301. Hypermutation: A rapid production of multiple mutations in a gene or genes through the activation of special mutator genes. The process may be deliberately used to maximize the possibility of creating desirable mutants.

302. Hyperthermophile: A bacterium that has its growth optimum between 80°C and about 113°C. Hyperthermophiles usually do not grow well below 55°C.

303. Hypha (hyphae): The unit of structure of most fungi and some bacteria; a tubular filament.

304. Identification: The process of determining that a particular, isolate or organism belongs to a recognized taxon.

305. Immobilization: The incorporation of a simple, soluble substance into the body of an organism, making it unavailable for use by other organisms.

306. Inclusion Bodies: Granules of organic or inorganic material lying in the cytoplasmic matrix of bacteria.

307. Inclusion Conjunctivitis: An infectitious disease that occurs worldwide. It is caused by *Chlamydia trachomatis* that infects the eye and causes inflammation and the occurrence of large inclusion bodies.

308. Incubation Period: The period after pathogen entry into a host and before signs and symptoms appear.

309. Incubatory Carrier: An individual who is incubating a pathogen but is not yet ill.

310. Indicator Organism: An organism whose presence indicates the condition of a substance or environment, for example, the potential presence of pathogens. Coliforms are used as indicators of fecal pollution.

311. Infection: The invasion of a host by a microorganism with subsequent establishment and multiplication of the agent. An infection may or may not lead to overt disease.

312. Infection Thread: A tubular structure formed during the infection of a root by nitrogen-fixing bacteria. The bacteria enter the root by way of the infection thread and stimulate the formation of the root nodule.

313. Infectious Disease Cycle (Chain of Infection): The chain or cycle of events that describes how an infectious organism grows, reproduces, and is disseminated.

314. Infectious Dose 50 (ID50): Refers to the dose or number of organisms that will infect 50% of an experimental group of hosts within a specified time period.

315. Infectivity: Infectiousness; the state or quality of being infectious or communicable.

316. Integration: The incorporation of one DNA segment into a second DNA molecule to form a new hybrid DNA. Integration occurs during such processes as genetic recombination, episome incorporation into host DNA, and prophage insertion into the bacterial chromosome.

317. Integrins: A large family of α/β heterodimers. Integrins are cellular adhesion receptors that mediate cell-cell and cell-substratum interactions. Integrins usually recognize linear amino acid sequences on protein ligands.

318. Integron: A genetic element with an attachment site for site-specific recombination and an integrase gene. It can capture genes and gene cassettes.

319. Intercalating Agents: Molecules that can be inserted between the stacked bases of a DNA double helix, thereby distorting the DNA and including insertion and deletion mutations.

320. Interferon (IFN): A glycoprotein that has nonspecific antiviral activity by stimulating cells to produce antiviral proteins, which inhibit the synthesis of viral RNA and proteins. Interferons also regulate the growth, differentiation, and/or function of a variety of immune system cells. Their production may be stimulated by virus infections, intracellular pathogens (chlamydiae and rickettsias), protozoan parasites, endotoxins, and other agents.

321. Interleukin: A glycoprotein produced by macrophages and T cells that regulates growth and differentiation, particularly of lymphocytes. Interleukins promote cellular and humoral immune responses.

322. Intermediate Filaments: Small protein filaments about 8 to 10 nm in diameter, in the cytoplasmic matrix of eucaryotic cells that are important in cell structure.

323. Interspecies Hydrogen Transfer: The linkage of hydrogen production from organic matter by anaerobic heterotrophic microorganisms to the use of hydrogen by other anaerobes in the reduction of carbon dioxide to methane. This avoids possible hydrogen toxicity.

324. Intertriginous Candidiasis: A skin infection caused by *Candida* species. Involves those areas of the body, usually opposed skin surfaces, that are warm and moist (axillae, groin, skin folds).

325. Intoxication: A disease that results from the entrance of a specific toxin into the body of a host. The toxin can induce the disease in the absence of the toxin producing organisms.

326. Intrinsic Factors: Food-related factors such as moisture, pH, and available nutrients that influence microbial growth.

327. Invasiveness: The ability of a microorganism to enter a host, grow and reproduce within the host, and spread throughout its body.

328. Kirby-Bauer Method: A disk diffusion test to determine the susceptibility of a microorganism to chemotherapeutic agents.

329. Koch's Postulates: A set of rules for proving that microorganism causes a particular disease.

330. Lactic Acid Fermentation: A fermentation that produces lactic acid as the sole or primary product.

331. Lager: Pertaining to the process of aging beers to allow flavor development.

332. Lag Phase: A period following the introduction of microorganisms into fresh culture medium when there is no increase in cell numbers or mass during batch culture.

333. Latent Period: The initial phase in the one-step growth experiment in which no phages are released.

334. Lectin Complement Pathway: The lectin pathway for complement activation is triggered by the binding of a serum lectin (mannan-binding lectin; MBL) to mannose-containing proteins or to carbohydrates on viruses or bacteria.

335. Leishmanias: Zooflagellates, members of the genus *Leishmania*, that cause the disease leishmaniasis.

336. Leishmaniasis: The disease caused by the protozoa called leishmanias.

337. Lepromatous (progressive) Leprosy. A relentless, progressive form of leprosy in which large numbers of *Mycobacterium leprae* develop in skin cells, killing the skin cells and resulting in the loss of features. Disfiguring nodules from all over the body.

338. Leprosy or Hansen's Disease: A severe disfiguring skin disease caused by *Mycobacterium leprae.*

339. Lethal Dose 50 (LD50): Refers to the dose or number of organisms that will kill 50% of an experimental group of hosts within a specified time period.

340. Leukemia: A progressive, malignant disease of blood-forming organs, marked by distorted proliferation and development of leukocytes and their precursors in the blood and bone marrow. Certain leukemias are caused by viruses (HTLV-1, HTLV-2).

341. Leukocidin: A microbial toxin that can damage or kill leukocytes.

342. Lichen: An organism composed of a fungus and either green algae or cyanobacteria in a symbiotic association.

343. Liebig's Law of the Minimum: Living organisms and populations will grow until lack of a resource begins to limit further growth.

344. Lipopolysaccharide (LPS): A molecule containing both lipid and polysaccharide, which is important in the outer membrane of the Gram-negative cell wall.

345. Listeriosis: A sporadic disease of animals and humans, particularly those who are immunocompromised or pregnant, caused by the bacterium *Listeria monocytogenes*.

346. Lithotroph: An organism that uses reduced inorganic compounds as its electron source.

347. Low Oxygen Diffusion Environment: An aquatic environment in which microorganisms are surrounded by deep water layers that limit oxygen-diffusion to the cell surface. In contrast, microorganisms in thin water films have good oxygen transfer from air to the cell surface.

348. LPS-Binding Protein: A special plasma protein that binds bacterial lipopolysaccharides and then attaches to receptors on monocytes, macrophages, and other cells. This triggers the release of IL-1 and other cytokines that stimulate the development of fever and additional endotoxin effects.

349. Lymphogranuloma Venereum (LGV): A sexually transmitted disease caused by *Chlamydia trachomatis* serotypes L1 - L3, which affect the lymph organs in the genital area.

350. Lysogens: Bacteria that are carrying a viral prophage and can produce bacteriophages under the proper conditions.

351. Lysogeny: The state in which a phage genome remains within the bacterial cell after infection and reproduces along with it rather than taking control of the host and destroying it.

352. Lysosome: A spherical membranous eucaryotic organelle that contains hydrolytic enzymes and is responsible for the intracellular digestion of substances.

353. Macrolide Antibiotic: An antibiotic containing a macrolide ring, a large lactone ring with multiple keto and hydroxyl groups, linked to one or more sugars.

354. Macromolecule Vaccine: A vaccine made of specific, purified macromolecules derived from pathogenic microorganisms.

355. Macronucleus: The larger of the two nuclei in ciliate protozoa. It is normally popyploid and directs the routine activities of the cell.

356. Macrophage: The name for a large mononuclear phagocytic cell, present in blood, lymph and other tissues. Macrophages are derived from monocytes. They phagocytose and destroy pathogens; some macrophages also activate B cells and T cells.

357. Maduromycosis: A subcutaneous fungal infection caused by Madurella mycetoma; also termed an eumycotic mycetoma.

358. Madurose: The sugar derivative 3-O-methyl-D-galactose, which is characteristic of several actinomycete genera that are collectively called maduromycetes.

359. Magnetosomes: Magnetite particles in magnetotactic bacteria that are tiny magnets and allow the bacteria to orient themselves in magnetic fields.

360. Malaria: A serious infectious illness caused by the parasitic protozoan *Plasmodium*. Malaria is characterized by bouts of high chills and fever that occur at regular intervals.

361. Mash: The soluble materials released from germinated grains and prepared as a microbial growth medium.

362. Mean Growth Rate Constant (k): The rate of microbial population growth expressed in terms of the number of generations per unit time.

363. Meiosis: The sexual process in which a diploid cell divides and forms two haploid cells.

364. Melting Temperature (Tm): The temperature at which double-standard DNA separates into individual strands; it is dependent on the G + C content of the DNA and is used to compare genetic material in microbial taxonomy.

365. Membrane Filter Technique: The use of a thin porous filter made from cellulose acetate or some other polymer to collect microorganisms from water, air and food.

366. Meningitis: A condition that refers to inflammation of the brain or spinal cord meninges (membranes). The disease can be divided into bacterial (septic) meningitis and aseptic meningitis syndrome (caused by nonbacterial sources).

367. Mesophile: A microorganism with a growth optimum around 20 to 45°C, a minimum of 15 to 20°C and a maximum about 45°C or lower.

368. Metachromatic Granules: Granules of polyphosphate in the cytoplasm of some bacteria that appear a different color when stained with a blue basic dye. They are storage reservoirs for phosphate. Sometimes called volutin granules.

369. Methanogens: Strictly anaerobic archaeons that derive energy by converting CO_2, H_2, formate, acetate, and other compounds to either methane or methane and CO_2.

370. Methylotroph: A bacterium that uses reduced one-carbon compounds such as methane and methanol as its sole source of carbon and energy.

371. Microaerophile: A microorganism that requires low levels of oxygen for growth, around 2 to 10%, but is damaged by normal atmospheric oxygen levels.

372. Microbial Ecology: The study of microorganisms in their natural environments, with a major emphasis on physical conditions, processes, and interactions that occur on the scale of individual microbial cells.

373. Microbial Loop: The mineralization of organic matter synthesized by photosynthetic phytoplankton through the activity of microorganisms such as bacteria and protozoa. This process "loops" minerals and carbon dioxide back for reuse by the primary producers and makes the organic matter unavailable to higher consumers.

374. Microbial Mat: A firm structure of layered microorganisms with complementary physiological activities that can develop on surfaces in aquatic environments.

375. Microbiology: The study of organisms that are usually too small to be seen with the naked eye. Special techniques are required to isolate and grow them.

376. Microbivory: The use of microorganisms as a food source by organisms that can ingest or phagocytose them.

377. Microenvironment: The immediate environment surrounding a microbial cell or other structure, such as a root.

378. Microorganism: An organism that is too small to be seen clearly with the naked eye.

379. Miliary Tuberculosis: An acute form of tuberculosis in which small tubercles are formed in a number of organs of the body because of dissemination of *M. tuberculosis* throughout the body by the bloodstream. Also known as reactivation tuberculosis.

380. Mineralization: The release of inorganic nutrients from organic matter during microbial growth and metabolism.

381. Minimal Inhibitory Concentration (MIC): The lowest concentration of a drug that will prevent the growth of a particular microorganism.

382. Minimal Lethal Concentration (MLC): The lowest concentration of a drug that will kill a particular microorganism.

383. Mitochondrion: The eucaryotic organelle that is the site of electron transport, oxidative phosphorylation, and pathways such as the Krebs cycle; it provides most of a nonphotosynthetic cell's energy under aerobic conditions. It is constructed of an outer membrane and an inner membrane, which contains the electron transport chain.

384. Mitosis: A process that takes place in the nucleus of a eucaryotic cell and results in the formation of two new nuclei, each with the same number of chromosomes as the parent.

385. Mixed Acid Fermentation: A type of fermentation carried out by members of the family Enterobacteriaceae in which ethanol and a complex mixture of organic acids are produced.

386. Mixotrophic: Refers to microorganisms that combine autotrophic and heterotrophic metabolic processes (they use inorganic electron sources and organic carbon sources).

387. Modified Atmosphere Packaging (MAP): Addition of gases such as nitrogen and carbon dioxide to packaged foods in order to inhibit the growth of spoilage organisms.

388. Mold: Any of a large group of fungi that cause mold or moldiness and that exist as multicellular filamentous colonies; also the deposit or growth caused by such fungi. Molds typically do not produce macroscopic fruiting bodies.

389. Most Probable Number (MPN): The statistical estimation of the probable population in a liquid by diluting and determining end points for microbial growth.

390. Mucociliary Blanket: The layer of cilia and mucus that lines certain portions of the respiratory system; it traps microorganisms up to 10 μm in diameter and then transports them by ciliary action away from the lungs.

391. Mucociliary Escalator: The mechanism by which respiratory ciliated cells move material and microorganisms, trapped in mucus, out of the pharynx, where it is spit out or swallowed.

392. Multi-drug-resistant Strains of Tuberculosis (MDR-TB): A multi-drug-resistant strain is defined as *Mycobacterium tuberculosis* resistant to isoniazid and rifampin, with or without resistance to other drugs.

393. Mutation: A permanent, heritable change in the genetic material.

394. Mutualist: An organism associated with another in an obligatory relationship that is beneficial to both.

395. Mycelium: A mass of branching hyphae found in fungi and some bacteria.

396. Mycolic Acids: Complex 60 to 90 carbon fatty acids with a hydroxyl on the β-carbon and an aliphatic chain on the α-carbon, found in the cell walls of mycobacteria.

397. Mycoplasma: Bacteria that are members of the class Mollicutes and order Mycoplasmatales; they lack cell walls and cannot synthesize peptidoglycan precursors; most require sterols for growth; they are the smallest organisms capable of independent reproduction.

398. Mycoplasma Pneumonia: A type of pneumonia caused by *Mycoplasma pneumoniae*. Spread involves airborne droplets and close contact.

399. Mycorrhizosphere: The region around ectomycorrhizal mantles and hyphae in which nutrients released from the fungus increase the microbial population and its activities.

400. Mycotoxicology: The study of fungal toxins and their effects on various organisms.

401. Myxobacteria: A group of Gram-negative, aerobic soil bacteria characterized by gliding motility, a complex life cycle with the production of fruiting bodies, and the formation of myxospores.

402. Myxospores: Special dormant spores formed by the myxobacteria.

403. Narrow-spectrum Drugs: Chemotherapeutic agents that are effective only against a limited variety of microorganisms.

404. Natural Classification: A classification system that arranges organisms into groups whose members share many characteristics and reflect as much as possible the biological nature of organisms.

405. Necrotizing Fasciitis: A disease that results from a severe invasive group A Streptococcus infection. Necrotizing fasciitis is an infection of the subcutaneous soft tissues, particularly of fibrous tissue, and is most common on the extremities. It begins with skin reddening, swelling, pain and cellulitis and proceeds to skin breakdown and gangrene after 3 to 5 days.

406. Negative Staining: A staining procedure in which a dye is used to make the background dark while the specimen is unstained.

407. Neurotoxin: A toxin that is poisonous to or destroys nerve tissue; especially the toxins secreted by *C. tetani, Corynebacterium diphtheriae, and Shigella dysenteriae.*

408. Neustonic: The microorganisms that live at the atmospheric interface of a water body.

409. Neutrophile: Microorganisms that grow best at a neutral pH range between pH 5.5 and 8.0.

410. Niche: The function of an organism in a complex system, including place of the organism, the resources used in a given location, and the time of use.

411. Nitrifying Bacteria: Chemolithotrophic, Gram-negative bacteria that are members of the family Nitrobacteriaceae and convert ammonia to nitrate and nitrite to nitrate.

412. Nitrogen Fixation: The metabolic process in which atmospheric molecular nitrogen is reduced to ammonia; carried out by cyanobacteria, Rhizobium and other nitrogen-fixing procaryotes.

413. Nitrogen Oxygen Demand (NOD): The demand for oxygen is sewage treatment, caused by nitrifying microorganisms.

414. Nocardioforms: Bacteria that resemble members of the genus *Nocardia*; they develop a substrate mycelium that readily breaks up into rods and coccoid elements (a quality sometimes called fugacity).

415. Nomenclature: The branch of taxonomy concerned with the assignment of names to taxonomic groups in agreement with published rules.

416. Nondiscrete Microorganism: A microorganism, best exemplified by a filamentous fungus, that does not have a defined and predictable cell structure or distinct edges and boundaries. The organism can be defined in terms of the cell structure and its cytoplasmic contents.

417. Normal Microbiota (also indigenous microbial population, microflora, microbial flora): The microorganisms normally associated with a particular tissue or structure.

418. Nucleoid: An irregularly shaped region in the procaryotic cell that contains its genetic material.

419. Nucleolus: The organelle, located within the eucaryotic nucleus and not bounded by a membrane, that is the location of ribosomal RNA synthesis and the assembly of ribosomal subunits.

420. Numerical Aperture: The property of a microscope lens that determines how much light can enter and how great a resolution the lens can provide.

421. Nutrient: A substance that supports growth and reproduction.

422. Nystatin: A polyene antibiotic from *Streptomyces noursei* that is used in the treatment of *Candida* infections of the skin, vagina and alimentary tract.

423. O Antigen: A polysaccharide antigen extending from the outer membrane of some gram-negative bacterial cell walls; it is part of the lipopolysaccharide.

424. Obligate Anaerobes: Microorganisms that cannot tolerate the presence of oxygen and die when exposed to it.

425. One-step Growth Experiment: An experiment used to study the reproduction of lytic phages in which one round of phage reproduction occurs and ends with the lysis of the host bacterial population.

426. Open Reading Frame (ORF): A reading frame sequence not interrupted by a stop codon; it is usually determined by nucleic acid sequencing studies.

427. Opportunistic Microorganism or Pathogen: A microorganism that is usually free-living or a part of the host's normal microbiota, but which may become pathogenic under certain circumstances, such as when the immune system is compromised.

428. Opsonization: The action of opsonins in making bacteria and other cells more readily phagocytosed. Antibodies, complement (especially C3b) and fibronectin are potent opsonins.

429. Optical Tweezer: The use of a focused laser beam to drag and isolate a specific microorganism from a complex microbial mixture.

430. Organotrophs: Organisms that use reduced organic compounds as their electron source.

431. Osmophilic Microorganisms: Microorganisms that grow best in or on media of high solute concentration.

432. Osmotolerant: Organisms that grow over a fairly wide range of water activity or solute concentration.

433. Outer Membrane: A special membrane located outside the peptidoglycan layer in the cell walls of Gram-negative bacteria.

434. Oxidative Burst: The generation of reactive oxygen species, primarily superoxide anion ($-O_2$) and hydrogen peroxide (H_2O_2) by a plant or an animal, in response to challenge by a potential bacterial, fungal, or viral pathogen.

435. Oxygenic Photosynthesis: Photosynthesis that oxidizes water to form oxygen; the form of photosynthesis characteristic of algae and cyanobacteria.

436. Parasite: An organism that lives on or within another organism (the host) and benefits from the association while harming its host. Often the parasite obtains nutrients from the host.

437. Parasitism: A type of symbiosis in which one organism benefits from the other and the host is usually harmed.

438. Parfocal: A microscope that retains proper focus when the objectives are changed.

439. Pasteur Effect: The decrease in the rate of sugar catobolism and change to aerobic respiration that occurs when microorganisms are switched from anaerobic to aerobic conditions.

440. Pasteurization: The process of heating milk and other liquids to destroy microorgnisms that can cause spoilage or disease.

441. Pathogen: Any virus, bacterium, or other agent that causes disease.

442. Pathogen-Associated Molecular Pattern (PAMP): Conserved molecular structures that occur in patterns on microbial surfaces. The structures and their patterns are unique to particular microorganisms and invariant among members of a given microbial group.

443. Pathogenicity: The condition or quality of being pathogenic, or the ability to cause disease.

444. Pathogenicity Island: A large segment of DNA in some pathogens that contains the genes responsible for virulence; often it codes for the type III secretion system that allows the pathogen to secrete virulence proteins and damage host cells. A pathogen may have more than one pathogenicity island.

445. Pathogenic Potential: The degree that a pathogen causes morbid signs and symptoms.

446. Ped: A natural soil aggregate, formed partly through bacterial and fungal growth in the soil.

447. Pencillins: A group of antibiotics containing a β-lactam ring, which are active against gram-positive bacteria.

448. Peptic Ulcer Disease: A gastritis caused by *Helicobacter pylori*.

449. Peptidoglycan: A large polymer composed of long chain of alternating N-acetyl-glucosamine and N-acetylmuramic acid residues. The polysaccharide chains are linked to each other through connections between tetrapeptide chains attached to the N-acetylmuramic acids. It provides much of the strength and rigidity possessed by bacterial cell walls.

450. Peptones: Water-soluble digests or hydrolysates of proteins that are used in the preparation of culture media.

451. Period of Infectivity: Refers to the time during which the source of an infectious disease is infectious or is disseminating the pathogen.

452. Periplasmic Space or Periplasm: The space between the plasma membrane and the outer membrane in gram-negative bacteria, and between the plasma membrane and the cell wall in gram-positive bacteria.

453. Pertussis: An acute, highly contagious infection of the respiratory tract, most frequently affecting young children, usually caused by *Bordetella pertussis* or *B. parapertussis*. Consists of peculiar paroxysms of coughing, ending in a prolonged crowing or whooping respiration; hence the name whooping cough.

454. Petri Dish: A shallow dish consisting of two round, overlapping halves that is used to grow microorganisms on solid culture medium; the top is larger than the bottom of the dish to prevent contamination of the culture.

455. Phase-contrast Microscope: A microscope that converts slight differences in refractive index and cell density into easily observed differences in light intensity.

456. Phenetic System: A classification system that groups organisms together based on the similarity of their observable characteristics.

457. Phenol Coefficient Test: A test to measure the effectiveness of disinfectants by comparing their activity against test bacteria with that of phenol.

458. Photolithotrophic Autotrophs: Organisms that use light energy, an inorganic electron source (e.g., H_2O, H_2, H_2S) and CO_2 as a carbon source.

459. Photoorganotrophic Heterotrophs: Microorganisms that use light energy and organic electron donors, and also employ simple organic molecules rather than CO_2 as their carbon source.

460. Phototrophs: Organisms that use light as their energy source.

461. Phycobiliproteins: Photosynthetic pigments that are composed of proteins with attached tetrapyrroles; they are often found in cyanobacteria and red algae.

462. Phycobilisomes: Special particles on the membranes of cyanobacteria that contain photosynthetic pigments and electron transport chains.

463. Phylogenetic Tree: A graph made of nodes and branches, much like a tree in shape, that shows phylogenetic relationships between groups of organisms and sometimes also indicates the evolutionary development of groups.

464. Phytoplankton: A community of floating photosynthetic organisms, largely composed of algae and cyanobacteria.

465. Phytoremediation: The use of plants and their associated microorganisms to remove, contain, or degrade environmental contaminants.

466. Plankton: Free-floating, mostly microscopic microorganisms that can be found in almost all waters; a collective name.

467. Plaque: 1. A clear area in a lawn of bacteria or a localized area of cell destruction in a layer of animal cells that results from the lysis of the bacteria by bacteriophages or the destruction of the animal cells by animal viruses, 2. The term also refers to dental plaque, a film of food debris, polysaccharides, and dead cells that cover the teeth.

468. Plasmid Fingerprinting: A technique used to identify microbial isolates as belonging to the same strain because they contain the same number of plasmids with the identical molecular weights and similar phenotypes.

469. Plasmodial (acellular) Slime Mold: A member of the devision Myxomycota that exists as a thin, streaming, multinucleate mass of protoplasm which creeps along in an amoeboid fashion.

470. Plasmodium (Pl. plasmodia): A stage in the life cycle of myxomycetes (plasmodial slime molds); a multinucleate mass of protoplasm surrounded by a membrane. Also, a parasite of the genus *Plasmodium*.

471. Plastid: A cytoplasmic organelle of algae and higher plants that contains pigments such as chlorophyll, stores food reserves, and often carries out processes such as photosynthesis.

472. Pleomorphic: Refers to bacteria that are variable in shape and lack a single, characteristic form.

473. Poly-β-hydroxybutyrate (PHB): A linear polymer of β-hydroxybutyrate used as a reserve of carbon and energy by many bacteria.

474. Polymerase Chain Reaction (PCR): An in vitro technique used to synthesize large quantities of specific nucleotide sequences from small amounts of DNA. It employs oligonucleotide primers complementary to specific sequences in the target gene and special heat-stable DNA polymerases.

475. Porin Proteins: Proteins that form channels across the outer membrane of gram-negative bacterial cell walls. Small molecules are transported through these channels.

476. Pour Plate: A petri dish of solid culture medium with isolated microbial colonies growing both on its surface and within the medium, which has been prepared by mixing microorganisms with cooled, still liquid medium and then allowing the medium to harden.

477. Primary (Frank) Pathogen: Any organism that causes a disease in the host by direct interaction with or infection of the host.

478. Primary Metabolites: Microbial metabolites produced during the growth phase of an organism.

479. Primary Producer: Photoautotrophic and chemoautotrophic organisms that incorporate carbon dioxide into organic carbon and thus provide new biomass for the ecosystem.

480. Primary Production: The incorporation of carbon dioxide into organic matter by photosynthetic organisms and chemoautotrophic bacteria.

481. Probiotic: A living organism that may provide health benefits beyond its nutritional value when it is ingested.

482. Procaryotic Cells: Cells that lack a true, membrane-enclosed nucleus; bacteria are procaryotic and have their genetic material located in a nucleoid.

483. Procaryotic Species: A collection of strains that share many stable properties and differ significantly from other groups of strains.

484. Propagated Epidemic: An epidemic that is characterized by a relatively slow and prolonged rise and then a gradual decline in the number of individuals infected. It usually results from the introduction of an infected individual into a susceptible population and the pathogen is transmitted from person to person.

485. Prostheca: An extension of a bacterial cell, including the plasma membrane and cell wall, that is narrower than the mature cell.

486. Protein Engineering: The rational design of proteins by constructing specific amino acid sequences through molecular techniques, with the objective of modifying protein characteristics.

487. Proteobacteria: A large group of bacteria, primarily gram-negative, that 16S rRNA sequence comparisons show to be phylogenetically related; proteobacteria contain the purple photosynthetic bacteria and their relatives and are composed of the α, β, γ, δ and ε subgroups.

488. Proteome: The complete collection of proteins that an organism produces.

489. Protists: Eukaryotes with unicellular organization, either in the form of solitary cells or colonies of cells lacking true tissues.

490. Protoplast: A bacterial or fungal cell with its cell wall completely removed. It is spherical in shape and osmotically sensitive.

491. Protoplast Fusion: The joining of cells that have had their walls weakened or completely removed.

492. Prototroph: A microorganism that requires the same nutrients as the majority of naturally occurring members of its species.

493. Protozoan or Protozoon (Pl. Protozoa): A microorganism belonging to the Protozoa subkingdom. A unicellular or acellular eukaryotic protist whose organelles have the functional role of organs and tissues in more complex forms. Protozoa vary greatly in size, morphology, nutrition and life cycle.

494. Protozoology: The study of protozoa.

495. Pseudopodium or Pseudopod: A non-permanent cytoplasmic extension of the cell body by which amoebae and amoeboid organisms move and feed.

496. Psittacosis (ornithosis): A disease due to a strain of *Chlamydia psittaci,* first seen in parrots and later found in other birds and domestic fowl (in which it is called ornithosis). It is transmissible to humans.

497. Psychrophile: A microorganisms that grows well at 0°C and has an optimum growth temperature of 15°C or lower and a temperature maximum around 20°C.

498. Psychrotroph: A microorganism that grows at 0°C, but has a growth optimum between 20 and 30°C and a maximum of about 35°C.

499. Puerperal Fever: An acute, febrile condition following childbirth; it is characterized by infection of the uterus and/or adjacent regions and is caused by streptococci.

500. Pulmonary Anthrax: A form of anthrax involving the lungs. Also known as Woolsorter's disease.

501. Pure Culture: A population of cells that are identical because they arise from a single cell.

502. Putrefaction: The microbial decomposition of organic matter, especially the anaerobic breakdown of proteins, with the production of foul-smelling compounds such as hydrogen sulfide and amines.

503. Quellung Reaction: The increase in visibility or the swelling of the capsule of a microorganism in the presence of antibodies against capsular antigens.

504. Quorum Sensing: The process in which bacteria monitor their own population density by sensing the levels of signal molecules that are released by the microorganisms. When these signal molecules reach a threshold concentration, quorum-dependent genes are expressed.

505. Rabies: An acute infectious disease of the central nervous system, which affects all warmblooded animals (including humans). It is caused by an ssRNA virus belonging to the genus Lyssavirus in the family Rhabdoviridae.

506. Radappertization: The use of gamma rays from a cobalt source for control of microorganisms in foods.

507. Radioimmunoassay (RIA): A very sensitive assay technique that uses a purified radioisotope labeled antigen or antibody to compete for antibody or antigen with unlabeled standard and samples to determine the concentration of a substance in the samples.

508. Recombinant DNA Technology: The techniques used in carrying out genetic engineering; they involve the identification and isolation of a specific gene, the insertion of the gene into a vector such as a plasmid to form a recombinant molecule, and the production of large quantities of the gene and its products.

509. Recombinant-vector Vaccine: The type of vaccine that is produced by the introduction of one or more of a pathogen's genes into attenuated viruses or bacteria. The attenuated virus or bacterium serves as a vector, replicating within the vertebrate host and expressing the gene(s) of the pathogen. The pathogen's antigens induce an immune response.

510. Recombination: The process in which a new recombinant chromosome is formed by combining genetic material from two organisms.

511. Red Tides: Red tides occur frequently in coastal areas and often are associated with population blooms of dinoflagellates. Dinoflagellate pigments are responsible for the red color of the water. Under these conditions, the dinoflagellates often produce saxitoxin, which can lead to paralytic shellfish poisoning.

512. Reductive Dehalogenation: The cleavage of carbon-halogen bonds by anaerobic bacteria that creates a strong electron-donating environment.

513. Regulatory Mutants: Mutant organisms that have lost the ability to limit synthesis of a product, which normally occurs by regulation of activity of an earlier step in the biosynthetic pathway.

514. Reservoir: A site, alternate host, or carrier that normally harbors pathogenic organisms and serves as a source from which other individuals can be infected.

515. Reservoir Host: An organism other than a human that is infected with a pathogen that can also infect humans.

516. Residuesphere: The region surrounding organic matter such as a seed or plant part in which microbial growth is stimulated by increased organic matter availability.

517. Resolution: The ability of a microscope to separate or distinguish between small objects that are close together.

518. Restricted Transduction: A transduction process in which only a specific set of bacterial genes are carried to another bacterium by a temperate phage; the bacterial genes are acquired because of a mistake in the excision of a prophage during the lysogenic life cycle.

519. Retroviruses: A group of viruses with RNA genomes that carry the enzyme reverse transcriptase and form a DNA copy of their genome during their reproductive cycle.

520. Ribotyping: Ribotyping is the use of *E. coli* rRNA to probe chromosomal DNA in Southern blots for typing bacterial strains. This method is based on the fact that rRNA genes are scattered throughout the chromosome of most bacteria and therefore polymorphic restriction endonuclease patterns result when chromosomes are digested and probed with rRNA.

521. Rocky Mountain Spotted Fever: A disease caused by *Rickettsia rickettsii.*

522. Root Nodule: Gall-like structures on roots that contain endosymbiotic nitrogen-fixing bacteria (e.g., Rhizobium or Bradyrhizobium is present in legume nodules).

523. Run: The straight line movement of a bacterium.

524. Salmonellosis: An infection with certain species of the genus *Salmonella,* usually caused by ingestion of food containing salmonellae or their products. Also known as *Salmonella gastroenteritis* or *Salmonella* food poisoning.

525. Sanitization: Reduction of the microbial population on an inanimate object to levels judged safe by public health standards; usually, the object is cleaned.

526. Saprophyte: An organism that takes up nonliving organic nutrients in dissolved form and usually grows on decomposing organic matter.

527. Saprozoic Nutrition: Having the type of nutrition in which organic nutrients are taken up in dissolved form; normally refers to animals or animal-like organisms.

528. Scanning Electron Microscope (SEM): An electron microscope that scans a beam of electrons over the surface of a specimen and forms an image of the surface from the electrons that are emitted by it.

529. Scanning Probe Microscope: A microscope used to study surface features by moving a sharp probe over the object's surface (e.g., the Scanning Tunneling Microscope).

530. Secondary Metabolites: Products of metabolism that are synthesized after growth has been completed.

531. Secondary Treatment: The biological degradation of dissolved organic matter in the process of sewage treatment ; the organic material is either mineralized or changed to settleable solids.

532. Selective Media: Culture media that favor the growth of specific microorganisms; this may be accomplished by inhibiting the growth of undesired microorganisms.

533. Selective Toxicity: The ability of a chemotherapeutic agent to kill or inhibit a microbial pathogen while damaging the host as little as possible.

534. Sepsis: Systemic response to infection. The systemic response is manifested by two or more of the following conditions as a result of infection : temperature > 38 or < 36 °C; heart rate > 90 beats per min; respiratory rate > 20 breaths per min, or pCO_2 < 32 mm Hg; leukocyte count > 12,000 cells per ml^3 or > 10% immature (band) forms. Sepsis also has been defined as the presence of pathogens or their toxins in blood and other tissues.

535. Septicemia: A disease associated with the presence in the blood of pathogens or bacterial toxins.

536. Septic Shock: Sepsis associated with severe hypotension despite adequate fluid resuscitation, along with the presence of perfusion abnormalities that may include, but are not limited to, lactic acidosis, oliguria, or an acute alternation in mental status. Gram-positive bacteria, fungi, and endotoxin-containing Gram-negative bacteria can initiate the pathogenic cascade of sepsis leading to septic shock.

537. Septum: A partition or crosswall that occurs between two cells in a bacterial, e.g. actinomycete or fungal filament, or which partitions off fungal structures such as spores. Septa also divide parent cells into two daughter cells during bacterial binary fission.

538. Serotyping: A technique or serological procedure that is used to differentiate between strains (serovars or serotypes) of microorganisms that have differences in the antigenic composition of a structure or product.

539. Serum (Pl. Serums or Sera): The clear, fluid portion of blood lacking both blood cells and fibrinogen. It is the fluid remaining after coagulation of plasma, the noncellular liquid faction of blood.

540. Serum Resistance: The type of resistance that occurs with bacteria such as *Neisseria gonorrhoeae* because the pathogen interferes with membrane attack complex formation during the complement cascade.

541. Settling Basin: A basin used during water purification to chemically precipitate out fine particles, microorganisms, and organic material by coagulation or flocculation.

542. Sex Pilus: A thin protein appendage required for bacterial mating or conjugation. The cell with sex pili donates DNA to recipient cells.

543. Sheath: A hollow tubelike structure surroundings a chain of cells and present in several genera of bacteria.

544. Shigellosis: The diarrheal disease that arises from an infection with Shigella spp. Often called bacillary dysentery.

545. Shine-Dalgarno Sequence: A segment in the leader of prokaryotic mRNA that binds to a special sequence on the 16S rRNA of the small ribosomal subunit. This helps properly orient the mRNA on the ribosome.

546. Shingles (Herpes Zoster): A reactivated form of chickenpox caused by the varicella-zoster virus.

547. Signal Peptide: The special amino-terminal sequence on a peptide destined for transport that delays protein folding and is recognized in bacteria by the Sec-dependent pathway machinery.

548. Silent Mutation: A mutation that does not result in a change in the organism's proteins or phenotype even though the DNA base sequence has been changed.

549. Simple Matching Coefficient (S SM): An association coefficient used in numerical taxonomy; the proportion of characters that match regardless of whether or not the attribute is present.

550. Site-specific Recombination: Recombination of nonhomologous genetic material with a chromosome at a specific site.

551. S-layer: A regularly structure layer composed of protein or glycoprotein that lies on the surface of many bacteria. It may protect the bacterium and help give it shape and rigidity.

552. Slime: The viscous extracellular glycoproteins or glycolipids produced by staphylococci and Pseudomonas aeruginosa bacteria that allows them to adhere to smooth surfaces such as prosthetic medical devices and catheters. More generally, the term often refers to an easily removed, diffuse, unorganized layer of extracellular material that surrounds a bacterial cell.

553. Slime Layer: A layer of diffuse, unorganized, easily removed material lying outside the bacterial cell wall.

554. Slow Sand Filter: A bed of sand through which water slowly flows the gelatinous microbial layer on the sand grain surface removes waterborne microorganisms, particularly Giardia, by adhesion to the gel. This type of filter is used in some water purification plants.

555. Sorocarp: The fruiting structure of the Acrasiomycetes.

556. Sorus: A type of fruiting structure composed of a mass of spores or sporangia.

557. Source: The location or object from which a pathogen is immediately transmitted to the host, either directly or through an intermediate agent.

558. Species: Species of higher organisms are groups of interbreeding or potentially interbreeding natural populations that are reproductively isolated. Bacterial species are collections of strains that have many stable properties in common and differ significantly from other groups of strains.

559. Spheroplast: A relatively spherical cell formed by the weakening or partial removal of the rigid cell wall component (e.g., by pencillin treatment of Gram-negative bacteria). Spheroplasts are usually osmotically sensitive.

560. Spirillum: A rigid, spiral-shaped bacterium.

561. Spirochete: A flexible, spiral-shaped bacterium with periplasmic flagella.

562. Spore: A differentiated, specialized form that can be used for dissemination, for survival of adverse conditions because of its heat and dessication resistance, and/or for reproduction. Spores are usually unicellular and may develop into vegetative organisms or gametes. They may be produced asexually or sexually and are of many types.

563. Sporulation: The process of spore formation.

564. Spread Plate: A petri dish of solid culture medium with isolated microbial colonies growing on its surface, which has been prepared by spreading a dilute microbial suspension evenly over the agar surface.

565. Stalk. A nonliving bacterial appendage produced by the cell and extending from it.

566. Staphylococcal Food Poisoning: A type of food poisoning caused by ingestion of improperly stored or cooked food in which *Staphylococcus aureus* has grown. The bacteria produce exotoxins that accumulate in the food.

567. Staphylococcal Scalded Skin Syndrome (SSSS): A disease caused by staphylococci that produce an exfoliative toxin. The skin becomes red (erythema) and sheets of epidermic may separate from the underlying tissue.

568. Starter Culture: An inoculum, consisting of a mixture of carefull selected microorganisms, used to start a commercial fermentation.

569. Stationary Phase: The phase of microbial growth in a batch culture when population growth ceases and the growth curve levels off.

570. Stem-nodulating Rhizobia: Rhizobia (members of the genera Rhizobium, Bradyrhizobium and Azorhizobium) that produce nitrogen-fixing structures above the soil surface on plant stems. These most often are observed in tropical plants and produced by Azorhizobium.

571. Sterilization: The process by which all living cells, viable spores, viruses, and viroids are either destroyed or removed from an objector habitat.

572. Strain: A population of organisms that descends from a single organism or pure culture isolate.

573. Streak Plate: A petri dish of solid culture medium with isolated microbial colonies growing on its surface, which has been prepared by spreading a microbial mixture over the agar surface, using an inoculating loop.

574. Streptococcal Pneumonia: A endogenous infection of the lungs caused by *Streptococcus pneumoniae* that occurs in predisposed individuals.

575. Streptococcal Sore Throat: One of the most common bacterial infections of humans. It is commonly referred to as "strep throat". The disease is spread by droplets of saliva or nasal secretions and is caused by *Streptococcus* spp. (particularly group A streptococci).

576. Streptolysin-O (SLO): A specific hemolysin produced by *Streptococcus pyogenes* that is inactivated by oxygen (hence the "O" in its name). SLO casuses beta-hemolysis of blood cells on agar plates incubated anaerobically.

577. Streptolysin-S (SLS): A product of *Streptococcus pyogenes* that is bound to the bacterial cell but may sometimes be released. SLS causes beta hemolysis on aerobically incubated blood-agar plates and can act as a leukocidin by killing leukocytes that phogocytose the bacterial cell to which it is bound.

578. Stromatolite: Dome-like microbial mat communities consisting of filamentous photosynthetic bacteria and occluded sediments (often calcareous or siliceous). They usually have a laminar structure. Many are fossilized, but some modern forms occur.

579. Superinfection: A new bacterial or fungal infection of a patient that is resistant to the drug(s) being used for treatment.

580. Swab: A wad of absorbent material usually wound around one end of a small stick and used for applying medication or for removing material from an area; also, a dacron-tipped polystyrene applicator.

581. Symbiosis: The living together or close association of two dissimilar organisms, each of these organisms being known as a symbiont.

582. Syntrophism: The association in which the growth of one organism either depends on, or is improved by, the provision of one or more growth factors or nutrients by a neighboring organism. Sometimes both organisms benefit.

583. Systematic Epidemiology: The field of epidemiology that focuses on the ecological and social factors that influence the development of emerging and re-emerging infectious disease.

584. Systematics: The scientific study of organisms with the ultimate objective being to characterize and arrange them in an orderly manner; often considered synonymous with taxonomy.

585. Taxon: A group into which related organisms are classified.

586. Taxonomy: The science of biological classification; it consists of three parts: classification, nomenclature and identification.

587. T-Cell or T Lymphocyte: A type of lymphocyte derived from bone marrow stem cells that matures into an immunologically competent cell under the influence of the thymus. T cells are involved in a variety of cell-mediated immune reactions.

588. T-Cell Antigen Receptor (TCR): The receptor on the T-cell surface consisting of two antigen binding peptide chains; it is associated with a large number of other glycoproteins. Binding of antigen to the TCR, usually in association with MHC, activates the T-cell.

589. Teichoic Acids: Polymers of glycerol or ribitol joined by phosphates they are found in the cell walls of Gram-positive bacteria.

590. Temperate Phages: Bacteriophages that can infect bacteria and establish a lysogenic relationship rather than immediately lysing their hosts.

591. Tetanolysin: A hemolysin that aids in tissue destruction and is produced by Clostridium tetani.

592. Tetrapartite Associations: A symbiotic association of the same plant with three different types of microorganisms.

593. Theory: A set of principles and concepts that have survived rigorous testing and that provide a systematic account of some aspects of nature.

594. Thermal Death Time (TDT): The shortest period of time needed to kill all the organisms in a microbial population at a specified temperature and under defined conditions.

595. Thermoacidophiles: A group of bacteria that grow best at acid pHs and high temperatures; they are members of the Archaea.

596. Thermophile: A microorganism that can grow at temperatures of 55°C or higher; the minimum is usually around 45°C.

597. Thrush: Infection of the oral mucous membrane by the fungus *Candila albicans*; also known as oral candidiasis.

598. Toxigenicity: The capacity of an organism to produce a toxin.

599. Toxin: A microbial product or component that injures another cell or organism. Often the term refers to a poisonous protein, but toxins may be lipids and other substances.

600. Transformation: A mode of gene transfer in bacteria in which a piece of free DNA is taken up by a bacterial cell and integrated into the recipient genome.

601. Transgenic Animal or Plant: An animal or plant that has gained new genetic information from the insertion of foreign DNA. It may be produced by such techniques as injecting DNA into animal eggs, electroporation of mammalian cells and plant cell protoplasts, or shooting DNA into plants cells with a gene gun.

602. Transmission Electron Microscope (TEM): A microscope in which an image is formed by passing an electron beam through a specimen and focusing the scattered electrons with magnetic lenses.

603. Transovarian Passage: The passage of a microorganisms such as a rickettsia from generation to generation of hosts through tick eggs. (No humans or other mammals are needed as reservoirs for continued propagation.)

604. Traveller's Diarrhea: A type of diarrhea resulting from ingestion of viruses, bacteria, or protozoa normally absent from the traveller's environment. A major pathogen is enterotoxigenic *Escherichia coli.*

605. Trichomoniasis: A sexually transmitted disease caused by the parasitic protozoan Trichomonas vaginalis.

606. Tripartite Associations: A symbiotic association of the same plant with two types of microorganisms.

607. Trophozoite: The active, motile feeding stage of a protozoan organism; in the malarial parasite, the stage of schizogony between the ring stage and the schizont.

608. Tropism: The movement of living organisms toward or away from a focus of heat, light, or other stimulus.

609. Tubercle: A small, rounded nodular lesion produced by *Mycobacterium tuberculosis.*

610. Tuberculoid (Neural) Leprosy: A mild, nonprogressive form of leprosy that is associated with delayed-type hypersensitivity to antigens on the surface of *Mycobacterium leprae.* It is characterized by early nerve damage and regions of the skin that have lost sensation and are surrounded by a border of nodules.

611. Tuberculosis (TB): An infectious disease of humans and other animals resulting from an infection by a species of Mycobacterium and characterized by the formation of tubercles and tissue necrosis, primarily as a result of host hypersensitivity and inflammation. Infection is usually by inhalation, and the disease commonly affects the lungs (pulmonary tuberculosis), although it may occur in any part of the body.

612. Tularemia: A plague-like disease of animals caused by the bacterium Francisella tularensis subsp. tularensis (Jellison type A), which may be transmitted to humans.

613. Tumble: Random turning or tumbling movements made by bacteria when they stop moving in a striaght line.

614. Turbidostat: A continuous culture system equipped with a photocell that adjusts the flow of medium through the culture vessel so as to maintain a constant cell density or turbidity.

615. Ultramicrobacteria: Bacteria that can exist normally in a miniaturized form or which are capable of miniaturization under low-nutrient conditions. They may be 0.2 μm or smaller in diameter.

616. Ultraviolet (UV) Radiation: Radiation of fairly short wavelength, about 10 to 400 nm, and high energy.

617. Vector-borne Transmission: The transmission of an infectious pathogen between hosts by means of a vector.

618. Vehicle: An inanimate substance or medium that transmits a pathogen.

619. Vibrio: A rod-shaped bacterial cell that is curved to form a comma or an incomplete spiral.

620. Virology: The branch of microbiology that is concerned with viruses and viral diseases.

621. Virulence: The degree or intensity of pathogenicity of an organism as indicated by case fatality rates and/or ability to invade host tissues and cause disease.

622. Virulence Factor: A bacterial product, usually a protein or carbohydrate, that contributes to virulence or pathogenicity.

623. Virus: An infectious agent having a simple acellular oganization with a protein coat and a single type of nucleic acid, lacking independent metabolism and reproducing only within living host cells.

624. Vitamin: An organic compound required by organisms in minute quantities for growth and reproduction because it cannot be synthesized by the organism; vitamins often serve as enzyme cofactors or parts of cofactors.

625. Whole-genome Shotgun Sequencing: An approach to genome sequencing in which the complete genome is broken into random fragments, which are then individually sequenced. Finally, the fragments are placed in the proper order using sophisticated computer programs.

626. Whole-organism Vaccine: A vaccine made from complete pathogens, which can be of four types: inactivated viruses; attenuated viruses; killed microorganisms; and live, attenuated microbes.

627. Widal Test: A test involving agglutination of typhoid bacilli when they are mixed with serum containing typhoid antibodies from an individual having typhoid fever; used to detect the presence of *Salmonella typhi* and *S. paratyphi*.

628. Winogradsky Column: A glass column with an anaerobic lower zone and an aerobic upper zone, which allows growth of microorganisms under conditions similar to those found in a nutrient-rich lake.

629. Xenograft: A tissue graft between animals of different species.

630. Xerophilic Microorganisms: Microorganisms that grow best under low aw conditions and may not be able to grow at high aw values.

631. Yellow Fever: An acute infectious disease caused by a flavivirus, which is transmitted to humans by mosquitoes. The liver is affected and the skin turns yellow in this disease.

632. YM Shift: The change in shape by dimorphic fungi when they shift from the yeast (Y) form in the animal body to the mold or mycelial form (M) in the environment.

Suggested Reading

1. Introduction to Microbiology: A Case-History Study Approach (with CD-ROM and InfoTrac) by John L. Ingraham, Catherine A. Ingraham, Publisher: Brooks Cole, 2003.
2. Microbiology: An Introduction, Eighth Edition by Gerard J. Tortora, Berdell R. Funke, Christine L. Case, Publisher: Benjamin Cummings, 2003.
3. Microbiology: A Laboratory Manual (7th Edition) by James Cappuccino, Natalie Sherman, Publisher: Benjamin Cummings, 2013.
4. Sherris Medical Microbiology: An Introduction to Infectious Diseases by Kenneth J. Ryan, C. George Ray, Publisher: McGraw-Hill Medical, 2011.
5. Mims' Medical Microbiology by Richard Goering, Publisher: Elsevier, 2012.
6. Clinical Microbiology Made Ridiculously simple by M Gladwin, Publisher: Medmaster, 2014.
7. Cellular and Molecular Immunology by Abul K. Abbas, Publisher: Saunders, 2011.
8. Microbiology: Lippincott Illustrated Reviews Series by Richard A. Harvey Cynthia Nau Cornelissen, Publisher: Lippincott Williams & Wilkins, 2012.
9. Medical Microbiology by Patrick R. Murray, Publisher: Elsevier, 2012.
10. Medical Microbiology and Infection at a Glance by Stephen Gillespie, Publisher: Wiley-Blackwell, 2012.
11. Jawetz Melnick & Adelbergs Medical Microbiology by Geo. F. Brooks, Publisher: McGraw-Hill Medical, 2013.

Index

Page numbers followed by *f* refer to figure, *fc* refer to flowchart, and *t* refer to table

B

C

D

E

F

G

H

I

M

N

Q

R

T